Early Child Development: From Measurement to Optimal Functioning and Evidence-Based Policy

Early Child Development: From Measurement to Optimal Functioning and Evidence-Based Policy

Editor

Verónica Schiariti

MDPI • Basel • Beijing • Wuhan • Barcelona • Belgrade • Manchester • Tokyo • Cluj • Tianjin

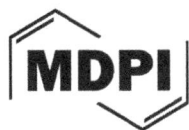

Editor
Verónica Schiariti
University of Victoria
Canada

Editorial Office
MDPI
St. Alban-Anlage 66
4052 Basel, Switzerland

This is a reprint of articles from the Special Issue published online in the open access journal *International Journal of Environmental Research and Public Health* (ISSN 1660-4601) (available at: https://www.mdpi.com/journal/ijerph/special_issues/early_child_development_measurement_optimal_functioning_evidence-based_policy).

For citation purposes, cite each article independently as indicated on the article page online and as indicated below:

LastName, A.A.; LastName, B.B., LastName, C.C. Article Title. *Journal Name* **Year**, *Volume Number*, Page Range.

ISBN 978-3-0365-1601-1 (Hbk)
ISBN 978-3-0365-1602-8 (PDF)

© 2021 by the authors. Articles in this book are Open Access and distributed under the Creative Commons Attribution (CC BY) license, which allows users to download, copy and build upon published articles, as long as the author and publisher are properly credited, which ensures maximum dissemination and a wider impact of our publications.

The book as a whole is distributed by MDPI under the terms and conditions of the Creative Commons license CC BY-NC-ND.

Contents

About the Editor vii

Preface to "Early Child Development: From Measurement to Optimal Functioning and
Evidence-Based Policy" ix

Verónica Schiariti
Introduction to the Special Issue on Early Child Development: From Measurement to Optimal
Functioning and Evidence-Based Policy
Reprinted from: *Int. J. Environ. Res. Public Health* **2021**, *18*, 5154, doi:10.3390/ijerph18105154 . . . 1

Magdalena Janus, Caroline Reid-Westoby, Noam Raiter, Barry Forer and Martin Guhn
Population-Level Data on Child Development at School Entry Reflecting Social Determinants
of Health: A Narrative Review of Studies Using the Early Development Instrument
Reprinted from: *Int. J. Environ. Res. Public Health* **2021**, *18*, 3397, doi:10.3390/ijerph18073397 . . . 5

Leah N. Isquith-Dicker, Andrew Kwist, Danae Black, Stephen E. Hawes, Jennifer Slyker,
Sharon Bergquist and Susanne P. Martin-Herz
Early Child Development Assessments and Their Associations with Long-Term Academic and
Economic Outcomes: A Systematic Review
Reprinted from: *Int. J. Environ. Res. Public Health* **2021**, *18*, 1538, doi:10.3390/ijerph18041538 . . . 21

Eun-Young Park
Stability of the Communication Function Classification System among Children with Cerebral
Palsy in South Korea
Reprinted from: *Int. J. Environ. Res. Public Health* **2021**, *18*, 1881, doi:10.3390/ijerph18041881 . . . 35

Silvana B. Napoli, María Paula Vitale, Pablo J. Cafiero, María Belén Micheletti,
Paula Pedernera Bradichansky, Celina Lejarraga, Maria Gabriela Urinovsky,
Anabella Escalante, Estela Rodriguez and Verónica Schiariti
Developing a Culturally Sensitive ICF-Based Tool to Describe Functioning of Children with
Autism Spectrum Disorder: TEA-CIFunciona Version 1.0 Pilot Study
Reprinted from: *Int. J. Environ. Res. Public Health* **2021**, *18*, 3720, doi:10.3390/ijerph18073720 . . . 45

Alessandra Schneider, Michelle Rodrigues, Olesya Falenchuk, Tiago N. Munhoz,
Aluisio J. D. Barros, Joseph Murray, Marlos R. Domingues and Jennifer M. Jenkins
Cross-Cultural Adaptation and Validation of the Brazilian Portuguese Version of an
Observational Measure for Parent–Child Responsive Caregiving
Reprinted from: *Int. J. Environ. Res. Public Health* **2021**, *18*, 1246, doi:10.3390/ijerph18031246 . . . 63

So Jin Yoon, Joohee Lim, Jung Ho Han, Jeong Eun Shin, Soon Min Lee, Ho Seon Eun,
Min Soo Park and Kook In Park
Identification of Growth Patterns in Low Birth Weight Infants from Birth to 5 Years of Age:
Nationwide Korean Cohort Study
Reprinted from: *Int. J. Environ. Res. Public Health* **2021**, *18*, 1206, doi:10.3390/ijerph18031206 . . . 79

Elena Pinero-Pinto, Verónica Pérez-Cabezas, Concepción De-Hita-Cantalejo,
Carmen Ruiz-Molinero, Estanislao Gutiérrez-Sánchez, José-Jesús Jiménez-Rejano,
José-María Sánchez-González and María Carmen Sánchez-González
Vision Development Differences between Slow and Fast Motor Development in Typical
Developing Toddlers: A Cross-Sectional Study
Reprinted from: *Int. J. Environ. Res. Public Health* **2020**, *17*, 3597, doi:10.3390/ijerph17103597 . . . 91

Magdalena Bendini and Lelys Dinarte
Does Maternal Depression Undermine Childhood Cognitive Development? Evidence from the Young Lives Survey in Peru
Reprinted from: *Int. J. Environ. Res. Public Health* **2020**, *17*, 7248, doi:10.3390/ijerph17197248 . . . **105**

Carien van Zyl and Carlien van Wyk
Exploring Factors That Could Potentially Have Affected the First 1000 Days of Absent Learners in South Africa: A Qualitative Study
Reprinted from: *Int. J. Environ. Res. Public Health* **2021**, *18*, 2768, doi:10.3390/ijerph18052768 . . . **123**

R. A. McWilliam, Tânia Boavida, Kerry Bull, Margarita Cañadas, Ai-Wen Hwang, Natalia Józefacka, Hong Huay Lim, Marisú Pedernera, Tamara Sergnese and Julia Woodward
The Routines-Based Model Internationally Implemented
Reprinted from: *Int. J. Environ. Res. Public Health* **2020**, *17*, 8308, doi:10.3390/ijerph17228308 . . . **143**

Verónica Schiariti, Rune J. Simeonsson and Karen Hall
Promoting Developmental Potential in Early Childhood: A Global Framework for Health and Education
Reprinted from: *Int. J. Environ. Res. Public Health* **2021**, *18*, 2007, doi:10.3390/ijerph18042007 . . . **163**

Egmar Longo, Ana Carolina De Campos, Amanda Spinola Barreto, Dinara Laiana de Lima Nascimento Coutinho, Monique Leite Galvão Coelho, Carolina Corsi, Karolinne Souza Monteiro and Samuel Wood Logan
Go Zika Go: A Feasibility Protocol of a Modified Ride-on Car Intervention for Children with Congenital Zika Syndrome in Brazil
Reprinted from: *Int. J. Environ. Res. Public Health* **2020**, *17*, 6875, doi:10.3390/ijerph17186875 . . . **179**

Yu-Hsin Hsieh, Maria Borgestig, Deepika Gopalarao, Joy McGowan, Mats Granlund, Ai-Wen Hwang and Helena Hemmingsson
Communicative Interaction with and without Eye-Gaze Technology between Children and Youths with Complex Needs and Their Communication Partners
Reprinted from: *Int. J. Environ. Res. Public Health* **2021**, *18*, 5134, doi:10.3390/ijerph18105134 . . . **191**

Melissa Gladstone, Gillian Lancaster, Gareth McCray, Vanessa Cavallera, Claudia R. L. Alves, Limbika Maliwichi, Muneera A. Rasheed, Tarun Dua, Magdalena Janus and Patricia Kariger
Validation of the Infant and Young Child Development (IYCD) Indicators in Three Countries: Brazil, Malawi and Pakistan
Reprinted from: *Int. J. Environ. Res. Public Health* **2021**, *18*, 6117, doi:10.3390/ijerph18116117 . . . **213**

Verónica Schiariti and Robin A. McWilliam
Crisis Brings Innovative Strategies: Collaborative Empathic Teleintervention for Children with Disabilities during the COVID-19 Lockdown
Reprinted from: *Int. J. Environ. Res. Public Health* **2021**, *18*, 1749, doi:10.3390/ijerph18041749 . . . **233**

About the Editor

Verónica Schiariti is a physician-scientist, and her work bridges clinical research and international child health. As a clinician, she has worked with children with developmental disabilities for over 10 years in community and tertiary level rehabilitation centers. As a researcher, her primary interest has been in promoting an ability-oriented approach in assessments and evaluations of children and youths with neurodevelopmental disabilities. Dr. Schiariti obtained her medical doctoral degree with honors at the University of Buenos Aires, Argentina. She trained in Pediatrics and completed a 3-year training program in Developmental Pediatrics at UBC, Canada. She obtained a Master of Health Science, a PhD and post-doctorate degrees at UBC. Dr. Schiariti is an international pediatric ICF scholar, helping to implement the ICF in different countries. She has led many knowledge translation initiatives to disseminate the application of the ICF in clinical practice globally. Her work has been recognized with many honors and awards.

Preface to "Early Child Development: From Measurement to Optimal Functioning and Evidence-Based Policy"

This textbook was first conceptualized during an invitation to create and edit a Special Issue dedicated to international child health. The Multidisciplinary Digital Publishing Institute gave me the freedom to propose a theme for the Special Issue that is of interest for a global audience. Although putting together a call for papers, editing, and contributing to a Special Issue as the only Guest Editor—during the COVID-19 pandemic—was a monumental task, I welcomed the challenge. The response from international colleagues and the quality of the papers made the Special Issue stood out. Consequently, I was invited to edit this textbook, including the content of the Special Issue entitled Early Child Development: From Measurement to Optimal Functioning and Evidence-Based Policy. The purpose of this textbook is to highlight the importance of focusing and investing in early child development. Following my clinical expertise and research interest, the guiding frameworks used in this textbook are the World Health Organization's International Classification of Functioning, Disability and Health (ICF) and the United Nations Convention on the Rights of the Child. As such, the content promotes a rights-based approach and a functioning-based approach in early child development, topics of global interest and application. As a developmental pediatrician, I am passionate about learning about the environmental factors influencing children's developmental trajectories, in particular identifying modifiable factors to promote optimal functioning of children with and without disabilities. This is crucial because early child development and overall children's developmental trajectories have long-term implications for health, functioning, and earning potential as these children become adults. Importantly, failing to reach developmental potential contributes to the global cycles of poverty, inequality, and social exclusion. In recent decades, the recognition of the close connection between the development of the child and the development of families and communities has served as the basis for national and global initiatives in health and education. Chapter 1 provides an overview of the content of this textbook, and it describes how the studies included in each chapter align with the core areas of Early Child Development, with a special focus on measurement, optimal functioning, and implications for evidence-based policy. The content of this textbook raises global awareness of the importance of a child's first years of life and the crucial role of child–environment interactions where the child lives, plays, and grows. The studies included in this textbook represent all the continents with diverse cultural and socioeconomic backgrounds. I am grateful to the international experts who generously shared information related to pivotal topics in early child development, including the need of culturally sensitive tools, successful transdisciplinary models of care, novel intersectoral frameworks, population-based data, and ongoing and upcoming environmental projects that invite positive change in practices. As such, I trust this text contributes—to the global community—novel information promoting optimal functioning in natural environments, ultimately guiding high-quality programs and evidence-based policies for young children around the world.

Verónica Schiariti
Editor

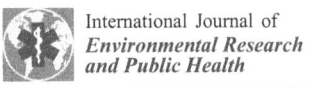

Editorial

Introduction to the Special Issue on Early Child Development: From Measurement to Optimal Functioning and Evidence-Based Policy

Verónica Schiariti

Division of Medical Sciences, University of Victoria, Victoria, BC V8W 2Y2, Canada; vschiariti@uvic.ca; Tel.: +1-250-472-5500

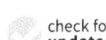

Citation: Schiariti, V. Introduction to the Special Issue on Early Child Development: From Measurement to Optimal Functioning and Evidence-Based Policy. *Int. J. Environ. Res. Public Health* **2021**, *18*, 5154. https://doi.org/10.3390/ijerph18105154

Received: 8 May 2021
Accepted: 9 May 2021
Published: 13 May 2021

Publisher's Note: MDPI stays neutral with regard to jurisdictional claims in published maps and institutional affiliations.

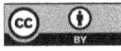

Copyright: © 2021 by the author. Licensee MDPI, Basel, Switzerland. This article is an open access article distributed under the terms and conditions of the Creative Commons Attribution (CC BY) license (https://creativecommons.org/licenses/by/4.0/).

The Importance of Early Child Development

Early child development and overall children's developmental trajectories have long-term implications for health, functioning, and earning potential as these children become adults. Importantly, failing to reach developmental potential contributes to the global cycles of poverty, inequality, and social exclusion. The recognition of the close connection between the development of the child and the development of families and communities has served as the basis for national and global initiatives in health and education in recent decades.

In 2015, for the first time, an international initiative—the 2030 Sustainable Development Goals (SDGs)—included an early childhood development goal. Specifically, SDG 4 is to ensure lifelong learning, early stimulation, increased length of schooling, school performance, and adult income. In addition, early childhood development is intricately linked to other SDG goals, poverty reduction, health and nutrition, equality for girls and women, and ending violence. Nevertheless, the risks for delay, disability and unmet potential in the early development of young children are still pervasive, particularly in low- and middle-income countries.

This editorial letter introduces the main contribution of this Special Issue and invites the readers to explore and share its content to benefit a wider audience. The Special Issue is dedicated to Early Child Development: from measurement to optimal functioning and evidence-based policy, it includes 15 open access papers addressing key topics of global interest and application.

From Measurement to Optimal Functioning and Evidence-Based Policy

Early child development measurement tools and their association with long-term outcomes were covered by many papers included in this issue [1–5]. Janus et al. [1] synthesized research using the Early Development Instrument (EDI), which was developed in Canada as a population-level assessment of children's developmental health at school entry. This narrative review shows the ability of the EDI to monitor children's developmental outcomes in various populations, how the EDI contributes to expanding the understanding of the impacts of social determinants on child development, and how it applies to special populations. Moreover, Isquith-Dicker et al. [2] examined the associations between the data obtained using child development assessment tools and educational attainment, academic achievement, or wealth. Their review demonstrates the potential for certain child development assessment tools to adequately assess long-term outcomes, but identifies that additional prospective studies using validated, culturally appropriate tools are needed. On the other hand, Napoli et al. [4] developed a novel International Classification of Functioning, Disability and Health-based tool for children with autism spectrum disorder (ASD) in Argentina, called TEA-CIFunciona. This is the first ASD culturally sensitive pediatric tool that guides the comprehensive description of functioning in Latin America. In addition, Schneide et al. [5] describe the cross-cultural validation of the responsive interactions for learning measure, the authors show that the Brazilian Portuguese version is a valid and reliable instrument for a brief assessment of responsive caregiving.

Different developmental trajectories of specific areas such as language development [3], nationwide growth patterns [6] and vision development [7] were covered by the original papers conducted in South Korea [3,6] and Spain [7]. Interestingly, Pinero-Pinto et al. [7] present the first study in a large sample of toddlers, describing the developmental correlations between visual and motor systems in typical developing toddlers.

Enabling optimal functioning, with special emphasis on child–environment interactions during early childhood, was addressed by several papers in this Special Issue. For example, Bendini & Dinarte [8] from The World Bank explored the effect of maternal depression on early childhood cognition in Peru using data from the Young Lives Survey [8]. Their findings make a strong case for recognizing maternal mental health problems as disorders of public health significance and guide maternal and infant health policies in Peru.

A qualitative study led by van Zyl, C [9] explored the environmental modifiable factors that could potentially have affected the first 1000 days of absent learners in the Western Cape of South Africa. The authors found six predominant themes that played a role during the first 1000 days of the lives of these absent learners, including health and nutrition of both the mothers and their children, substance use/abuse during pregnancy, toxic stress, support received by the mothers and their children, attachment, attentive care, and stimulation and play.

Professor McWilliam R.A and his international collaborators from 10 countries contributed to a project report on the global implementation of the Routines-Based Model (RBM) [10], sharing implementation challenges and successes, the group concluded that support-based visits with families—an RBM hallmark—can shape excellent early intervention practices for international use.

A narrative review [11], co-authored by professor Simeonsson R., synthesizes key global initiatives driving the international agenda on early child development. Furthermore, this paper proposes a universal assessment and intervention framework promoting the developmental potential in early childhood to be adopted across sectors [11].

Lastly, a study protocol by Longo et al., entitled GO-ZIKA-GO, describes a promising child-friendly environmental intervention for children affected by congenital Zika syndrome in Brazil [12].

A special mention to the paper led by Yu Hsin et al. [13], a collaboration between Sweden, U.S.A, and Dubai, which investigates the impact of using assistive technology (video-coding approach) to facilitate communication and social participation for all children with complex needs in day-to-day functioning. As such, the topic of this study enhances the content of this Special Issue, particularly how to promote optimal functioning in children and youths who need it the most. The study advocates for children's rights to express their opinions regardless of their physical limitations.

The implication of contributing quality early child development data that can ultimately guide evidence based-policy was covered by many papers [8,9,11,13–15]. Notably, Gladstone et al. [14] report on the psychometric properties of the World Health Organization (WHO) indicators of Infant and Young Child Development (IYCD). Specifically, the study validates the IYCD in Brazil, Malawi and Pakistan, showing that the IYCD performed well in cognitive testing, had similar developmental trajectories and high reliability across countries. Importantly, the IYCD initiative creates a set of global population-based developmental indicators for the currently overlooked population of children aged 0 to 3 years of age, a major contribution that will provide data/evidence of the developmental status and needs of this population, a crucial step for creating evidence-based polices globally.

Finally, a paper by Schiariti & McWilliam [15] focuses on innovative strategies promoting collaborative empathic teleintervention for children with disabilities during and post the COVID-19 lockdown. This perspective paper proposes to apply principles of RBM beyond the age of five in combination with novel rights and ability-oriented approach e-tools—e.g., My Abilities First [15].

Contributions of This Special Issue to the International Community

This Special Issue raises global awareness of the importance of children's first years of life and the crucial role of child–environment interactions where the child lives, plays, and grows. The papers included in this Special Issue represent all the continents with diverse cultural and socioeconomic backgrounds. International experts generously shared information related to pivotal topics in early child development, including the need of culturally sensitive tools, successful transdisciplinary models of care, novel intersectoral frameworks, population-based data, and ongoing and upcoming environmental projects that invite positive change in practices. As such, this Special Issue contributes—to the global community—novel information promoting optimal functioning in natural environments, ultimately guiding high-quality programs and evidence-based policies for young children around the world.

Funding: This research received no external funding.

Institutional Review Board Statement: This editorial letter did not require ethics review.

Informed Consent Statement: This editorial did not require informed consent.

Data Availability Statement: Data sharing is not applicable to this article as no new data were created in this editorial. The data supporting the author's comments are available within the reference list.

Acknowledgments: Special gratitude and appreciation is extended to all the authors for their high-quality submissions and the anonymous reviewers for volunteering their time and expertise to evaluate the scientific merit of the submitted papers. Additionally, the Special Issue managing editor, Miya Zhang, deserves special thanks for her great effort and support in making this Special Issue successful.

Conflicts of Interest: The author has no conflicts to declare.

References

1. Janus, M.; Reid-Westoby, C.; Raiter, N.; Forer, B.; Guhn, M. Population-Level Data on Child Development at School Entry Reflecting Social Determinants of Health: A Narrative Review of Studies Using the Early Development Instrument. *Int. J. Environ. Res. Public Health* **2021**, *18*, 3397. [CrossRef] [PubMed]
2. Isquith-Dicker, L.; Kwist, A.; Black, D.; Hawes, S.; Slyker, J.; Bergquist, S.; Martin-Herz, S. Early Child Development Assessments and Their Associations with Long-Term Academic and Economic Outcomes: A Systematic Review. *Int. J. Environ. Res. Public Health* **2021**, *18*, 1538. [CrossRef] [PubMed]
3. Park, E.-Y. Stability of the Communication Function Classification System among Children with Cerebral Palsy in South Korea. *Int. J. Environ. Res. Public Health* **2021**, *18*, 1881. [CrossRef] [PubMed]
4. Napoli, S.; Vitale, M.; Cafiero, P.; Micheletti, M.; Bradichansky, P.; Lejarraga, C.; Urinovsky, M.; Escalante, A.; Rodriguez, E.; Schiariti, V. Developing a Culturally Sensitive ICF-Based Tool to Describe Functioning of Children with Autism Spectrum Disorder: TEA-CIFunciona Version 1.0 Pilot Study. *Int. J. Environ. Res. Public Health* **2021**, *18*, 3720. [CrossRef] [PubMed]
5. Schneider, A.; Rodrigues, M.; Falenchuk, O.; Munhoz, T.; Barros, A.; Murray, J.; Domingues, M.; Jenkins, J. Cross-Cultural Adaptation and Validation of the Brazilian Portuguese Version of an Observational Measure for Parent–Child Responsive Caregiving. *Int. J. Environ. Res. Public Health* **2021**, *18*, 1246. [CrossRef] [PubMed]
6. Yoon, S.; Lim, J.; Han, J.; Shin, J.; Lee, S.; Eun, H.; Park, M.; Park, K. Identification of Growth Patterns in Low Birth Weight Infants from Birth to 5 Years of Age: Nationwide Korean Cohort Study. *Int. J. Environ. Res. Public Health* **2021**, *18*, 1206. [CrossRef] [PubMed]
7. Pinero-Pinto, E.; Pérez-Cabezas, V.; De-Hita-Cantalejo, C.; Ruiz-Molinero, C.; Gutiérrez-Sánchez, E.; Jiménez-Rejano, J.-J.; Sánchez-González, J.-M.; Sánchez-González, M.C. Vision Development Differences between Slow and Fast Motor Development in Typical Developing Toddlers: A Cross-Sectional Study. *Int. J. Environ. Res. Public Health* **2020**, *17*, 3597. [CrossRef] [PubMed]
8. Bendini, M.; Dinarte, L. Does Maternal Depression Undermine Childhood Cognitive Development? Evidence from the Young Lives Survey in Peru. *Int. J. Environ. Res. Public Health* **2020**, *17*, 7248. [CrossRef] [PubMed]
9. van Zyl, C.; van Wyk, C. Exploring Factors That Could Potentially Have Affected the First 1000 Days of Absent Learners in South Africa: A Qualitative Study. *Int. J. Environ. Res. Public Health* **2021**, *18*, 2768. [CrossRef] [PubMed]

10. McWilliam, R.A.; Boavida, T.; Bull, K.; Cañadas, M.; Hwang, A.-W.; Józefacka, N.; Lim, H.H.; Pedernera, M.; Sergnese, T.; Woodward, J. The Routines-Based Model Internationally Implemented. *Int. J. Environ. Res. Public Health* **2020**, *17*, 8308. [CrossRef] [PubMed]
11. Schiariti, V.; Simeonsson, R.J.; Hall, K. Promoting Developmental Potential in Early Childhood: A Global Framework for Health and Education. *Int. J. Environ. Res. Public Health* **2021**, *18*, 2007. [CrossRef] [PubMed]
12. Longo, E.; De Campos, A.C.; Barreto, A.S.; Coutinho, D.L.D.L.N.; Coelho, M.L.G.; Corsi, C.; Monteiro, K.S.; Logan, S.W. Go Zika Go: A Feasibility Protocol of a Modified Ride-on Car Intervention for Children with Congenital Zika Syndrome in Brazil. *Int. J. Environ. Res. Public Health* **2020**, *17*, 6875. [CrossRef]
13. Hsieh, Y.-H.; Borgestig, M.; Gopalarao, D.; McGowan, J.; Granlund, M.; Hwang, A.-W.; Hemmingsson, H. Communicative Interaction with and without Eye-Gaze Technology between Children and Youths with Complex Needs and Their Communication Partners. *Int. J. Environ. Res. Public Health* **2021**, *18*, 5134. [CrossRef]
14. Gladstone, M.; Lancaster, G.; McCray, G.; Cavallera, V.; Dua, T.; Lindgren Alves, C.R.; Malawichi, L.; Rasheed, M.; Janus, M.; Karige, P. Validation of the W.H.O Indicators of Infant and Young Child Development (IYCD) in three countries; Brazil, Malawi and Pakistan. *Int. J. Environ. Res. Public Health* **2021**, in press.
15. Schiariti, V.; McWilliam, R.A. Crisis Brings Innovative Strategies: Collaborative Empathic Teleintervention for Children with Disabilities during the COVID-19 Lockdown. *Int. J. Environ. Res. Public Health* **2021**, *18*, 1749. [CrossRef] [PubMed]

Review

Population-Level Data on Child Development at School Entry Reflecting Social Determinants of Health: A Narrative Review of Studies Using the Early Development Instrument

Magdalena Janus [1,2,*], Caroline Reid-Westoby [1], Noam Raiter [3], Barry Forer [2] and Martin Guhn [2]

[1] Offord Centre for Child Studies, Department of Psychiatry and Behavioural Neurosciences, McMaster University, Hamilton, ON L8S 4L8, Canada; reidwc@mcmaster.ca

[2] Human Early Learning Partnership, School of Population and Public Health, University of British Columbia, Vancouver, BC V6T 1Z3, Canada; barry.forer@ubc.ca (B.F.); martin.guhn@ubc.ca (M.G.)

[3] Michael G. DeGroote School of Medicine, McMaster University, Hamilton, ON L8P 1H6, Canada; noam.raiter@gmail.com

* Correspondence: janusm@mcmaster.ca; Tel.: +1-905-525-9140 (ext. 21418)

Abstract: Background: The Early Development Instrument (EDI) was developed as a population-level assessment of children's developmental health at school entry. EDI data collection has created unprecedented opportunities for population-level studies on children's developmental outcomes. The goal of this narrative review was to synthesize research using the EDI to describe how it contributes to expanding the understanding of the impacts of social determinants on child development and how it applies to special populations. Methods: Select studies published in peer-reviewed scientific journals between 2015 and 2020 and incorporating the social determinants of health perspectives were chosen to highlight the capability of the EDI to monitor children's developmental health and contribute knowledge in the area of early childhood development. Results: A number of studies have examined the association between several social determinants of health and children's developmental outcomes, including hard-to-reach and low-frequency populations of children. The EDI has also been used to evaluate programs and interventions in different countries. Conclusions: The ability of the EDI to monitor children's developmental outcomes in various populations has been consistently demonstrated. The EDI, by virtue of its comprehensive breadth and census-like collection, widens the scope of research relating to early childhood development and its social determinants of health.

Keywords: Early Development Instrument; developmental health; social determinants of health

1. Introduction

Over 20 years ago, Dan Keating and Clyde Hertzman formulated a framework connecting early child development with the wealth and health of nations [1], introducing the term "developmental health." This term was created to emphasize the intersection between different aspects of health, operationalizing the World Health Organization's definition of health, described as more than just the absence of illness. The idea is that health includes components of physical, mental, and social well-being, which are linked and intertwined, whereby improvements in abilities in one area require the promotion and support of other areas [2]. It is now widely recognized that developmental health extends beyond cognitive abilities and combines children's physical, mental, social, and emotional well-being [1,3]. Until early in the 21st century, much of the research on child development at school entry focused on cognitive abilities or a concept of school readiness that rarely went beyond the academic aspects [4]. Longitudinal studies show that measuring children's cognitive abilities leaves significant variance in later academic achievement unexplained [5]; other childhood characteristics—factors such as motivation, sociality, self-regulation, and physical capacities—influence success in school [6,7]. More importantly, however, the strongest predictors of school success are often social context factors, such as poverty, opportunities for learning, and environments in which children learn [8].

In the early 2000s, researchers began examining developmental health from a more holistic perspective. One tool developed in Canada in the late 1990s was designed to do just this—the Early Development Instrument (EDI) [9]. The EDI was developed as a population-level assessment of children's developmental health at school entry, taking a developmental epidemiology approach [10,11], which is used to characterize the distribution of children's developmental health in kindergarten children and examine factors that might be associated with their developmental vulnerabilities. Its implementation in jurisdictions across Canada and internationally has led to many population-level studies on children's developmental outcomes, including the examination of the associations with social determinants of health. The population-level approach is achieved through assessment of all children in a jurisdiction; in the case of the EDI, data are collected for each child in kindergarten [12].

Through this approach, the EDI has enabled researchers to examine hard-to-reach, low-frequency populations of children. Representative research evidence on minority groups is needed to effectively plan and implement large-scale interventions to improve children's developmental health. To create universal change and lower the burden of developmental vulnerability for all children, widespread monitoring using valid instruments and reliable reporting is required [13]. The EDI has been a valuable tool in providing empirical evidence on the status of kindergarten children's developmental outcomes, something that has led to the implementation of various child-related policies. Before the development of the EDI, the majority of developmental research was sample-based. While sample-based studies are informative, they are unable to examine certain associations that population-level studies can, and thus are limited in terms of their ability to provide comprehensive answers [14,15]. In contrast, population-level studies allow for comprehensive representativeness, including subpopulations of children, such as minority groups, which tend to be much less represented in sample-based studies.

The EDI has also enabled researchers to examine the impacts of early childhood programs and interventions meant to help improve developmental outcomes for children, for example by evaluating the effectiveness of preschools [16,17] or in-home interventions [18,19]. As the understanding of the pervasive influence of social determinants of health on children development increased, it has also become more evident that they may moderate the impacts of interventions [20]. Targeted interventions, such as Head Start in the USA for example [21], often by default address social determinants of health, as they focus on children in families experiencing poverty. In contrast, universal interventions, such as provision of preschool or full-day learning in kindergarten, are intended to reach everyone, but may have differential impacts depending on social determinants, such as neighborhood or family socioeconomic status [17,22].

In Canada, the EDI has been used for over 20 years, providing a population-wide view of early childhood development at school entry for over 1.2 million children. The EDI has been adapted and validated in many countries, including Australia, Ireland, Scotland, Sweden, Brazil, Chile, Estonia, Peru, Jordan, Mexico, and the United States [9]. Its utilization of teacher ratings makes the EDI a cost-effective way to gather population-level data and has allowed the collection of data from a variety of jurisdictions across the full spectrum of wealth and health. The EDI encompasses five developmental domains and provides a well-grounded, holistic view of early child development.

Although the benefits of population-level data may seem obvious in theory, it is necessary to examine the extent to which population-level data on child development have indeed contributed to the research discourse relevant to implementation science and policy [14]. This article is part of a Special Issue entitled "Early Child Development: From Measurement to Optimal Functioning and Evidence-based Policy." This article represents a narrative review of select policy-relevant studies that have involved an internationally widely used population-based tool for measurement of early child development outcomes—

the EDI. In the United Nations Children's Fund (UNICEF) Report Card #11 published in 2013 [23], the EDI was mentioned as being the only population-based tool that can be used to understand early child development outcomes in different national contexts—providing unique opportunities to study trends over time of childhood development outcomes, as well as variability in childhood development outcomes in connection with social context factors (e.g., poverty, access to resources, socioeconomic status).

In this article, we examine the ways in which research studies using population-based EDI measurement have been able to contribute to the discourse on "evidence-based policies" that seeks to enhance "optimal functioning" (e.g., positive health and education outcomes) of children. In the following, we will provide background information that situates the EDI within a context of linking international early child development research to social determinants of health and policy or decision-making that seeks to enhance population health. We then provide a narrative review of select studies using EDI data to address three questions related to the theme of the Special Issue and discuss remaing gaps and limitations, as well as future opportunities for population-based developmental health and social determinants of health (SDOH) research, in order to inform policy-making that enhances population health. In this narrative review, we synthesize selected published research on child development, conducted using the EDI as one of the measures. Our aim was to identify and describe the areas of research in which the EDI has:

(1) Widened the scope of understanding of the magnitude of the impacts of social determinants of health on child development by including large populations of children and hard-to-reach subgroups;
(2) Extended the understanding of how the social determinants of health impact developmental health in special populations of children;
(3) Contributed to the understanding of the impacts of early interventions on child development.

2. Materials and Methods

This paper represents a "narrative review" [24], as we conducted a directed synthesis of select studies using population-level EDI data to illustrate the themes of this paper. In the following, we describe the study selection process and criteria for inclusion in this review.

2.1. Paper Selection Process

This qualitative overview started by looking at all peer-reviewed papers published between 2015 and 2020 that used EDI data as an outcome measure (included in the EDI Bibliography page, https://edi.offordcentre.com/resources/bibliography-of-the-edi/ (accessed on 23 February 2021). These papers ($n = 133$) were summarized based on the research question, population studied, analyses conducted, results, and new knowledge created. The summaries were then reviewed for suitability to the three research areas listed in the introduction. Papers had to describe an empirical study (either prospective or secondary data analysis), include research questions that could be categorized as addressing social determinants of health (including prevention or intervention programs), and identify the EDI as the main outcome measure. As a result, papers that represented study protocols or data repository profiles, straightforward validation studies, commentaries, or reviews were excluded. No restrictions were put on country or region of origin or sample size. The authors each selected five papers they considered as most relevant for each area of research and then agreed upon selection criteria for inclusion in this review via consensus. Once we reached a relative saturation level for a specific topic [25], we limited further inclusion of papers. During the process of writing the sections, the list of papers included in the review was expanded to incorporate papers published prior to 2015, resulting in an addition of two papers: one published in 2010 addressing intersectionality [26] and one published in 2013 [27], including data from Scotland to increase geographical coverage. Where possible, for each category, we included work that addressed diverse populations, represented several geographic regions, and was authored by researchers from a range of institutions. The findings of the 33 included papers are described and summarized in the results (13, 13, and 7 papers in each of the three areas of research, respectively). The limitations of this approach are addressed in the Discussion.

2.2. Measures

Early Development Instrument

The EDI [9] is a population-level measure of children's developmental health at school entry. It is a teacher-completed questionnaire that assesses children's age-appropriate abilities in five different areas of development: physical health and well-being, social competence, emotional maturity, language and cognitive development, and communication skills and general knowledge. While teachers complete the EDI for every child in their class, the results are never interpreted at the individual level. Rather, they are aggregated and analyzed for groups of children (e.g., school, neighborhood, sex). For example, reports are provided to school authorities at the school- and district-level, to communities at the municipality-level, and to provinces or territories at the jurisdictional level. For research purposes, children are often grouped into various categories of interest (e.g., sex, age, illness, special needs, immigrant status) and results are compared between groups [9].

The EDI's validity, reliability, and consistency has been extensively tested in a number of countries. In Canada, the EDI has shown internal consistency values in the range of 0.84 to 0.94 for the various domains, while an assessment of test–retest reliability showed values in the range of 0.80 to 0.90 [9]. Additionally, international studies have reported similar values of internal validity and test–retest reliability. A comparison across Canada, Australia, Jamaica, and the United States showed internal consistency values ranging between 0.62 to 0.94 [28]. Evidence of predictive validity has been provided by studies from Canada and Australia [6,29,30]. Additionally, studies have shown that EDI teacher ratings align well with those of parents and with other forms of developmental assessments [31–33]. Moreover, developmental vulnerability indicated by any of the five EDI domains in kindergarten is predictive of academic, emotional, and social incompetence in later elementary school years in Canada [30], Australia [29], and the USA [34].

3. Results

3.1. Social Determinants of Health and Early Childhood Development

It was evident early in the history of published EDI literature that it provided a new and useful vehicle for widening the scope of research on the effects of SDOH on children's development, fulfilling and expanding the promise of such data predicted by Keating and Hertzman [1]. Indeed, by 2007, when the first peer-reviewed paper was published on the development and psychometric properties of the EDI [9], there were already seven papers published on the relationship between neighborhood-level EDI scores and their associated socioeconomic and demographic contexts. Most of these appeared in the first EDI-focused Special Issue in the journal "Early Education and Development" [32,35–37].

EDI literature examining SDOH contexts has demonstrated a steady output over time of over 60 articles, with at least five published in any two-year period going back to 2007, likely because of the EDI's usefulness in studying the social determinants of health (SDOH) from a population perspective. In contrast, the majority of peer-reviewed literature on EDI psychometric properties was published in 2011 or earlier.

Population-level studies, such as those made possible by the EDI, help to illustrate the fundamental and enduring impacts of SDOH on children's health. Population-level studies commonly focus on modeling the effects of SDOH as the key variables of interest [38]. In psychological child development studies, it is common to relegate SDOH variables, such as parental education and household income, to the role of controlling for selection effects. When SDOH variables are explicitly modeled, studies have shown that they have stronger effects on children's outcomes than child-level "risk factors". For example, using population-level data in Manitoba, Brownell et al. found that family risk factors (e.g., being on income assistance) and neighborhood socioeconomic status (SES) indicators (e.g., proportion not completing high school) were more strongly associated with language and cognitive outcomes in kindergarten than were factors influencing child health at birth (e.g., low birth weight) [39]. Guhn et al. found similar findings for population-level linked data in British Columbia for mental health outcomes [40]. While several birth-related factors were significantly associated with conditions such as hyperactivity and anxiety for kindergarten-age children, as well as for children up to age 15, the largest associations with these outcomes were seen with family-level poverty.

3.1.1. Area-level Socioeconomic Status and Early Child Development

Given its emphasis on area-level interpretations of whole populations, the EDI has naturally spurred research interests in examining area-level SDOH in ways that capture the breadth of available socioeconomic and demographic variables, and yet also attend to the particular context of families with young children. As Kershaw and Forer [26] point out, pan-Canadian administrative data, such as the census and income tax file data, provide a treasure trove of SDOH indicators to model area-level developmental outcomes in children. However, the choice of such indicators in the neighborhood effects literature has not been sufficiently informed by considerations relating to the intersectionality of race, class, and sex for families with young children. Kershaw and Forer's models of EDI outcomes using custom-tabulated administrative data demonstrated the usefulness of including intersectional variables (e.g., percentage of couples with female-only earners, income inequality for lone mothers) that are rarely included in other studies of neighborhood effects.

This dual analytic strategy of widening the scope of SDOH predictors being modeled while building in intersectionality concerns has been applied recently to the development of a pan-Canadian, neighborhood-level SES index [41]. This index is a composite of 10 variables taken from the census and income tax files that accounts for almost twice as much of the variance in overall pan-Canadian vulnerability rates as other existing SES indices [42]. Most of the new index's variables are specific to families with children under age six, with some specific to single-parent families of young children.

Having an efficient SES index tailored to the developmental outcomes of young children in Canada is crucial in order to examine SDOH–child development associations in a variety of contexts relevant to our first research question and described in the next section. For example, Webb et al. used this new SES index to examine how EDI–SES gradients vary by children's sex [43]. They found that the gradients were steeper for boys than girls, consistently across all developmental domains and across all Canadian provinces. More generally, it is a goal of international EDI research activities to examine the patterns of associations between SDOH and child development outcomes. Understanding the extent to which similar or different mechanisms and factors may be related to child development outcomes in different contexts and subpopulations will establish a more differentiated evidence base for identifying which actionable, changeable conditions may be addressed to enhance child development and well-being [44].

3.1.2. Social Gradients in Child Development

Examining SES gradients in child development has been a ubiquitous analytic approach to demonstrating the effects of social determinants and has been employed by researchers from many countries [1,45]; we describe three examples herein using the EDI to examine such associations. In Canada, using a newly developed pan-Canadian SES index and based on EDI scores from almost 300,000 kindergarten children from essentially all Canadian jurisdictions, Forer et al. found that children in the lowest SES quintile were developmentally vulnerable at 1.5 to 1.8 times the rate of those in the highest quintile, depending on the jurisdiction [41]. Ip et al., in a study of 567 preschool children in Hong Kong, found a strong EDI–SES gradient at the child and family level of analysis [46]. The family SES index was composed of variables relating to parental education, parental occupation, family income, and family material assets. In Scotland, Woolfson et al. used the

EDI to study developmental vulnerability in a sample of all 1090 Primary 1 children in one Scottish school district [27]. Using the Scottish Index of Multiple Deprivation as their index of socioeconomic status, they found that children in the lowest SES quintile were at least twice as likely as those in the highest quintile to be developmentally vulnerable.

3.1.3. Contributions of Social Determinants of Health to Prediction of Risk for Later Outcomes

Due to the population-wide implementation of the index, the EDI data, when linked with other data sources, offer the opportunity to examine developmental outcomes at kindergarten in relation to later outcomes for otherwise "undiagnosed" populations—for mental health outcomes, academic outcomes, or both.

Two sets of studies, one from Canada and one from Australia, provide examples of this opportunity. Thomson et al. studied the mental health of over 35,000 kindergarten-age children in British Columbia using EDI data. The study examined the patterns of children's emotional maturity and social competence (based on the subdomains of the EDI) and investigated the degree to which sociodemographic variables were related to these patterns [47]. Using latent profile analysis, six distinct social–emotional profile groups were found, with membership in the lowest functioning groups associated with being male, having English as a second language, and lower household income. In a subsequent study, children were followed up to age 14 using administrative health databases [48]. The latent socioemotional functioning profiles were applied once again and were found to be associated with early-onset mental health conditions. An examination of sociodemographic characteristics revealed that boys, children in households with unmarried parents, younger mothers, and those receiving subsidies were overrepresented in the lower socioemotional functioning groups.

These findings were reflected in Australian research [49,50]. In a study by Green and colleagues, four developmental profiles were identified using the EDI domains and subdomains that were hypothesized to present varied levels of risk for future development of mental health disorders [49]. The authors found that the odds of being in the risk groups were related to several SDOH (e.g., socioeconomic disadvantage, maltreatment) and non-SDOH (e.g., parental history of mental illness and criminal offending) variables. In a study by Piotrowska and colleagues [50] linking kindergarten data to educational, health, and protection records up to 11 years of age, researchers explored the context of transition from competence to vulnerability and found that only about 22% of children deemed as typically competent on the EDI transitioned to later vulnerability; 42% of those identified with a cluster of emotional vulnerabilities in kindergarten were also vulnerable later and 41% of children with cognitive vulnerabilities remained vulnerable. Demographic factors that have been shown to impact child development and mental health, such as parental mental illness, parental offending, and evidence of use of child protection services, were powerful determinants in influencing a child's transition between developmental profiles.

3.1.4. Racial Inequalities and Early Child Development

Only a few studies using EDI data examined racial inequalities in child development. Race is a complex construct to study, and is almost impossible to study in Canada, where race and ethnicity data are rarely collected. EDI results from the US point to racism as the root cause of observed racial inequalities. Halfon et al. [51], based on a sample of over 180,000 kindergarten children in the United States, found large differences in developmental vulnerability between racial groups; specifically, vulnerability on one or more domains was 32% for Black children, 26% for Latinx children, 19% for White children, and 18% for Asian children. All groups showed the familiar gradient by neighborhood income, although it was steepest for White children and least steep for Black children. Halfon et al. concluded that equity from the start was required, and "must consider the services, supports, and interventions that children and families need to promote optimal health development" (p. 1708).

3.2. Studying Social Determinants of Health among Special Populations of Children

Hard-to-reach, vulnerable populations tend to be under-represented in research. As Brownell and colleagues reported in 2004, children living in lower socioeconomic (SES) neighborhoods tend to be less represented in educational data than those in higher SES neighborhoods [52]. In their analyses of Grade 3 standardized test outcomes, they found that greater percentages of children from lower SES neighborhoods either did not complete the provincial standardized tests, received an exemption from writing them, or were absent during the time the test was being written [52]. Due to the population-level reach of the EDI, it has been possible to examine associations between SDOH and developmental outcomes in a number of different special populations of children. In this section, we will focus on research involving immigrant and refugee children, children with health disorders, and children who experience maltreatment or who are placed in out-of-home care.

3.2.1. Immigrant and Refugee Children

Immigrant and refugee children represent a socially, culturally, and economically diverse group, which in Canada is a growing percentage of the population. To date, the literature on child development outcomes of immigrant and refugee children tends to be sample-based and relies on parent reports, which while an important source of data on children, may not provide a representative picture, as families who do not speak the study language fluently are often excluded and there may be mistrust towards researchers. Recently, a group of Canadian researchers started examining the associations between the SDOH and developmental outcomes using EDI data linked with a range of other datasets. For example, guided by Bronfenbrenner's bioecological model [44,53], Milbrath and Guhn [54] examined the relationship between immigrant children's cultural background, neighborhood-level socioeconomic factors and cultural composition, and their developmental outcomes. Their study used EDI data linked with administrative immigration records and census data to examine the effects of family and neighborhood poverty, neighborhood cultural density (in terms of being similar or not to the child's culture), and immigrant generational status on children's developmental health at school entry among Cantonese, Mandarin, Punjabi, and Filipino children in comparison to non-immigrant, English-speaking children. In line with previous studies, they found a negative association between family and neighborhood socioeconomic disadvantage and children's EDI scores. They also found differences in the associations between a neighborhood's cultural diversity and children's developmental outcomes based on neighborhood SES indicators and children's cultural backgrounds, with Mandarin-speaking children having lower developmental outcomes in neighborhoods with greater cultural density and Punjabi-speaking children having better developmental outcomes in poorer neighborhoods with greater cultural density.

Another Canadian study by Gagné and colleagues [55] investigated the relationships between income and literacy and numeracy trajectories from kindergarten to Grade 7 for various groups of migrant children living in the Canadian province of British Columbia. They examined the three official categories of migrant children: economic, family, and refugee categories. They found that similarly to non-migrant children, lower income was associated with lower literacy and numeracy trajectories in all but one group of migrant children. Migrant children who were in the high-achieving economic class group were less impacted by low income. Gagné et al. [55] found that parental education levels and children's abilities in English predicted high literacy and numeracy trajectories, despite low income.

3.2.2. Children with Health Disorders

Until recently, Canada has lacked nationally representative data pertaining to social indicators of young children's developmental health, especially for those with health disorders. The ability to link EDI data with other datasets has allowed researchers to conduct studies on children with health disorders that were not possible before, either because of non-representative samples or because of a lack of data on certain key variables. Here, we will describe some studies from Canada and Australia that have examined SDOH in kindergarten children with health disorders.

Using pan-Canadian EDI data linked to a custom,-built neighborhood-level SES index [41], Zeraatkar and colleagues [56] examined the relationships between neighborhood-level SES and developmental health in children with disabilities, as identified in the EDI. Their results showed that all developmental domains were positively correlated with neighborhood-level SES, with the strongest relationship evident in the language and cognitive development domain. This association had already been noted in typically developing children (e.g., [41]), however this was the first Canadian population-level study to examine this link in children with disabilities. Relatedly, in Australia, O'Connor and colleagues [57] found a link between neighborhood-level SES and the odds of having an established or emerging special health-care need, with children living in the most disadvantaged neighborhoods having the highest odds of having a special health-care need.

Other studies have focused on specific health disorders, such as autism spectrum disorder [58–60], fetal alcohol spectrum disorder (FASD) [61,62], and unaddressed dental needs in kindergarten [63]. These studies consistently demonstrated the relationships between children's diagnoses, health needs, and SDOH, such as indicators of socioeconomic status at the neighborhood level.

3.2.3. Child Maltreatment and Children in Care

Developmental information on children in out-of-home care or those who experience maltreatment has been hard to come by without the opportunities to link administrative data with the EDI. Studies in Australia found that more children who have been maltreated tended to be vulnerable in all domains of their development than those who were not [64,65]. Green and colleagues [64] found that children exposed to two or more types of maltreatment and those with reported maltreatment before the age of 3 years had greater odds of being vulnerable on the EDI compared to their non-maltreated peers. Similarly, for children who were reported to child services by 5 years of age, those with the highest number of reports of maltreatment had the highest odds of being vulnerable on three or more developmental domains [65]. Maltreated children placed in the care of child protection services had slightly better developmental health in three domains (physical health and well-being, language and cognitive development, and communication skills and general knowledge) compared to maltreated children not placed in care. The authors also found that children with reports of maltreatment before the age of 18 months had the highest odds of being vulnerable in at least three domains compared to those with no maltreatment. A Canadian study reported somewhat different results. In a population-based cohort of 53,477 children living in the province of Manitoba, Wall-Weiler and colleagues [66] found that children placed in out-of-home care by child protection services were more likely to be vulnerable than children not placed in care. They also examined vulnerability levels in a subcohort of children for whom one sibling was taken into care while another one was not, as well as for discordant cousins, and did not find any differences in vulnerability between the discordant siblings or cousins. The discrepancy between the findings in the Australian and Canadian studies indicates that while children who experienced maltreatment are at risk for poor developmental outcomes, it is the larger, systemic, environmental, and social factors intersecting with microsystem characteristics (e.g., family environment) that contribute to shaping children's developmental trajectories and that require action at policy levels.

3.3. Using the EDI to Evaluate Programs and Interventions

3.3.1. Preschool Programs

EDI data collected in countries across the globe, such as Canada, Australia, Ireland, and Ethiopia, have been used to implement and evaluate programs meant to improve children's developmental health at school entry [16–18,67]. One of the most important and ubiquitous programs put in place to help support early child development is preschool. Worldwide, up to 50% of children aged 3–5 years attend preschool [68], and preschool attendance has been associated with better school readiness and academic achievement [69,70]. An Australian study of over 250,000 children showed that preschool attendance was associated with reduced odds of developmental vulnerability during children's first year of formal schooling, as reported by teachers in the EDI. Children who attended preschool had higher scores than those who did not in all developmental domains except emotional maturity, regardless of a child's socioeconomic status [17]. Goldfeld and colleagues' study emphasized most specifically the importance of continued attendance. In contrast, in a study conducted in Ireland [67], socioeconomic factors were stronger predictors of child development at school entry than preschool attendance. Children attended one year of a free preschool at any time between ages 3 years and 2 months and 4 years and 7 months, and teachers used the EDI to evaluate their development in the first year of school. Although children who participated in preschool had better social and emotional skills, and to a lesser extent better cognitive and language skills, other factors such as a child's home life and socioeconomic status had stronger effects than preschool attendance. In addition, developmental health was relatively stable over time for most children: children starting the program with higher EDI scores tended to have higher scores than their peers at the end of the program [67]. Another recent study in Mozambique evaluated the impacts of a community-based preschool program and saw increases in all EDI domains correlated with attendance [71]. Similarly to the Ireland study, children with higher initial levels showed greater academic progress in the program. The EDI has also been utilized to evaluate the effectiveness of a comprehensive preschool curriculum in Addis Ababa, Ethiopia [16]. In one of very few randomized control intervention trials that utilized the EDI as an outcome, this study assigned children to either the regular basic preschool curriculum or to a new comprehensive preschool curriculum. The authors found that children attending the comprehensive preschool curriculum scored higher on the social competence, emotional maturity, language skills, cognitive development, communication skills, and general knowledge domains of the EDI compared to their peers receiving the basic curriculum [16]. However, the recency of this study does not allow consideration of whether this effect lasted beyond school entry.

3.3.2. Early Interventions

In addition to preschool evaluations, the EDI has also been used to explore the impacts of early child development programs. One such program is the *Primeira Infância Melhor* (Better Early Childhood), a home-visiting program held in Rio Grande do Sul State, Brazil, involving regularly scheduled visits to pregnant women in their home, which continue after the child is born. The goal of this program was to help women promote their child's health and holistic development. The EDI was used to assess the efficacy of this program. The results showed that the earlier a child exited the program, the more vulnerable they were in all five developmental domains of the EDI [19], suggesting the program was effective at improving children's developmental health; however, a multivariate analysis found no overall difference among the study groups in terms of EDI outcomes. Many other countries have attempted to use early at-home interventions to improve developmental outcomes for marginalized communities before entering preschool [18,72]. A study by Enns et al. [18] focused specifically on the Families First Home Visiting (FFHV) program available to indigenous populations in Manitoba. An analysis of data for over 4000 families showed no significant difference in a child's likelihood of being vulnerable in one or more domains of the EDI in comparison to non-participants. Another study of early intervention was conducted in Australia and explored the efficacy of a nurse home visiting (NHV) program, in which mothers from disadvantaged populations received home visits by a registered nurse during the immediate postnatal period. The children enrolled in this program were followed up at age five and did not show any improvement in EDI scores in comparison to children who were not involved in the NHV program [72].

4. Discussion

In this narrative review, we integrated insights from select studies that allowed us to examine the ways in which the population-based EDI data have been useful for exploring the questions raised by the Special Issue theme; that is, the extent to which population-based measurements can inform evidence-based policy in support of enhancing children's optimal functioning [73]. In this regard, our review highlighted several points. Importantly, the population-level collection of EDI data in numerous jurisdictions internationally has provided unique opportunities to systematically examine the variability in child development outcomes in relation to social determinants of health, and to do so for subpopulations that are commonly either unrepresented or under-represented in sample-based research. The EDI has helped investigators widen the scope of research relating to the social determinants of health by virtue of its comprehensive breadth, both conceptually and analytically, in addition to as a result of the census-like nature of the data collected. The EDI also offers researchers and policy-makers the opportunity to address systemic differences in children's development. The studies investigating the impacts of early programs and interventions using the EDI have shown inconsistent results. These inconsistences suggest that these interventions and programs may be ineffective for these children or for the domains measured with the EDI, or that the impacts of the program might be evident only in the long term.

Studies utilizing the EDI have contributed to our understanding of the role of social context factors at multiple ecological levels (e.g., community, family) in the early development of a child. By linking the EDI with administrative data, researchers have been able to examine associations between children's developmental health and the social determinants of health at the population level, which were previously difficult to examine. This type of research has allowed us to gain a better understanding of the socioeconomic disparities across various jurisdictions, such as with the work conducted by Forer and colleagues [41]. The EDI has also facilitated the monitoring of child developmental trajectories over time, which combined with other indicators, can inform future research and child-related policies about early developmental outcomes and predictors of later health and development.

Another advantage of the population-level data collected using the EDI is that researchers are able to study special populations of children, for whom numbers are typically low in sample-based research. Using the EDI, researchers have been able to examine the developmental health of children with autism spectrum disorder, fetal alcohol spectrum disorder, unaddressed dental needs, and children with disabilities in relation to social determinants of health. These studies have consistently demonstrated an association between neighborhood-level socioeconomic status and children's developmental health. These studies have also been able to identify jurisdictional differences in either the prevalence of a given disorder or developmental vulnerabilities in these children. This research is vital for policy-makers, as it offers information that can help improve our ability to identify children earlier in order to provide early intervention and access to services. Some of this work is already being translated into policy briefs and recommendations (e.g., [74]).

The EDI has also been used to evaluate early programs and interventions meant to improve children's developmental health. Our review indicates that the results are mixed, with some studies showing a large effect (e.g., [17]), small effect (e.g., [19]), or no effect (e.g. [72]). The research examining the impacts of home visiting in particular has not shown advantages for child development at school entry. There are many potential possibilities, not the least of which is that home visiting rarely leads to overall better cognitive or behavioral outcomes in children [75]. The impacts of participating in preschool in the year prior to school entry also showed mixed results. While conceptually a sound strategy, such an intervention may not be enough to deflect the strong influence of other early social determinants, such as socioeconomic status. These studies add not only to our understanding of the limited reach of the early interventions and short preschool programs, but also to the methodological considerations in terms of evaluating their outcomes. A recent meta-analysis of early parenting interventions with a specific focus on reducing children's disruptive behavior failed to show any evidence to support the argument for the better effectiveness of programs implemented for younger rather than older children, even though they were mostly effective [76].

This also gives us an opportunity to focus on the EDI's characteristics as an instrument that provides evidence suitable for policy-level use. The EDI detects variability in early child development outcomes in a population; population-level monitoring may be the best way of capturing and examining how social determinants of health and macrosystem factors (such as implementation of preschool, variability in poverty and income, or minority status) are related to early childhood outcomes and early child development trajectories. Population-level developmental health monitoring may, thus, be an ideal tool providing evidence of the extent to which policies that significantly affect SDOH and macrosystem factors achieve lasting positive effects on developmental health outcomes, and whether such policies help to reduce inequities that exist in our societies.

Overall, results from the studies discussed in this paper show that the social determinants of health show a strong association with children's developmental outcomes at an early age, and that the SDOH have a much stronger association than child characteristics. These findings also suggest that program interventions alone, such as preschool or home visiting, will often not be enough to compensate for the detrimental effects of poor SDOH on children's development without addressing the more fundamental social determinants, such as poverty.

Limitations and Future Opportunities

It is important to acknowledge several limitations. One limitation relates to the authors' personal preferences, which could have influenced the selection of studies reviewed in this paper. In some cases, several papers addressed the same or similar issues, and the final selection could have been swayed by the authors' own research interests or unconscious preferences for a certain methodology, despite a thorough review of the final included papers and all authors' consensus. All papers using the EDI are listed on the EDI bibliography website, which is constantly updated and may be easily reviewed by readers. We have not included in this review research including indigenous children, since our author team did not include indigenous members. We recognize that this is a limitation and aspire to rectify this in future reviews. Finally, the focus of this review has been on potentially unique contributions of population-based measurements of child development to inform policy-making in order to enhance children's optimal functioning. However, a population-based lens is not a substitute for in-depth, developmental, longitudinal child development studies or evaluation studies of early interventions; rather, the different disciplinary lenses ideally complement and inform each other. We anticipate that future developmental research that draws from population-level data linkages may be able to integrate population-level data on child development at different stages of the life course—and eventually follow child cohorts intergenerationally—involving comprehensive data on children's social context (e.g., family, community, school, socioeconomic factors, policy) and also measured during different life periods (e.g., childhood, youth, adulthood). Such comprehensive socioecological, developmental, population-based monitoring and data linkages would realize the type of developmental science that has been proposed by Urie Bronfenbrenner, in his influential formulation of the "bioecological model of human development". In fact, this trend is already noticeable in the EDI literature, as the papers using individual-level linkages between EDI and other data sources constitute 59% of articles published within the past five years.

5. Conclusions

One of the major characteristics of the EDI that lends itself well towards the population-wide studies reviewed in this paper is its holistic nature. Research demonstrates that the EDI is an effective tool for monitoring children's developmental health, both in typically developing children and those with health disorders. Thus far, the research using the EDI has contributed to the expansion of our knowledge on the associations between SDOH and children's developmental health, and mostly through linkages with other databases has opened many possibilities for further investigation of early childhood development.

Author Contributions: Conceptualization, M.J. and M.G.; writing—original draft preparation, N.R., C.R.-W., M.J., and B.F.; writing—review and editing, N.R., C.R.-W., M.J., B.F., and M.G. All authors have read and agreed to the published version of the manuscript.

Funding: This research received no external funding.

Institutional Review Board Statement: Not applicable.

Informed Consent Statement: Not applicable.

Data Availability Statement: No new data were created or analyzed in this study. Data sharing is not applicable to this article.

Acknowledgments: We would like to acknowledge the contributions of the late Dan Offord, Clyde Hertzman, and Fraser Mustard to the development of the idea of population-level measures of early child development in service of improving the odds for optimal development of all children.

Conflicts of Interest: The authors declare no conflict of interest.

References

1. Keating, D.P.; Hertzman, C. *Developmental Health and the Wealth of Nations: Social, Biological, and Educational Dynamics*; The Guildford Press: New York, NY, USA, 1999.
2. National Research Council (USA); Institute of Medicine (USA). *Committee on Integrating the Science of Early Childhood Development, from Neurons to Neighborhoods: The Science of Early Childhood Development*; National Academies Press: Washington, DC, USA, 2000.
3. Hair, E.; Halle, T.; Terry-Humen, E.; Lavelle, B.; Calkins, J. Children's school readiness in the ECLS-K: Predictions to academic, health, and social outcomes in first grade. *Early Child. Res. Q.* **2006**, *21*, 431–454. [CrossRef]
4. Janus, M.; Gaskin, A. School Readiness. In *Encyclopedia of Quality of Life and Well-Being Research*; Metzler, J.B., Ed.; Springer: Dordrecht, The Netherlands, 2014; pp. 5703–5706.
5. Cerda, C.A.; Im, M.H.; Hughes, J.N. Learning-related skills and academic achievement in academically at-risk first graders. *J. Appl. Dev. Psychol.* **2014**, *35*, 433–443. [CrossRef]
6. Davies, S.; Janus, M.; Duku, E.; Gaskin, A. Using the Early Development Instrument to examine cognitive and non-cognitive school readiness and elementary student achievement. *Early Child. Res. Q.* **2016**, *35*, 63–75. [CrossRef]
7. Romano, E.; Babchishin, L.; Pagani, L.S.; Kohen, D. School readiness and later achievement: Replication and extension using a nationwide Canadian survey. *Dev. Psychol.* **2010**, *46*, 995–1007. [CrossRef] [PubMed]
8. Ray, K.; Smith, M.C. The Kindergarten Child: What Teachers and Administrators Need to Know to Promote Academic Success in all Children. *J. Fam. Econ. Issues* **2010**, *38*, 5–18. [CrossRef]
9. Janus, M.; Offord, D.R. Development and psychometric properties of the Early Development Instrument (EDI): A measure of children's school readiness. *Can. J. Behav. Sci. Rev. Can. Sci. Comport.* **2007**, *39*, 1–22. [CrossRef]
10. Costello, E.J.; Angold, A. Developmental Epidemiology. In *Developmental Psychopathology*; American Cancer Society: New York, NY, USA, 2016; pp. 1–35.
11. McLaughlin, K.A. Developmental Epidemiology. In *Handbook of Developmental Psychopathology*; Lewis, M., Rudolph, K.D., Eds.; Springer: Boston, MA, USA, 2014; pp. 87–107.
12. Janus, M. *The Early Development Instrument: A Population-Based Measure for Communities. A Handbook on Development, Properties, and Use*; Offord Centre for Child Studies: Hamilton, ON, USA, 2007; Available online: https://edi-offordcentre.s3.amazonaws.com/uploads/2015/07/2007_12_FINAL.EDI_.HANDBOOK.pdf (accessed on 23 February 2021).
13. Offord, D.R.; Kraemer, H.C.; Kazdin, A.E.; Jensen, P.S.; Harrington, R. Lowering the Burden of Suffering From Child Psychiatric Disorder: Trade-Offs Among Clinical, Targeted, and Universal Interventions. *J. Am. Acad. Child Adolesc. Psychiatry* **1998**, *37*, 686–694. [CrossRef] [PubMed]
14. Keating, D.P. Formative Evaluation of the Early Development Instrument: Progress and Prospects. *Early Educ. Dev.* **2007**, *18*, 561–570. [CrossRef]
15. Vernon-Feagans, L.; Blair, C. Measurement of School Readiness. *Early Educ. Dev.* **2006**, *17*, 1–5. [CrossRef]
16. Deyessa, N.; Webb, S.; Duku, E.; Garland, A.; Fish, I.; Janus, M.; Desta, M. Epidemiological study of a developmentally and culturally sensitive preschool intervention to improve school readiness of children in Addis Ababa, Ethiopia. *J. Epidemiol. Community Health* **2020**, *74*, 489–594. [CrossRef] [PubMed]
17. Goldfeld, S.; O'Connor, E.; O'Connor, M.; Sayers, M.; Moore, T.; Kvalsvig, A.; Brinkman, S. The role of preschool in promoting children's healthy development: Evidence from an Australian population cohort. *Early Child. Res. Q.* **2016**, *35*, 40–48. [CrossRef]

18. Enns, J.E.; Chartier, M.; Nickel, N.; Chateau, D.; Campbell, R.; Phillips-Beck, W.; Sarkar, J.; Burland, E.; Lee, J.B.; Katz, A.; et al. Association between participation in the Families First Home Visiting programme and First Nations families' public health outcomes in Manitoba, Canada: A retrospective cohort study using linked administrative data. *BMJ Open* **2019**, *9*, e030386. [CrossRef]
19. Gonçalves, T.R.; Duku, E.; Janus, M. Developmental health in the context of an early childhood program in Brazil: The "Primeira Infância Melhor" experience. *Cadernos de Saúde Pública* **2019**, *35*, e00224317. [CrossRef]
20. Brooks-Gunn, J. Do You Believe In Magic? What We Can Expect From Early Childhood Intervention Programs. *Soc. Policy Rep.* **2003**, *17*, 1–16. [CrossRef]
21. Deming, D. Early Childhood Intervention and Life-Cycle Skill Development: Evidence from Head Start. *Am. Econ. J. Appl. Econ.* **2009**, *1*, 111–134. [CrossRef]
22. Brownell, M.; Nickel, N.; Chateau, D.; Martens, P.; Taylor, C.; Crockett, L.; Katz, A.; Sarkar, J.; Burland, E.; Goh, C. Long-term benefits of full-day kindergarten: A longitudinal population-based study. *Early Child Dev. Care* **2014**, *185*, 291–316. [CrossRef] [PubMed]
23. Adamson, P. Child Well-being in Rich Countries: A comparative overview. In *Innocenti Report Card*; no. 11; UNICEF Office of Research: Florence, Italy, 2013.
24. Ferrari, R. Writing narrative style literature reviews. *Med. Writ.* **2015**, *24*, 230–235. [CrossRef]
25. Fusch, P.I.; Ness, L.R. Are We There Yet? Data Saturation in Qualitative Research. *Qual. Rep.* **2015**, *20*, 1408–1416.
26. Kershaw, P.; Forer, B. Selection of area-level variables from administrative data: An intersectional approach to the study of place and child development. *Health Place* **2010**, *16*, 500–511. [CrossRef]
27. Woolfson, L.M.; Geddes, R.; McNicol, S.; Booth, J.N.; Frank, J. A cross-sectional pilot study of the Scottish early development instrument: A tool for addressing inequality. *BMC Public Health* **2013**, *13*, 1187. [CrossRef]
28. Janus, M.; Brinkman, S.A.; Duku, E.K. Validity and Psychometric Properties of the Early Development Instrument in Canada, Australia, United States, and Jamaica. *Soc. Indic. Res.* **2011**, *103*, 283–297. [CrossRef]
29. Brinkman, S.; Gregory, T.; Harris, J.; Hart, B.; Blackmore, S.; Janus, M. Associations between the Early Development Instrument at Age 5, and Reading and Numeracy Skills at Ages 8, 10 and 12: A Prospective Linked Data Study. *Child Indic. Res.* **2013**, *6*, 695–708. [CrossRef]
30. Guhn, M.; Gadermann, A.M.; Almas, A.; Schonert-Reichl, K.A.; Hertzman, C. Associations of teacher-rated social, emotional, and cognitive development in kindergarten to self-reported wellbeing, peer relations, and academic test scores in middle childhood. *Early Child. Res. Q.* **2016**, *35*, 76–84. [CrossRef]
31. Forget-Dubois, N.; Lemelin, J.-P.; Boivin, M.; Dionne, G.; Séguin, J.R.; Vitaro, F.; Tremblay, R.E. Predicting Early School Achievement With the EDI: A Longitudinal Population-Based Study. *Early Educ. Dev.* **2007**, *18*, 405–426. [CrossRef]
32. Janus, M.; Duku, E. The School Entry Gap: Socioeconomic, Family, and Health Factors Associated with Children's School Readiness to Learn. *Early Educ. Dev.* **2007**, *18*, 375–403. [CrossRef]
33. Lloyd, J.E.; Hertzman, C. From Kindergarten readiness to fourth-grade assessment: Longitudinal analysis with linked population data. *Soc. Sci. Med.* **2009**, *68*, 111–123. [CrossRef] [PubMed]
34. Duncan, R.J.; Duncan, G.J.; Stanley, L.; Aguilar, E.; Halfon, N. The kindergarten Early Development Instrument predicts third grade academic proficiency. *Early Child. Res. Q.* **2020**, *53*, 287–300. [CrossRef]
35. Lesaux, N.K.; Rupp, A.A.; Siegel, L.S. Growth in reading skills of children from diverse linguistic backgrounds: Findings from a 5-year longitudinal study. *J. Educ. Psychol.* **2007**, *99*, 821–834. [CrossRef]
36. Lapointe, V.R.; Ford, L.; Zumbo, B.D. Examining the Relationship between Neighborhood Environment and School Readiness for Kindergarten Children. *Early Educ. Dev.* **2007**, *18*, 473–495. [CrossRef]
37. Kershaw, P.; Forer, B.; Irwin, L.G.; Hertzman, C.; Lapointe, V. Toward a Social Care Program of Research: A Population-Level Study of Neighborhood Effects on Child Development. *Early Educ. Dev.* **2007**, *18*, 535–560. [CrossRef]
38. Guhn, M.; Goelman, H. Bioecological Theory, Early Child Development and the Validation of the Population-Level Early Development Instrument. *Soc. Indic. Res.* **2011**, *103*, 193–217. [CrossRef]
39. Brownell, M.D.; Ekuma, O.; Nickel, N.C.; Chartier, M.J.; Koseva, I.; Santos, R.G. A population-based analysis of factors that predict early language and cognitive development. *Early Child. Res. Q.* **2016**, *35*, 6–18. [CrossRef]
40. Guhn, M.; Emerson, S.D.; Mahdaviani, D.; Gadermann, A.M. Associations of Birth Factors and Socio-Economic Status with Indicators of Early Emotional Development and Mental Health in Childhood: A Population-Based Linkage Study. *Child Psychiatry Hum. Dev.* **2020**, *51*, 80–93. [CrossRef] [PubMed]
41. Forer, B.; Minh, A.; Enns, J.; Webb, S.; Duku, E.; Brownell, M.; Muhajarine, N.; Janus, M.; Guhn, M. A Canadian Neighbourhood Index for Socioeconomic Status Associated with Early Child Development. *Child Indic. Res.* **2019**, *13*, 1133–1154. [CrossRef]
42. Webb, S.; Janus, M.; Duku, E.; Raos, R.; Brownell, M.; Forer, B.; Guhn, M.; Muhajarine, N. Neighbourhood socioeconomic status indices and early childhood development. *SSM Popul. Health* **2017**, *3*, 48–56. [CrossRef]
43. Webb, S.; Duku, E.; Brownell, M.; Enns, J.; Forer, B.; Guhn, M.; Minh, A.; Muhajarine, N.; Janus, M. Sex differences in the socioeconomic gradient of children's early development. *SSM Popul. Health* **2020**, *10*, 100512. [CrossRef] [PubMed]
44. Bronfenbrenner, U.; Morris, P.A. The Bioecological Model of Human Development. In *Handbook of Child Psychology*; John Wiley & Sons Inc.: Hoboken, NJ, USA, 2006; Volume 1, pp. 793–828.
45. Marmot, M. Social determinants of health inequalities. *Lancet* **2005**, *365*, 1099–1104. [CrossRef]

46. Ip, P.; Rao, N.; Bacon-Shone, J.; Li, S.L.; Ho, F.K.-W.; Chow, C.-B.; Jiang, F. Socioeconomic gradients in school readiness of Chinese preschool children: The mediating role of family processes and kindergarten quality. *Early Child. Res. Q.* **2016**, *35*, 111–123. [CrossRef]
47. Thomson, K.C.; Guhn, M.; Richardson, C.G.; Ark, T.K.; Shoveller, J. Profiles of children's social–emotional health at school entry and associated income, gender and language inequalities: A cross-sectional population-based study in British Columbia, Canada. *BMJ Open* **2017**, *7*, e015353. [CrossRef] [PubMed]
48. Thomson, K.C.; Richardson, C.G.; Gadermann, A.M.; Emerson, S.D.; Shoveller, J.; Guhn, M. Association of Childhood Social-Emotional Functioning Profiles at School Entry With Early-Onset Mental Health Conditions. *JAMA Netw. Open* **2019**, *2*, e186694. [CrossRef]
49. Green, M.J.; Tzoumakis, S.; Laurens, K.R.; Dean, K.; Kariuki, M.; Harris, F.; O'Reilly, N.; Chilvers, M.; A Brinkman, S.; Carr, V.J. Latent profiles of early developmental vulnerabilities in a New South Wales child population at age 5 years. *Aust. N. Z. J. Psychiatry* **2018**, *52*, 530–541. [CrossRef] [PubMed]
50. Piotrowska, P.J.; Whitten, T.; Tzoumakis, S.; Laurens, K.R.; Katz, I.; Carr, V.J.; Harris, F.; Green, M.J. Transitions between socio-emotional and cognitive vulnerability profiles from early to middle childhood: A population study using multi-agency administrative records. *Eur. Child Adolesc. Psychiatry* **2020**, *29*, 1659–1670. [CrossRef] [PubMed]
51. Halfon, N.; Aguilar, E.; Stanley, L.; Hotez, E.; Block, E.; Janus, M. Measuring Equity From The Start: Disparities In The Health Development Of US Kindergartners. *Health Aff.* **2020**, *39*, 1702–1709. [CrossRef]
52. Brownell, M. *How Do Educational Outcomes Vary with Socioeconomic Status?: Key Findings from the Manitoba Child Health Atlas 2004*; Manitoba Centre for Health Policy, Dept. of Community Health Sciences, Faculty of Medicine, University of Manitoba: Winnipeg, MB, USA, 2004.
53. Bronfenbrenner, U. *The Ecology of Human Development: Experiments by Nature and Design*; Harvard University Press: Cambridge, MA, USA, 1979.
54. Milbrath, C.; Guhn, M. Neighbourhood culture and immigrant children's developmental outcomes at kindergarten. *Early Child. Res. Q.* **2019**, *48*, 198–214. [CrossRef]
55. Gagné, M.; Janus, M.; Muhajarine, N.; Gadermann, A.; Duku, E.; Milbrath, C.; Minh, A.; Forer, B.; Magee, C.; Guhn, M. Disentangling the role of income in the academic achievement of migrant children. *Soc. Sci. Res.* **2020**, *85*, 102344. [CrossRef] [PubMed]
56. Zeraatkar, D.; Duku, E.; Bennett, T.; Guhn, M.; Forer, B.; Brownell, M.; Janus, M. Socioeconomic gradient in the developmental health of Canadian children with disabilities at school entry: A cross-sectional study. *BMJ Open* **2020**, *10*, e032396. [CrossRef] [PubMed]
57. O'Connor, M.; O'Connor, E.; Quach, J.; Vashishtha, R.; Goldfeld, S. Trends in the prevalence and distribution of teacher-identified special health-care needs across three successive population cohorts. *J. Paediatr. Child Health* **2018**, *55*, 312–319. [CrossRef] [PubMed]
58. Janus, M.; Mauti, E.; Horner, M.; Duku, E.; Siddiqua, A.; Davies, S. Behavior profiles of children with autism spectrum disorder in kindergarten: Comparison with other developmental disabilities and typically developing children. *Autism Res.* **2018**, *11*, 410–420. [CrossRef]
59. Siddiqua, A.; Duku, E.; Georgiades, K.; Mesterman, R.; Janus, M. Neighbourhood-level prevalence of teacher-reported Autism Spectrum Disorder among kindergarten children in Canada: A population level study. *SSM Popul. Health* **2020**, *10*, 100520. [CrossRef] [PubMed]
60. Siddiqua, A.; Duku, E.; Georgiades, K.; Mesterman, R.; Janus, M. Association between neighbourhood socioeconomic status and developmental vulnerability of kindergarten children with Autism Spectrum Disorder: A population level study. *SSM Popul. Health* **2020**, *12*, 100662. [CrossRef]
61. Brownell, M.; Enns, J.E.; Hanlon-Dearman, A.; Chateau, D.; Phillips-Beck, W.; Singal, D.; MacWilliam, L.; Longstaffe, S.; Chudley, A.; Elias, B.; et al. Health, Social, Education, and Justice Outcomes of Manitoba First Nations Children Diagnosed with Fetal Alcohol Spectrum Disorder: A Population-Based Cohort Study of Linked Administrative Data. *Can. J. Psychiatry* **2019**, *64*, 611–620. [CrossRef]
62. Pei, J.; Reid-Westoby, C.; Siddiqua, A.; Elshamy, Y.; Rorem, D.; Bennett, T.; Birken, C.; Coplan, R.; Duku, E.; Ferro, M.A.; et al. Teacher-Reported Prevalence of FASD in Kindergarten in Canada: Association with Child Development and Problems at Home. *J. Autism Dev. Disord.* **2021**, *51*, 433–443. [CrossRef] [PubMed]
63. Janus, M.; Reid-Westoby, C.; Lee, C.; Brownell, M.; Maguire, J.L. Association between severe unaddressed dental needs and developmental health at school entry in Canada: A cross-sectional study. *BMC Pediatr.* **2019**, *19*, 1–9. [CrossRef]
64. Green, M.J.; Tzoumakis, S.; McIntyre, B.; Kariuki, M.; Laurens, K.R.; Dean, K.; Chilvers, M.; Harris, F.; Butler, M.; Brinkman, S.A.; et al. Childhood Maltreatment and Early Developmental Vulnerabilities at Age 5 Years. *Child Dev.* **2017**, *89*, 1599–1612. [CrossRef] [PubMed]
65. Rossen, L.; Tzoumakis, S.; Kariuki, M.; Laurens, K.R.; Butler, M.; Chilvers, M.; Harris, F.; Carr, V.J.; Green, M.J. Timing of the first report and highest level of child protection response in association with early developmental vulnerabilities in an Australian population cohort. *Child Abus. Negl.* **2019**, *93*, 1–12. [CrossRef]
66. Wall-Wieler, E.; Roos, L.L.; Lee, J.B.; Urquia, M.L.; Roos, N.P.; Bruce, S.; Brownell, M. Placement in Care in Early Childhood and School Readiness: A Retrospective Cohort Study. *Child Maltreatment* **2019**, *24*, 66–75. [CrossRef] [PubMed]

67. McKeown, K.; Haase, T.; Pratschke, J. Determinants of child outcomes in a cohort of children in the Free Pre-School Year in Ireland, 2012/2013. *Ir. Educ. Stud.* **2015**, *34*, 245–263. [CrossRef]
68. UNICEF. *A World Ready to Learn Prioritizing Quality Early Childhood Education*; United Nations Children's Fund: New York, NY, USA, 2019.
69. Barnett, W.S.; Frede, E. The Promise of Preschool: Why We Need Early Education for All. *Am. Educ.* **2010**, *34*, 21.
70. Nores, M.; Belfield, C.R.; Barnett, W.S.; Schweinhart, L. Updating the Economic Impacts of the High/Scope Perry Preschool Program. *Educ. Eval. Policy Anal.* **2005**, *27*, 245–261. [CrossRef]
71. Martinez, S.; Naudeau, S.; Pereira, V.A. *Preschool and Child Development Under Extreme Poverty: Evidence from a Randomized Experiment in Rural Mozambique*; Social Science Research Network: Rochester, NY, USA, 2017; Available online: https://papers.ssrn.com/abstract=3092440 (accessed on 18 December 2020).
72. Sawyer, A.C.; Le Kaim, A.; Mittinity, M.N.; Jeffs, D.; Lynch, J.W.; Sawyer, M.G. Effectiveness of a 2-year post-natal nurse home-visiting programme when children are aged 5 years: Results from a natural experiment. *J. Paediatr. Child Health* **2018**, *55*, 1091–1098. [CrossRef]
73. Janus, M.; Reid-Westoby, C. Monitoring the development of all children: The Early Development Instrument. In *Early Childhood Matters*; Moreno, T., Ed.; Bernard van Leer Foundation: The Hague, The Netherlands, 2016; pp. 40–45.
74. Canadian Autism Spectrum Disorder Alliance. Policy Compendium: The Development of a National Autism Strategy through Community and Stakeholder Engagement; Canadian Autism Spectrum Disorder Alliance; 2020. Available online: https://kidsbrainhealth.ca/wp-content/uploads/2021/01/CASDA-KBHN-Briefs-Compendium-_28102020-.docx-1.pdf (accessed on 20 February 2021).
75. Peacock, S.; Konrad, S.; Watson, E.; Nickel, D.; Muhajarine, N. Effectiveness of home visiting programs on child outcomes: A systematic review. *BMC Public Health* **2013**, *13*, 17. [CrossRef] [PubMed]
76. Gardner, F.; Leijten, P.; Melendez-Torres, G.; Landau, S.; Harris, V.; Mann, J.; Beecham, J.; Hutchings, J.; Scott, S. The Earlier the Better? Individual Participant Data and Traditional Meta-analysis of Age Effects of Parenting Interventions. *Child Dev.* **2018**, *90*, 7–19. [CrossRef] [PubMed]

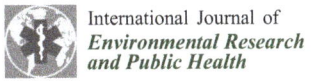

Review

Early Child Development Assessments and Their Associations with Long-Term Academic and Economic Outcomes: A Systematic Review

Leah N. Isquith-Dicker [1,2,†], Andrew Kwist [1,3,†], Danae Black [1,3], Stephen E. Hawes [1,3], Jennifer Slyker [1,3], Sharon Bergquist [4] and Susanne P. Martin-Herz [5,*]

1. Department of Global Health, University of Washington START Center, Seattle, WA 98195, USA; leahiuw@gmail.com (L.N.I.-D.); andrew.kwist@gmail.com (A.K.); danaesb@uw.edu (D.B.); hawes@uw.edu (S.E.H.); jslyker@uw.edu (J.S.)
2. Department of Anthropology, School of Public Health, University of Washingto, Seattle, WA 98195, USA
3. Department of Epidemiology, School of Public Health, University of Washington, Seattle, WA 98195, USA
4. Bill & Melinda Gates Foundation, 500 5th Ave N, Seattle, WA 98109, USA; sharon.bergquist@gatesventures.com
5. Department of Pediatrics, University of California San Francisco, 1825 Fourth St., 6th Floor, UCSF Box 4054, San Francisco, CA 94143, USA
* Correspondence: susanne.martinherz@ucsf.edu; Tel.: +1-415-502-1338
† Leah N. Isquith-Dicker and Andrew Kwist are co-first authors and contributed equally to this project and manuscript preparation.

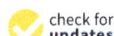

Citation: Isquith-Dicker, L.N.; Kwist, A.; Black, D.; Hawes, S.E.; Slyker, J.; Bergquist, S.; Martin-Herz, S.P. Early Child Development Assessments and Their Associations with Long-Term Academic and Economic Outcomes: A Systematic Review. *Int. J. Environ. Res. Public Health* **2021**, *18*, 1538. https://doi.org/10.3390/ijerph18041538

Academic Editor: Verónica Schiariti
Received: 25 December 2020
Accepted: 30 January 2021
Published: 5 February 2021

Publisher's Note: MDPI stays neutral with regard to jurisdictional claims in published maps and institutional affiliations.

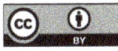

Copyright: © 2021 by the authors. Licensee MDPI, Basel, Switzerland. This article is an open access article distributed under the terms and conditions of the Creative Commons Attribution (CC BY) license (https://creativecommons.org/licenses/by/4.0/).

Abstract: Developmental screening instruments were designed as diagnostic tools, but there is growing interest in understanding whether select tools can also be used systematically in research to examine intervention impacts on long-term outcomes. As such, this systematic review aims to examine associations between child development assessment tools and educational attainment, academic achievement, or wealth. We included studies identified in PubMed, PsycINFO, and Educational Resources Information Center if they reported an association between at least one tool from a pre-established list and one outcome of interest after age 10. Of 597 studies identified, 11 met inclusion criteria; three examined educational attainment as the outcome of interest, six examined academic achievement, one wealth, and one both educational attainment and wealth. Intelligence tests were utilized in five of the included studies, neuropsychological/executive function or behavior tools were used in five, and one study used tools across the domains. High-quality studies were identified across all three of the domains, but educational attainment and wealth had the greatest proportion of high-quality studies, as compared to academic achievement. Our review demonstrates the potential for certain child development assessment tools to adequately assess long-term outcomes of interest, but additional prospective studies using validated, culturally appropriate tools are needed. PROSPERO registration number: CRD42018092292.

Keywords: child development; functioning; outcomes; education; measurement; child development assessment; academic achievement; educational attainment; wealth/socioeconomic status

1. Introduction

Recent findings from the *Lancet* series on early childhood development estimate that over 250 million children under five years of age in low-and middle-income countries are at risk of not achieving their full developmental potential [1]. Children in low- and middle-income countries may face a variety of adversities, including recurrent illness, malnutrition, and trauma, with long-term consequences for their health, productivity, and overall well-being [2]. It has been previously estimated that children not reaching their full developmental potential results in an average adult annual income deficit of 19.8% [3]. In addition to income loss, developmental delays have also been associated with considerable academic underachievement [4–6]. These factors have led to increased interest in child development assessment tools that are adequately associated with long-term academic, economic, and human capital outcomes from a young age. However, existing child development assessment tools were generally designed to assess risk or developmental status at the time of testing [7–10]. Limited research focused on this topic suggests that available tools may not have strong predictive potential for later outcomes [1,4], highlighting the need for additional investigation to determine if specific tools or developmental domains may be useful for both prediction of outcome without intervention or in evaluation of intervention programs.

This systematic review was conducted to identify child development assessment tools that are associated with the long-term outcomes of educational attainment, academic achievement, and wealth. Given that an assessment of study quality is also included in this review, this synthesis provides information to aid researchers in the selection and prioritization of tools or domains for further research in this area.

2. Materials and Methods

2.1. Data Sources

A literature search was conducted in PubMed, PsycINFO, and Educational Resources Information Center (ERIC) on March 30, 2018. Publication date was restricted to manuscripts published in 1990 or later, due to differences in assessment tools and publication standards in comparison to more recent literature (Document S1). A search template was created that was applied to all 3 databases with minimal tailoring (Document S2). The search yielded 597 unique results that were exported into the Covidence (Melbourne, Australia) systematic review software [11]. This systematic review was conducted in accordance with PRISMA (Preferred Reporting Items for Systematic Reviews and Meta-Analyses) guidelines and preregistered at PROSPERO: CRD42018092292.

2.2. Development Tool Selection

The search template contained a list of 104 child development assessment tools (Table S1). An initial list of 1398 tools was generated from a search of the PsycTEST database, a repository of assessment tools indexed from articles in peer-reviewed journals and books by experts at the American Psychological Association [12]. The PsycTEST search utilized the search terms, "child development, executive function, school, education, academic, readiness, reading, literacy" and excluded the terms "sexual behaviors and divorce." As many tools were not relevant to study objectives, one of the authors (SMH) manually filtered the list and added additional relevant assessment tools absent from PsycTEST database to assemble the final list. Tools were retained in the final list if they measured at least one of the five most common domains of development (gross motor, fine motor, language, cognitive, and social emotional), or examined reading/pre-reading skills or executive function. Tools were required to show some indication of psychometric properties, since it was felt that at least some evidence of reliability and validity were prerequisites to adequate association between the tools and future educational and economic outcomes, even if this was obtained from cross-sectional as opposed to longitudinal research. Tools were excluded if they examined only sublevels of developmental domains, were specific to second language learning, were designed explicitly to evaluate gender differences, were specific to health or mental health diagnoses, were specific to a particular study context, examined child or caregiver attitudes toward a developmental domain or skill set rather than the child's development (e.g., child reading attitude), or focused specifically on theory of the mind, math achievement, or home literacy environment.

2.3. Study Inclusion and Exclusion Criteria

Studies were included in this review on the basis of the following criteria: (1) the study was conducted using an experimental or observational design; (2) the study used at least one of the assessment tools in the list with children under the age of 18; (3) the study reported at least one outcome related to educational attainment, academic achievement, or wealth and assessed this outcome after the age of 10 years; educational attainment was defined by the highest-grade level completed at the time of data collection, while academic achievement was defined as performance in one or more subject areas; (4) articles were published in English or French; French-language articles were included in an attempt to ensure inclusion of articles that were conducted in Francophone Africa.

Cross-sectional studies were excluded because the study objective was to identify tools that were associated with long-term academic and socioeconomic outcomes. Studies conducted with children who were hospitalized or had severe neurologic injuries, genetic conditions, or autism spectrum disorder were excluded, because the use of a tool in such a sample could not easily be generalizable to the larger pediatric population. The age of 10 was chosen as a lower bound for long-term outcomes due to concern that children in some low-and middle-income countries may terminate formal schooling near this age. There were no exclusion criteria related to the length of time between tool assessment and outcome evaluation or the specific geographic location. Detailed inclusion and exclusion criteria can be found in the study's PROPSERO preregistration.

2.4. Research Processes

Title and abstract screening were completed for all identified studies independently by two reviewers (LNID and AK), and discordance was resolved by a third reviewer (JS). Full text screening was also completed by two reviewers (LNID and AK), with discordance resolved by a third reviewer (DB). For studies excluded by full-text review, reviewers selected one primary reason for exclusion, and discordance in study exclusion rationale was resolved by a third reviewer (JS). The exclusion hierarchy was as follows, in order of priority: outcome not of interest, cross-sectional study design, outcome assessed at younger than 10 years of age, population with medical/developmental condition, assessment tool not on list. A PRISMA flowchart is provided in Figure 1.

In addition to this structured search, targeted searching was conducted in two ways. First, publications identified from a list of cohort studies recommended by subject matter experts (SMH and SB) were evaluated for their adherence to study inclusion criteria [13–16]. Second, an additional search using cohort studies identified during the initial stages of the title and abstract screening process was undertaken, and three potentially relevant studies were added to the total pool for title and abstract screening (additional studies identified through other sources in Figure 1). These additional steps were taken in an effort to broaden the scope of the review in the event that the search terms missed relevant studies.

2.5. Data Abstraction

The following information was abstracted from the articles identified in the full-text review: author, publication year, sample size, sampling method, time between assessment tool and outcome, assessment tool(s) used, age at which assessment tool was used, outcome(s), age at which outcome was evaluated, and measure(s) of association. For studies that used an assessment tool at multiple time points without separate effect measures, we only reported the greater duration from child development assessment to outcome (e.g., for tool applied at age 11 and age 16 and outcome measured at age 19, we only reported association between age 11 to age 19). In some studies, more than one assessment tool was used, including some child development assessment tools that were not on our pre-specified list. In these cases, only the associations between the tools on the list and our outcomes of interest were reported. Effect measures are presented adjusted for standard sociodemographic factors (i.e., parent education, sex, and wealth) unless otherwise stated. Regression coefficients and odds ratios are presented with statistical significance, and confidence intervals when measures of statistical significance were unavailable.

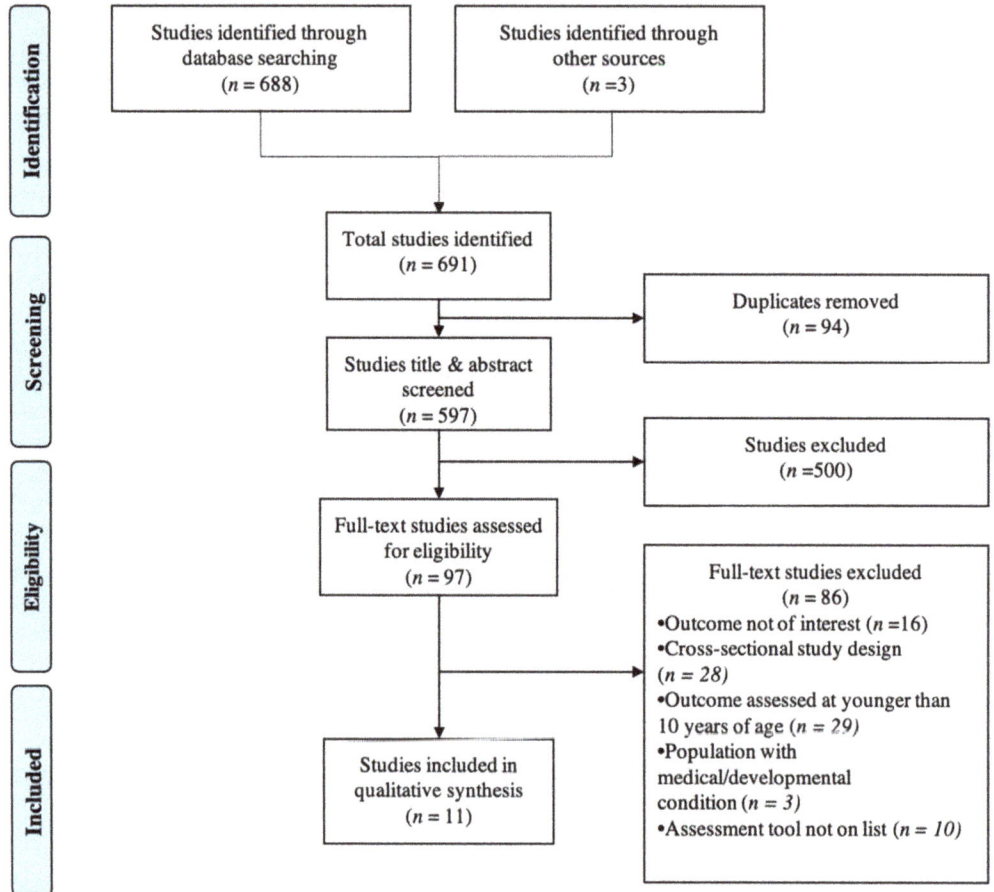

Figure 1. A Preferred Reporting Items for Systematic Reviews and Meta-Analyses (PRISMA) flowchart of the selection process of published studies.

2.6. Data Synthesis

We used a narrative approach to data synthesis, which is the preferred method when empirical approaches and variables are highly varied across studies [17]. Tools were then categorized by the domain or construct area they assessed. This classification was initially made by a developmental-behavioral pediatrician (SMH) and then independently by 3 volunteer neuropsychologists. We used outcome, tool domain, and a study quality assessment as the classification schemes for synthesizing data.

2.7. Quality Assessment

A quality assessment was conducted to determine the rigor of study methods and relevance of the effect measures reported, in the context of the objectives of our study. For the quality assessment, five criteria were evaluated by the two authors (DB and LID) who completed the data extraction. These criteria were adapted from the Cochrane Collaboration Risk of Bias Tool, usually applied to evaluations of quantitative evidence from systematic reviews [18]. The authors of this tool recommended the assessment of five specific categories of bias and one category for other types of bias as needed in accordance with study objectives. Detail on bias categories is provided below; other categories were not considered given the sufficient coverage provided by those applied. The authors evaluated the criteria on these categories independently by maintaining separate data sheets that were shared only when evaluations were complete. Discordance was discussed and resolved by a third reviewer (JS). Each criterion is defined below and was assigned a designation of, low, high, or unclear quality with point values of −1, 1, and 0, respectively. Criteria were weighted equally because each category of bias was deemed of equal importance to study quality. An overall assessment of study quality was ascertained by the sum of the point values, termed the "cumulative quality assessment", which was used to categorize studies as of high, low, or neutral quality. The unclear designation was assigned when information regarding a criterion were not provided in the article itself and was not possible to ascertain from supplemental materials or earlier publications describing study methods. Quality assessment criteria were as follows:

(1) Selection: Evaluated how participants were selected for inclusion in the study. A study with a random sample or an attempted census was designated high quality and a convenience sample was designated as low quality.
(2) Sample size: Examined the adequacy of the sample size. A total sample size of >100 participants was designated high quality for the current review, as smaller studies may have very limited statistical power.
(3) Attrition: Assessed loss to follow up, withdrawal, or exclusion from analysis. Studies with a rate of attrition of < 25% were designated high quality.
(4) Duration: Evaluated the length of time between child development assessment and outcome. Studies with durations >5 years were considered to be high quality.
(5) Outcome reporting: Evaluated the extent to which authors provided information on how outcomes were measured. Standardized tests, registries, or assessment tools and those reported by teachers or trained experts (e.g., psychologist) were designated high quality, and self-report (child or parent) was designated low quality.
(6) Cumulative quality assessment: Sum of point values for criterion 1–5.

3. Results

3.1. Overview of Studies

Of 597 unique articles identified, 500 were excluded during the title and abstract screening phase, largely due to being cross-sectional in nature, not assessing an outcome of interest, or having the outcome of interest but assessing it prior to 10 years of age. During this phase, none of the publications identified by subject matter experts for targeted searching met criteria for full-text review. Of the 97 articles included in the full text review phase, 11 met study criteria for inclusion (Table S2); the number of articles excluded for each criterion is documented in Figure 1. All included studies were observational cohort studies, with a follow-up duration range from 2 years to greater than 20 years. Six studies were sampled from a school setting [19–24], two from birth cohorts [25,26], one via an adoption agency [27], and two through larger population-based studies [28,29]. Sample sizes varied widely, with smaller cohorts (<50) among special populations (e.g., low-income families) and larger population-based cohorts (>6000).

3.2. Assessment Tool Domains of Studies Included for Review

The child development assessment tools utilized in the 11 included studies were classified into three categories: neuropsychological/executive function and behavior, intelligence, and general development and achievement (Table 1). Figure 2 displays the distribution of studies by the domain of the tool used. Neuropsychological/executive function and behavior tools were employed in five studies; intelligence tests in five studies, and multiple tools from both the general development/achievement and intelligence domains were used in one study (see Figure 2 notes for details). Studies that analyzed multiple tools independently were counted separately for each tool.

Table 1. Child development assessment tools utilized in included studies, by domain.

Domain	Tools
Neuropsychological/ executive function and behavior	CBCL—Child Behavior Checklist RINT—Reitan-Indiana Neuropsychological Battery for Children SDQ—Strengths and Difficulties Questionnaire SMFQ—Short Mood and Feelings Questionnaire YSR—Youth Self Report of the Child Behavior Checklist CAAS—Children's Attention and Adjustment Survey
Intelligence	Stanford-Binet FE (Fourth Edition) Stanford-Binet: LM (Form LM) WISC-R—Weschler Intelligence Scale for Children-Revised WISC Verbal IQ WISC Performance IQ
Development/achievement	PIAT—Peabody Individual Achievement Test-Reading subscale PPVT-R—Peabody Picture Vocabulary Test-Revised

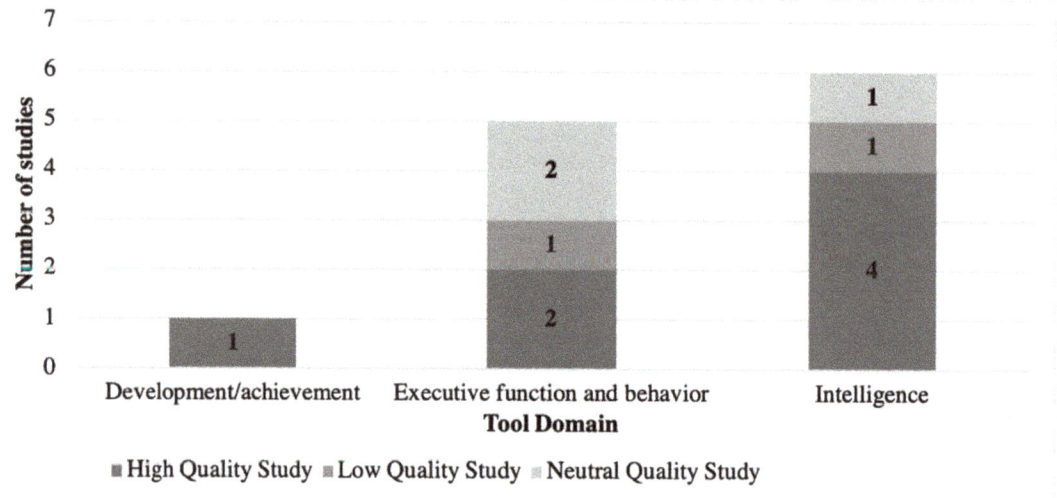

Figure 2. Included studies by domain of child development assessment tool. The total number of studies listed exceeds the number of studies included in this review because [27] included 2 child development assessment tools of interest in 2 domains (Development/achievement and Intelligence). A detailed explanation for the high/neutral/low quality designation is provided in Section 3.4 below.

3.3. Outcomes

The association between a child development assessment tool of interest and educational attainment was measured by four of the 11 selected studies, as shown in Figure 3 [25,27–29]. Educational attainment was determined either by self-report of the number of school years completed or national registries that included school completion information. Six studies reported associations between a tool of interest and academic achievement [19–24]. There was more heterogeneity in the measurement of academic achievement, including standardized tests that were named (e.g., Iowa Test of Basic Skills, Metropolitan Achievement Test, and General Certificate of Secondary Education) or unnamed, as well as school grade point averages, either from school records or by self-report. Only two studies assessed outcomes related to wealth, income, or socioeconomic status [25,26].

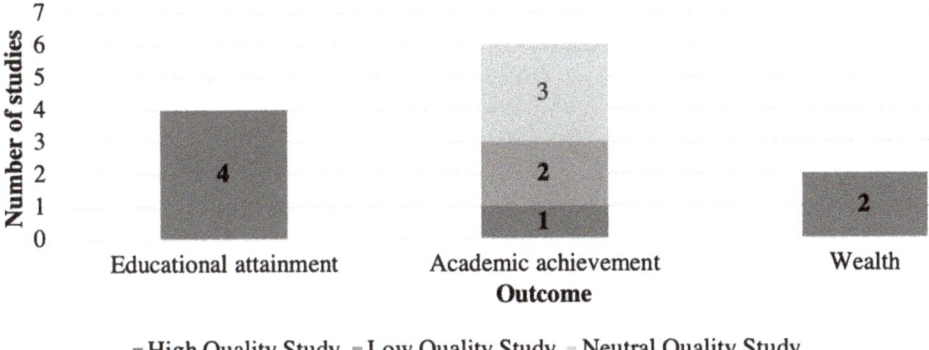

Figure 3. Included studies by outcome of interest. NOTES: The total number of studies listed exceeds the number of studies included in this review because [25] assessed both educational attainment and wealth. A detailed explanation for the high/neutral/low quality designation is provided in Section 3.4 below.

3.4. Quality Assessment

Table 2 displays the results of the quality assessment, which identified two low quality studies, four neutral quality studies, and five high quality studies. The low-quality studies were published in 1995 and 2017 and represented small samples of children attending a residential school in Canada (N = 20) and an elementary school in Switzerland (N = 103), respectively [20,21]. These studies reported non-significant effect estimates for outcomes and had short duration of follow-up (≤3 years). The high-quality studies were published between 2001 and 2014, included large cohorts (>1000) from New Zealand, Norway, and The Netherlands, and a smaller cohort from the United States [22,25,26,28,29]. The effect measures for the high-quality studies were almost all significant (except one effect measure from a study that used the Youth Self Report & Child Behavior Checklist [29] and had greater length of follow up (range 5 to 29 years). The five high quality studies are summarized below:

- Moffitt, 2011 [26]

A prospective cohort study from the participants in the Dunedin Multidisciplinary Health and Development Study Cohort in New Zealand assessed childhood self-control, socioeconomic factors, and IQ using the Wechsler Intelligence Scales for Children, Revised (WISC-R; repeat measures at ages 3, 5, 7, 9, and 11), and the association with wealth at age 32. Statistical models included adjustment for socioeconomic factors and fixed-effects modeling applied to dizygotic same-gender twins to compare outcomes of siblings with differential self-control levels and thus isolate the effect of self-control. The study found that the intelligence assessment was significantly associated with four measures of wealth: socioeconomic status, income, financial planfulness, and financial issues (regression estimates −0.400, −0.291, −0.160, and 0.029, respectively; all $p < 0.05$).

- Sagatun, 2014 [28]

A retrospective cohort study that utilized data from a Norwegian registry to assess the association between the Strengths and Difficulties Questionnaire administered to 15- to 16-year-olds and academic attainment as recorded in the national registry of school completion at age 20–21. Statistical models included adjustments for children's ethnic background, county of residence, parents' education, income, and marital status. The study found that this tool was significantly associated with odds of non-completion of school (ORs 1.11–1.48, all $p < 0.001$).

- Lamp, 2001 [22]

A prospective cohort study among families enrolled in the Head Start Program in the United States assessed intelligence using the Stanford Binet Intelligence scale at age 4 and its correlation with academic achievement at ages 5 to 10 years, measured by the Metropolitan Achievement Test. No information regarding the factors used for adjustment in statistical models was provided. The study found that intelligence as measured by this tool was significantly correlated with academic achievement (correlation coefficients 0.39–0.62, all $p < 0.01$).

- Fergusson, 2005 [25]

A retrospective cohort study involving participants from the Christchurch Child Development Study in New Zealand assessed intelligence using the WISC-R in 8 to 9-year-olds and analyzed its association with wealth, educational outcomes, and obtaining a university degree between the ages of 18 and 25 years. Statistical models included adjustment for a series of covariate factors including measures of childhood social and family disadvantage and behavior. The study found that intelligence was significantly associated with gross income (regression coefficient 1.595, $p < 0.05$) and gaining school or university qualifications (regression coefficients 0.67–0.82, $p < 0.01$).

- Veldman, 2014 [29]

A prospective cohort study to determine likelihood of educational attainment (measured by number of years of schooling completed) by age 19, using data from the Tracking Adolescent's Individual Lives Survey in The Netherlands, assessed 11 year-olds using the Child Behavior Checklist and its Youth Self Report. Statistical models included adjustment for children's sex, age, IQ, parental educational status, and physical health status. The study found that externalizing, internalizing, and attention problems, as assessed by these combined tools, were associated with higher odds of low (primary, lower vocational and lower secondary education) vs. medium (intermediate vocational and intermediate secondary) educational attainment at age 19 (OR 1.25–1.78; statistical significance varied—see Table S3 for details).

Table 2. Study quality assessment.

Author, Year	Selection	Attrition	Outcome Reporting	SAMPLE SIZE	Duration	Cumulative Assessment
Moffitt, 2011 [26]	High	High	High	High	High	5 (High)
Sagatun, 2014 [28]	High	High	High	High	High	5 (High)
Lamp, 2001 [22]	High	High	High	Low	High	3 (High)
Fergusson, 2005 [25]	High	High	Low	High	High	3 (High)
Veldman, 2014 [29]	High	High	Low	High	High	3 (High)
Clarren, 1993 [19]	Low	Low	High	High	High	1 (Neutral)
Rothon, 2009 [23]	High	Low	High	High	Low	1 (Neutral)
Samuels, 2016 [24]	Unclear	Unclear	High	Unclear	Low	0 (Neutral)
McClelland, 2013 [27]	Low	Low	Low	High	High	−1 (Neutral)
Richards, 1995 [20]	Low	Unclear	High	Low	Low	−2 (Low)
Gygi, 2017 [21]	Unclear	Low	Low	Low	Low	−4 (Low)

Each criterion was evaluated with the following numerical values: high quality = 1; low quality = −1, unclear quality = 0. Each study could receive up to a cumulative assessment value of 5. Studies with values > 1 were designated high quality studies, values of 1, 0 and −1 neutral quality, and < −1 low quality studies. See Section 2.7 (Materials and Methods: Quality Assessment) for additional detail.

4. Discussion

4.1. Overview of Key Findings

This study sought to examine the evidence base for the association between child development assessment tools and longer-term outcome. After applying a rigorous set of inclusion criteria on 597 studies identified from our initial search, we retained 11 observational cohort studies in this systematic review that investigated the association between a child development assessment tool of interest and a long-term outcome of interest. Although the studies were distributed across all three outcomes of interest, and three development tool domains, the majority of these studies investigated the outcome of academic achievement and used intelligence or neuropsychological/executive function and behavioral tools as predictors. Five of the eleven studies were determined to be high quality and reported measures of association that were almost all significant; given that these studies had at least 100 participants, and a minimum of 5 years duration of follow-up, these would have more statistical power to show a significant effect size. These findings suggest that child development assessment tools across a range of development domains may have predictive potential for various types of outcomes later in life, but several limitations of the available literature and limitations of our study suggest that further research is needed as described below.

4.2. Limitations of the Available Literature

The evidence base supporting the ability of child development assessment tools to predict long-term outcomes remains limited to remarkably few studies, with a need for more high-quality studies that are adequately powered and have follow-up sufficient to reveal associations with adult-life outcomes. Figures 2 and 3 illustrate that there are high quality studies distributed across the three outcomes of interest and all three assessment tool domains. However, the included studies were heterogeneous with respect to study design, assessment tools, outcome measures, and statistical models. This heterogeneity precludes direct comparison, even between studies that used the same tool (e.g., WISC-R) to determine whether these associations are repeatable, and the effect sizes are consistent across populations. Our quality assessment suggests that issues related to attrition remain a challenge in longitudinal studies; continuing to engage and track study participants over decades is a common challenge in longitudinal studies, so this finding is not all together surprising. However, it is notable that two studies did not clearly describe attrition, which threatens both evaluation of sample size and effect measures [20,24].

All included studies in this review were observational cohort studies, which are susceptible to several limitations. Cohort studies are prone to differential loss to follow-up of participants with medical or financial challenges, which can bias findings. While many studies accounted for confounding with adjusted effect estimates, additional sources of residual confounding likely remained, including family and community contextual factors, the impact of developmental interventions, and children's physical health. Longitudinal studies that document and control for these contextual factors are needed.

Additionally, the use of multiple or composite assessment tools was framed as a "best fit" approach by some authors. However, the utilization of multiple predictors can diminish the statistical validity of significant results due to the increased probability of a significant result due solely to chance, given the large number of hypothesis tests. A priori assertions grounded in theoretical rationale for the utility of composite or multiple domain assessment tools can help to mitigate this issue and provide better evidence as to whether composite assessments improve prediction of outcomes; alternatively, the assessment of predictors separately would help to isolate the effect of individual tools.

Finally, the generalizability of findings from this review is limited by the fact that all of the studies took place in high-income countries among relatively homogenous racial and ethnic groups. Few of the tools assessed in this review have been validated for use in African, Asian, and South American populations. The absence of studies from low- and middle-income countries may be a reflection of the small number of tools validated for use in these populations, and limits generalizability of findings to populations from low-income countries, and populations with high rates of malnutrition or limited access to education.

4.3. Limitations of Present Study

There are several limitations to this review. First, the study was designed with a specific purpose to identify developmental assessment tools that predict long term outcomes related to academic and economic potential of individuals and communities and did not include research assessing other long-term outcomes with high relevance for health and quality of life. Despite efforts to be comprehensive in its inclusion of tools by completing a broad search of the PsycTESTS database and reviewing almost 1400 tools, some studies were excluded at full-text review because they did not include an assessment tool from the original search list (e.g., a study that examined educational attainment among three large cohorts from Finland, the UK, and the Philippines and found significant positive associations between cognitive development scores at early ages and attainment in adulthood [30]). Despite a thorough search of three robust databases, there is likely additional relevant research that was not captured. In particular, grey literature, such as non-peer reviewed organizational reports, and economics literature (e.g., EconLit database) were not considered and may be a source of additional information regarding the socioeconomic outcome of interest. Additionally, only English and French literature was reviewed due to the linguistic capacity of the research team, and thus there may be additional literature in other languages that may be particularly relevant to address the issue mentioned above related to generalizability of findings to the low-and middle-income country context.

Next, this review was completed in 2018; to remediate the concern of additional published literature not being reflected in this review, in January 2021 we conducted post-hoc abstract screening of articles published in 2018–2021 in all three databases (PubMed, Educational Resources Information Center (ERIC), and PsycINFO), using the same search terms. Of 158 results across the three databases, five articles passed abstract screening and were full-text reviewed, and only two additional studies met inclusion criteria [31,32]. First, Samuels et al., 2019 found that the Behavior Rating Inventory of Executive Function (BRIEF) and BRIEF Self-Report (BRIEF-SR) were significantly associated with the upcoming cumulative grade point average in a diverse population of 259 New York middle and high school students, independent of gender, free/reduced lunch, and special education status [31]. However, it is unclear whether this instrument predicts longer-term academic performance because the time interval between tool assessment and outcome assessment was notably short. Second, Kosik et al., 2018 found in a U.S based birth cohort that the WISC at age seven was significantly associated with educational attainment, employment, and wealth in adulthood [32]. Despite the identification of these two additional studies, of which likely only Kosik et al., 2018 would be considered high-quality, we are confident that the findings reported in our main review remain relevant and continue to fill a needed gap in the literature. These studies' findings do not conflict with findings of the five high-quality studies in the main review, and in fact only further support our review's overall conclusions.

Finally, all of the high-quality studies reviewed reported positive associations, suggesting publication bias and potential underreporting of null findings. Coupled with the small sample sizes and shorter follow-up of the low and neutral quality studies reviewed, additional research is needed to support the associations identified between tools and outcomes studied herein.

4.4. Recommendations for Future Research

Additional research evaluating regionally-validated tools, conducted in large and diverse study populations with adequate follow-up, including low-and middle-income countries, are needed to understand whether these tools can be used to predict long term outcomes and assess the impact of interventions. Existing data from large cohort studies in these low-and middle-income countries, either ongoing or already completed, could also be leveraged to contribute to this field of work. Many of the tools evaluated in our review were proprietary, and there is growing interest in developing tools that are valid across multiple populations and that can be administered by medical staff or community health workers [33]. Additionally, to address the limitation of the inability to capture all potentially relevant development tools of interest, researchers conducting future research on this topic could consider not restricting their search to specific tools, but instead develop a detailed search string on keywords related developmental domains.

5. Conclusions

Our review identified 11 studies investigating associations between early childhood assessment tools and long-term economic and academic outcomes of interest. Five of these studies were determined to be high-quality and reported mostly statistically significant associations, suggesting that certain child development assessment tools are associated with the long-term outcomes of interest. Given that child development assessment tools were designed to identify children with developmental delay at the time of assessment, our study addresses a key need to characterize the potential for these tools to be sensitive to intervention effects and to potentially predict longer-term outcomes. The high-quality literature reviewed was primarily conducted in high-resource contexts and was relatively sparse; as such, additional prospective studies, engaging large, diverse populations in both high-income and low-and middle-income countries are needed to adequately address remaining gaps in this evidence base.

Supplementary Materials: The following are available online at https://www.mdpi.com/1660-4601/18/4/1538/s1, Document S1, Document S2: PubMed, PyscINFO, and ERIC database search strings, Table S1: Child development assessment tools included in search string, Table S2. Details of studies included in the review.

Author Contributions: S.P.M.-H. and S.B. conceptualized and designed the study, reviewed, and revised the manuscript. L.N.I.-D., A.K., D.B. and J.S. designed the study, collected the data, carried out the analyses, drafted the initial manuscript, and reviewed and revised the manuscript. S.E.H. critically reviewed the manuscript for important intellectual content and reviewed and revised the manuscript. All authors have read and agreed to the published version of the manuscript.

Funding: This research was funded by the Bill & Melinda Gates Foundation through a grant with the University of Washington Strategic Analysis, Research and Training (START) Center.

Institutional Review Board Statement: Not Applicable.

Informed Consent Statement: Not Applicable.

Data Availability Statement: Not Applicable.

Acknowledgments: We appreciate the three volunteer neuropsychologists who assisted in domain classification of the childhood development assessment tools of interest: Shannon Lundy, Stephany Cox, and Gina Pfeifle. The majority of the content of this paper was included in some form in a report for the Bill & Melinda Gates Foundation; further refinement of the quality assessment methodology and Discussion section was conducted after the report was delivered.

Conflicts of Interest: Sharon Bergquist was employed by and Susanne Martin-Herz was a consultant to the Bill & Melinda Gates Foundation during the course of the review. The content is solely the responsibility of the authors and does not necessarily represent the official views of the Bill & Melinda Gates Foundation. All other authors have no conflict of interest to declare.

References

1. Black, M.M.; Walker, S.P.; Fernald, L.C.H.; Andersen, C.T.; DiGirolamo, A.M.; Lu, C.; McCoy, D.C.; Fink, G.; Shawar, Y.R.; Shiffman, J.; et al. Early childhood development coming of age: Science through the life course. *Lancet* **2017**, *389*, 77–90. [CrossRef]
2. Elder, J.P.; Pequegnat, W.; Ahmed, S.; Bachman, G.; Bullock, M.; Carlo, W.A.; Chandra-Mouli, V.; Fox, N.A.; Harkness, S.; Huebner, G.; et al. Caregiver Behavior Change for Child Survival and Development in Low- and Middle-Income Countries: An Examination of the Evidence. *J. Health Commun.* **2014**, *19*, 25–66. [CrossRef] [PubMed]

3. Grantham-McGregor, S.; Cheung, Y.B.; Cueto, S.; Glewwe, P.; Richter, L.; Strupp, B. Developmental potential in the first 5 years for children in developing countries. *Lancet* **2007**, *369*, 60–70. [CrossRef]
4. Dornelas, L.D.F.; Magalhães, L.D.C. Functional performance of school children diagnosed with developmental delay up to two years of age. *Rev. Paul. Pediatr.* **2016**, *34*, 78–85. [CrossRef]
5. Perna, R. Early Developmental Delays: A Cross Validation Study. *J. Psychol. Abnorm. Child.* **2013**, *1*. [CrossRef]
6. Willoughby, M.T.; Magnus, B.; Vernon-Feagans, L.; Blair, C.B. Developmental Delays in Executive Function from 3 to 5 Years of Age Predict Kindergarten Academic Readiness. *J. Learn. Disabil.* **2017**, *50*, 359–372. [CrossRef]
7. Dumont, R.; Cruse, C.L.; Alfonso, V.; Levine, C. Book Review: Mullen Scales of Early Learning: AGS Edition. *J. Psychoeduc. Assess.* **2000**, *18*, 381–389. [CrossRef]
8. Harman, T.M.; Smith-Bonahue, J.L. The Bayley-III Adaptive Behavior Scale. In *Bayley-III Clinical Use and Interpretation*, 1st ed.; Aylward, T.O., Glen, L.W., Eds.; Elsevier: Amsterdam, The Netherlands, 2010; pp. 177–200.
9. Laher, K.; Cockcroft, S. (Eds.) *Psychological Assessment in South Africa: Research and Application*; Wits University Press: Johannesburg, South Africa, 2013.
10. Prado, E.L.; Abbeddou, S.; Adu-Afarwuah, S.; Arimond, M.; Ashorn, P.; Ashorn, U.; Bendabenda, J.; Brown, K.H.; Hess, S.Y.; Kortekangas, E.; et al. Predictors and pathways of language and motor development in four prospective cohorts of young children in Ghana, Malawi, and Burkina Faso. *J. Child Psychol. Psychiatry* **2017**, *58*, 1264–1275. [CrossRef] [PubMed]
11. Covidence Systematic Review Software. Veritas Health Innovation. Available online: www.covidence.org (accessed on 25 April 2018).
12. American Psychological Association. PsycTESTS. 2018. Available online: http://www.apa.org/pubs/databases/psyctests/index.aspx%0D (accessed on 15 May 2018).
13. Fall, C.H.; Sachdev, H.S.; Osmond, C.; Restrepo-Mendez, M.C.; Victora, C.; Martorell, R.; Stein, A.D.; Sinha, S.; Tandon, N.; Adair, L.; et al. Association between maternal age at childbirth and child and adult outcomes in the offspring: A prospective study in five low-income and middle-income countries (COHORTS collaboration). *Lancet Glob. Health* **2015**, *3*, e366–e377. [CrossRef]
14. Martorell, R.; Horta, B.L.; Adair, L.S.; Stein, A.D.; Richter, L.; Fall, C.H.D.; Bhargava, S.K.; Biswas, S.K.D.; Perez, L.; Barros, F.C.; et al. Weight Gain in the First Two Years of Life Is an Important Predictor of Schooling Outcomes in Pooled Analyses from Five Birth Cohorts from Low- and Middle-Income Countries. *J. Nutr.* **2010**, *140*, 348–354. [CrossRef] [PubMed]
15. Richter, L.; Victora, C.G.; Hallal, P.C.; Adair, L.S.; Bhargava, S.K.; Fall, C.H.; Lee, N.; Martorell, R.; A Norris, S.; Sachdev, H.S.; et al. Cohort Profile: The Consortium of Health-Orientated Research in Transitioning Societies. *Int. J. Epidemiol.* **2012**, *41*, 621–626. [CrossRef] [PubMed]
16. Stein, A.D.; Barros, F.C.; Bhargava, S.K.; Hao, W.; Horta, B.L.; Lee, N.; Kuzawa, C.W.; Martorell, R.; Ramji, S.; Stein, A.; et al. Birth status, child growth, and adult outcomes in low- and middle-income countries. *J. Pediatr.* **2013**, *163*, 1740–1746. [CrossRef] [PubMed]
17. Popay, J.; Roberts, H.; Sowden, A.; Petticrew, M.; Arai, L.; Rodgers, M.; Britten, N.; Roen, K.; Duffy, S. *Guidance on the Conduct of Narrative Synthesis in Systematic Reviews*; ESRC Methods Programme: Lancaster, UK, 2006.
18. Cochrane. Chapter 8: Assessing Risk of Bias in Included Studies. In Cochrane Handbook for Systematic Reviews of Interventions Version 5.0.; 2008. Available online: http://www.cochrane-handbook.org (accessed on 25 April 2018).
19. Clarren, S.B.; Martin, D.C.; Townes, B.D. Academic achievement over a decade: A neuropsychological prediction study. *Dev. Neuropsychol.* **1993**, *9*, 161–176. [CrossRef]
20. Richards, T.N.; Symonsa, D.; Greene, C.A.; Szuszkiewicz, T.A. The Bidirectional Relationship between Achievement and Externalizing Behavior Problems of Students with Learning Disabilities. *J. Learn. Disabil.* **1995**, *28*, 8–17. [CrossRef] [PubMed]
21. Gygi, J.T.; Arx, P.H.-V.; Schweizer, F.; Grob, A. The Predictive Validity of Four Intelligence Tests for School Grades: A Small Sample Longitudinal Study. *Front. Psychol.* **2017**, *8*. [CrossRef]
22. Lamp, R.E.; Krohn, E.J. A Longitudinal Predictive Validity Investigation of the Sb:Fe and K-Abc With At-Risk Children. *J. Psychoeduc. Assess.* **2001**, *19*, 334–349. [CrossRef]
23. Rothon, C.; Head, J.; Clark, C.; Klineberg, E.; Cattell, V.; Stansfeld, S. The impact of psychological distress on the educational achievement of adolescents at the end of compulsory education. *Soc. Psychiatry Psychiatr. Epidemiol.* **2009**, *44*, 421–427. [CrossRef]
24. Samuels, W.E.; Tournaki, N.; Blackman, S.; Zilinski, C. Executive functioning predicts academic achievement in middle school: A four-year longitudinal study. *J. Educ. Res.* **2016**, *109*, 1–13. [CrossRef]
25. Fergusson, D.M.; Horwood, L.J.; Ridder, E.M. Show me the child at seven II: Childhood intelligence and later outcomes in adolescence and young adulthood. *J. Child Psychol. Psychiatry* **2005**, *46*, 850–858. [CrossRef]
26. Moffitt, T.E.; Arseneault, L.; Belsky, D.W.; Dickson, N.; Hancox, R.J.; Harrington, H.; Houts, R.; Poulton, R.; Roberts, B.W.; A Ross, S.; et al. A gradient of childhood self-control predicts health, wealth, and public safety. *Proc. Natl. Acad. Sci. USA* **2011**, *108*, 2693–2698. [CrossRef] [PubMed]
27. McClelland, M.M.; Acock, A.C.; Piccinin, A.M.; Rhea, S.A.; Stallings, M.C. Relations between preschool attention span-persistence and age 25 educational outcomes. *Early Child. Res. Q.* **2013**, *28*, 314–324. [CrossRef] [PubMed]
28. Sagatun, Å.; Heyerdahl, S.; Wentzel-Larsen, T.; Lien, L. Mental health problems in the 10thgrade and non-completion of upper secondary school: The mediating role of grades in a population-based longitudinal study. *BMC Public Health* **2014**, *14*, 16. [CrossRef]
29. Veldman, K.; Bültmann, U.; Stewart, R.E.; Ormel, J.; Verhulst, F.C.; Reijneveld, S.A. Mental Health Problems and Educational Attainment in Adolescence: 9-Year Follow-Up of the TRAILS Study. *PLoS ONE* **2014**, *9*, e101751. [CrossRef]

30. Peet, E.D.; McCoy, D.C.; Danaei, G.; Ezzati, M.; Fawzi, W.; Järvelin, M.-R.; Pillas, D.; Fink, G. Early Childhood Development and Schooling Attainment: Longitudinal Evidence from British, Finnish and Philippine Birth Cohorts. *PLoS ONE* **2015**, *10*, e0137219. [CrossRef] [PubMed]
31. Samuels, W.E.; Tournaki, N.; Sacks, S.; Sacks, J.; Blackman, S.; Byalin, K.; Zilinski, C. Lavelle Preparatory Charter School Predicting GPAs with Executive Functioning Assessed by Teachers and by Adolescents Themselves. *Eur. Educ. Res.* **2019**, *2*, 173–194. [CrossRef]
32. Kosik, R.; Mandell, G.; Fan, A.; Nguyen, T.; Chen, J.; Eaton, W. The association between childhood educational attainment and adult mental health and status: A thirty-year longitudinal follow up study. *Eur. J. Psychiatry* **2018**, *32*, 53–62. [CrossRef]
33. Black, M.M.; Bromley, K.; Cavallera, V.A.; Cuartas, J.; Dua, T.; Eekhout, I.; Fink, G.; Gladstone, M.; Hepworth, K.; Janus, M.; et al. The Global Scale for Early Development (GSED). *Early Child. Matters* **2019**, *14*, 80–84. Available online: https://earlychildhoodmatters.online/2019/the-global-scale-for-early-development-gsed/ (accessed on 25 April 2018).

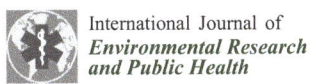

Article

Stability of the Communication Function Classification System among Children with Cerebral Palsy in South Korea

Eun-Young Park

Department of Secondary Special Education, College of Education, Jeonju University, Jeonju 55069, Korea; eunyoung@jj.ac.kr; Tel.: +82-63-220-3186

Abstract: Interest in the prognosis of skill levels has been an important issue among children with cerebral palsy (CP). This study aimed to verify the stability of the Communication Function Classification System (CFCS) in 2- to 18-year-old children with CP. Data collected from 171 children with CP who received rehabilitation therapy in hospitals or attended special elementary schools in South Korea were reviewed. They were divided into two groups, children <4 years and children ≥4 years. Participants were evaluated over 1-year and 2-year intervals from the first rating. Agreement between the three measurements and the weighted kappa were analyzed. At the 1-year interval, results demonstrated a high agreement rate of the CFCS in children ≥4 years old, and during the 2-year interval the study revealed a low agreement rate in children aged 2–4 years. The results indicated the stability of the CFCS in children ≥4 years old but some change of the CFCS in 2- to 4-year-old children. Moreover, the findings suggested that the change of the CFCS varied with time and age. Based on these results, it is recommended that the CFCS assessments be performed periodically, especially among 2- to 4-year-old children with CP.

Keywords: children with cerebral palsy; agreement; stability; communication function classification system

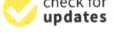

Citation: Park, E.-Y. Stability of the Communication Function Classification System among Children with Cerebral Palsy in South Korea. *Int. J. Environ. Res. Public Health* **2021**, *18*, 1881. https://doi.org/10.3390/ijerph18041881

Academic Editors: Byoung-Hee Lee and Verónica Schiariti
Received: 22 December 2020
Accepted: 10 February 2021
Published: 15 February 2021

Publisher's Note: MDPI stays neutral with regard to jurisdictional claims in published maps and institutional affiliations.

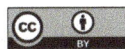

Copyright: © 2021 by the author. Licensee MDPI, Basel, Switzerland. This article is an open access article distributed under the terms and conditions of the Creative Commons Attribution (CC BY) license (https://creativecommons.org/licenses/by/4.0/).

1. Introduction

For children with cerebral palsy (CP), it is essential to assess their communication abilities to better support their needs. However, evaluating the communication function of children with CP is difficult to do accurately with a single evaluation system. In the case of children with CP, evaluating items included in communication measures poses many challenges, including practicality and familiarity with the content of assessment and/or evaluation measures. Therefore, there is a need for a comprehensive assessment that uses an informal evaluation based on direct observation or parent and teacher feedback [1] and comprehensive tools in a natural setting.

Communication among children with CP is one of relevant activities identified by the International Classification of Functioning, Disability, and Health's (ICF) conceptual frameworks. Communication activities include the transmission and reception of messages such as speaking, listening, reading, writing, and the use of alternative and augmentative communications [2,3]. The incidence of communication disorders in children with CP has been reported to vary widely. The Communication Function Classification System (CFCS) [4] that is used to classify the communication level in individuals with CP was developed based on the Gross Motor Function Classification System (GMFCS) [5] and the Manual Ability Classification System (MACS) [6] as part of a growing trend in classifying the activities and impairments proposed by the ICF [4]. Since they were developed, the psychometric properties of the classification systems have been actively studied. The reliability and validity of the GMFCS and MACS have been reported, and studies on the validity of the CFCS [4] have also been reported. Sixty-one experts evaluated 68 children with CP and aged 2 to 18 years on the CFCS and reported a reliability of

0.66 (95% CI = 0.55–0.78), a test-retest reliability of 0.82 (CI = 0.74–0.90), and an inter-rater reliability of 0.49 (95% CI = 0.40–0.59) [4].

The Korean translation of the CFCS [7] was used to evaluate its reliability. The results showed that the test-retest reliability among professionals was 0.991 (95% CI = 0.979–1.00), the inter-rater reliability among professionals was 0.905 (95% CI = 0.864–0.946), and the inter-rater reliability between the professional and parent groups was 0.882 (95% CI = 0.837–0.927) [7]. One of the important psychometric properties of the classification systems is stability over time. In the case of the GMFCS, 610 children with CP were confirmed to be stable [8]. The MACS also confirmed the stability of 1267 children with CP over five years and confirmed the stability of the MACS level over time [9]. In the case of the first GMFCS, research has been conducted on whether the classification system is stable over time [10,11], and subsequent studies on the MACS provide information on the change [9]. However, the relatively recent developments in the CFCS have not been tested for stability or change as children grow. Recently, one study [12] examined the stability of the CFCS with GMFCS and MACS in 664 children with CP (with ages ranging from 18 months to 12 years). It was reported that the kappa coefficients varied from 0.76–0.88 for the GMFCS, 0.59–0.73 for the MACS, and 0.57–0.77 for the CFCS. Whether or not the child's skill level will change because of a change in prognosis, decision making and counseling with parents is an important issue, and the degree of stability of the classification system can provide information regarding the possibility of changes in functioning in the child. The stability of the classification system indicates whether children with CP maintain the same level of functioning over time or whether they can be reclassified to different levels over time [13]. Considering the lack of related information on the stability of the CFCS, this study aimed to determine its stability over a second rating and third rating from the first rating.

2. Materials and Methods

2.1. Participants

Totally, 171 children with CP (mean = 10.9 years, SD = 4.6 years) participated in this study. Participants attended a convalescent or rehabilitation center for disabled individuals or a special school for physical disabilities in South Korea. There were 99 boys (57.9%) and 72 girls (42.1%). The age range was 2 to 18 years. Totally, 21 children with CP were below 4 years and 150 were older. The parents of all children agreed to participate in this study. The types of CP in the children were spastic (81.0%), dyskinetic/athetotic (6.8%), ataxic (3.4%), and hypotonic (8.8%). The participants were classified using the GMFCS: 19 (11.1%) were classified into Level I, 24 (14.0%) into Level II, 18 (10.5%) into Level III, 24 (14.0%) into Level IV, and 86 (50.3%) into Level V. The present study was approved by the Research Ethics Board of Jeonju University (Jeonju University IRB-1041042-2013-1).

2.2. Measurement

To classify their communication function, the CFCS was used. CFCS is a tool developed with support from the National Institute of Health (NIH), the Cerebral Palsy International Research Foundation, and The Hearst Foundation. We used the Korean version of the CFCS (http://cfcs.us/wp-content/uploads/2018/11/CFCS_Korean.pdf) [7] developed by Hidecker and her colleagues [4]. The CFCS content was as follows: Level 1 child with CP is an effective sender and receiver with unfamiliar and familiar partners. Level 2 child with CP is an effective but slower paced sender and/or receiver with unfamiliar and familiar partners. Level 3 child with CP is an effective sender and receiver with familiar partners. Level 4 child with CP is sometimes an effective sender and receiver with familiar partners. Level 5 child with CP is seldom an effective sender and receiver even with familiar partners. The inter-rater reliability of CFCS has been reported from 0.66–0.98 [4,14]. Hidecker et al. [15] reported the validity of the CFCS in preschool children with speech and language disorders. The stability of the CFCS was reported by previous studies. Palisano et al. [12] reported the kappa coefficients to be 0.57–0.77 in 664 children with CP.

2.3. Raters

Data regarding the CFCS were collected by 18 occupational therapists who had treated children with CP for more than 6 months. One occupational therapist evaluated 3–9% of the children with CP. Although occupational therapists met the eligibility requirements for administering the CFCS evaluations, all therapists were trained specifically for using these evaluation tools. They were encouraged to seek clarification from the investigators regarding any question or problem arising during the assessments. The amount of time it took to complete the CFCS was less than 5 min because the occupational therapists were familiar with children with CP. The same evaluators performed the assessments across the three measurements and were blinded to the previous CFCS ratings.

2.4. Data Collection Procedure

The data were collected once a year over two years during the same month. For example, if data were collected on 1 September of the first year, data were collected between 1 September and 31 September the next year. After the third measurement of evaluation, all collected data were subjected to central statistical monitoring.

2.5. Statistical Method

Agreement rate of the CFCS and weighted kappa were used in this study to examine the stability of the CFCS in three repetitive ratings in two years. Weighted kappa was performed to investigate the change of the CFCS across three times measurements. In general, the criteria for the weighted kappa are: a slight agreement between 0 and 0.20, a fair agreement between 0.21 and 0.40, a moderate agreement between 0.41 and 0.60, a substantial agreement between 0.61 and 0.80, and 0.81 to 1.00 interprets as an almost perfect agreement [16]. Agreement rate of stability above 80% was of acceptable value [17].

Based on a previous study on CFCS's stability, here the CFCS stability was verified by evaluating data for children ≥ 4 years versus children <4 years [12]. The analysis was completed for about 171 children (whole group) with 21 being below 4 years (younger group) and 150 above 4 years (older group). The age criterion for dividing two subgroups was set to 4 years with reference to the first study to find out the stability of the CFCS [12]. The age reference point for dividing the groups was 4 years at first rating.

3. Results

3.1. Agreement Rate across Three Measurement Points

The agreement rate between the first and second ratings according to age ranges is shown in Table 1. In the whole group, the agreement rate between the first and second ratings was 69.9% (n = 118). In total, 30 children with CP (17.6%) were rated in the more severe functional level and 23 (13.5%) were rated in the less severe functional level during the second rating than in the first rating. Regarding the younger group, the change rate was 33.3% (n = 7). Three children with CP (14.3%) were rated in the more severe functional level and four children with CP (19.0%) were rated in the less severe functional level during the second rating than in the first rating. Regarding the older group, the change rate was 30.7% (n = 46). Totally, 27 children with CP (18.0%) were rated in the more severe functional level and 19 (12.7%) were rated in the less severe functional level.

Table 1. The CFCS levels between the first rating and second rating.

Category		Second Rating					
		Level I	Level II	Level III	Level IV	Level V	Total
Whole group (Age from 2 to 18)							
First rating	I	20	4	0	0	0	24
	II	3	21	5	2	0	31
	III	3	2	9	9	0	23
	IV	0	2	2	25	10	39
	V	0	0	2	9	43	54
	Total	26	29	18	45	53	171
	Percentage agreement 69.9%, Weighted kappa 0.775 (95% CI 0.717~0.833)						
Younger subgroup (Age below 4)							
First rating	I	1	0	0	0	0	1
	II	0	5	1	1	0	7
	III	0	2	2	0	0	4
	IV	0	0	0	2	1	3
	V	0	0	1	1	4	6
	Total	1	7	4	4	5	21
	Percentage agreement 66.7%, Weighted kappa 0.702 (95% CI 0.492~0.913)						
Older subgroup (Age above 4)							
First rating	I	19	4	0	0	0	23
	II	3	16	4	1	0	24
	III	3	0	7	9	0	19
	IV	0	2	2	23	9	36
	V	0	0	1	8	39	48
	Total	25	22	14	41	48	150
	Percentage agreement 69.3%, Weighted kappa 0.782 (95% CI 0.722~0.842)						

The agreement rates between the first and third ratings among different age groups are shown in Table 2. In the whole group, the agreement rate between the first rating and ratings was 66.1% ($n = 113$). In total, 21 children with CP (12.3%) were rated in the more severe functional level and 37 (21.6%) were rated in the less severe functional level during the third rating than in the first rating. Regarding the younger group, the change rate was 42.9% ($n = 9$). Four children with CP (19.0%) were rated in the more severe functional level and five children with CP (23.9%) were rated in the less severe functional level during the third rating than in the first rating. Regarding the older group, the change rate was 28.7% ($n = 49$). Totally, 26 children with CP (17.4%) were rated in the more functional severe level and 23 (15.3%) were rated in the less severe functional level.

The agreement rate between the second and third ratings according to age ranges is shown in Table 3. In the whole group, the agreement rate between the second and third ratings was 80.1% ($n = 137$). In total, 13 children with CP (7.6%) were rated in the more severe functional level and 21 (13.3%) were rated in the less severe functional level during the third rating than in the second rating. Regarding the younger group, the change rate was 33.3% ($n = 7$). Two children with CP (9.5%) were rated in the more severe functional level and five children with CP (23.8%) were rated in the less severe functional level during the third rating than in the second rating. Regarding the older group, the change rate was 18.0% ($n = 27$). Totally, 11 children with CP (7.3%) were rated in the more severe functional level and 26 (10.7%) were rated in the less severe functional level.

Table 2. The CFCS levels between the first rating and second rating.

Category		Third Rating					
		Level I	Level II	Level III	Level IV	Level V	Total
Whole group (Age from 2 to 18)							
First rating	I	20	4	0	0	0	24
	II	5	17	8	1	0	31
	III	4	2	9	8	0	23
	IV	0	2	1	27	9	39
	V	0	0	2	12	40	54
	Total	29	25	20	48	49	171
	Percentage agreement 66.1%, Weighted kappa 0.757 (95% CI 0.699~0.815)						
Younger subgroup (Age below 4)							
First rating	I	1	0	0	0	0	1
	II	0	5	2	0	0	7
	III	2	0	1	1	0	4
	IV	0	0	0	2	1	3
	V	0	0	1	2	3	6
	Total	3	5	4	5	4	21
	Percentage agreement 57.1%, Weighted kappa 0.620 (95% CI 0.410~0.831)						
Older subgroup (Age above 4)							
First rating	I	19	4	0	0	0	23
	II	5	12	6	1	0	24
	III	2	2	8	7	0	19
	IV	0	2	1	25	8	36
	V	0	0	1	10	37	48
	Total	26	20	16	43	45	150
	Percentage agreement 67.3%, Weighted kappa 0.774 (95% CI 0.714~0.833)						

Table 3. The CFCS levels between the second rating and third rating.

Category		Third Rating					
		Level I	Level II	Level III	Level IV	Level V	Total
Whole group (Age from 2 to 18)							
Second rating	I	24	2	0	0	0	26
	II	5	20	3	1	0	29
	III	0	3	11	4	0	18
	IV	0	0	6	36	3	45
	V	0	0	0	7	46	53
	Total	29	25	20	48	49	171
	Percentage agreement 80.1%, Weighted kappa 0.873 (95% CI 0.832~0.914)						
Younger subgroup (Age below 4)							
Second rating	I	1	0	0	0	0	1
	II	2	4	1	0	0	7
	III	0	1	2	1	0	4
	IV	0	0	1	3	0	4
	V	0	0	0	1	4	5
	Total	3	5	4	5	4	21
	Percentage agreement 66.7%, Weighted kappa 0.774 (95% CI 0.628~0.920)						
Older subgroup (Age above 4)							
Second rating	I	23	2	0	0	0	25
	II	3	16	2	1	0	22
	III	0	2	9	3	0	14
	IV	0	0	5	33	3	41
	V	0	0	0	6	42	48
	Total	26	20	16	43	45	150
	Percentage agreement 82.0%, Weighted kappa 0.885 (95% CI 0.843~0.927)						

3.2. Agreement across Three Ratings

In terms of the CFCS levels' stability, the weighted kappa coefficients were 0.757 to 0.873 in the whole group (Tables 1–3). The lowest coefficient was between the first and third ratings measurement points in the younger group. The highest coefficient was between the second and third ratings in the older group. Appearance patterns of the weighted kappa were the same in all age groups.

4. Discussion

The functional classification systems in children with CP are widely used not only in research, but also in clinical practice. This aligns with a WHO proposed functioning and disability assessment approach focused on activities and participation restrictions [18]. The CFCS for functional classification of communicative ability in children with CP has been recently developed and has been built on five levels to correspond to the well-known GMFCS for motor performance. Our study was conducted to evaluate the stability of the CFCS, which was developed to classify the level of communication function in children with CP. Possessing information on the functional state of children with CP can help in improving the quality of life of these children and their families, ensuring them a promising future [19].

The weighted kappa coefficients, the primary measure of stability in our study, provide evidence of the stability of the CFCS for 4-year to 18-year-old children with CP in one and two-year intervals and for children below 4 years and with CP between the first and third ratings based on the above 0.75 value. There was no stability of the CFCS for children below 4 years and with CP between the first rating and second rating and the first rating and third rating. According to the criterion, the results of this study showed the almost perfect agreement of the CFCS for children above 4 years and with CP between the second and third ratings. The weighted kappa results showed higher value than in previous studies that examined the stability of the CFCS for children with CP. Palisano et al. [12] reported that the linear weighted kappa was 0.57 for children below 4 years and with CP in a 12 month visit and 0.77 for children above 4 years and with CP.

The weighted kappa for the CFCS was lower than the GMFCS and MACS. Over 0.80 weighted kappa for the GMFCS have been reported by previous studies. The weighted kappa of 0.895 was reported in 103 participants aged 17–38 years [11], and Palisano et al. [8] reported that the weighted kappa coefficient for the GMFCS between the first and last measurements was 0.84 and 0.89 for children <6 years old and at least 6 years old, respectively. Palisano et al. [12] reported that the weighted kappa was 0.76 to 0.95 from the GMFCS and 0.59 to 0.73 from the MACS. The first reason for the lower weighted kappa might be due to the characteristics of the CFCS. The CFCS derives one overall rating based on subjective judgments about how well your child sends messages, how quickly you communicate, and how well your child receives or understands your messages [4]. The need to resolve a single CFCS score to account for these skills is inconsistent between the level of expressiveness and capacity-communication, or there is an expressive repertoire of skills, but it is problematic for children with slow communication due to motorized speech or augmentative and alternative communication (AAC) access [20]. The second reason might be due to the characteristics of communication. Since communication is not a single function, it is not possible to capture the multidimensional nature of communication with a single five-stage measurement, suggesting a breakdown of the communication classification into component functions [21]. The findings of this study on the CFCS suggest a challenge for further studies that need to find out why the kappa is lower than other classification systems and what is the way to increase it.

The agreement rate of this study was 66.9% between the first and third ratings and 80.1% between the second and third ratings. This rate showed a different agreement rate in relation to previous studies. The agreement rate of children below 4 years and with CP between the first and third ratings (57.1%) was higher than in the study by Palisano et al. [12] (51.6%). Similarly, the agreement rate of children above 4 years and with CP between the first and second ratings (67.3%) was higher than in the study by Palisano et al. [12] (64.5%). The agreement rate results were context with the linearly weighted kappa results, which was lower than other classification systems. The original CanChild study of the GMFCS stability had a higher agreement of 76% and 83% for children younger and older than 6 years, respectively [8]. One of the possible reasons that the results of this study are not completely consistent with previous studies could be the environmental impact of communication. The level of CFCS changed to a more severe functional level and a less severe functional level. In this study, the number of children with CP that moved into a 2-level difference was seven both between the first and second rating and also between the first and third rating. The number of children with a 2-level difference between the second and third rating was five. The case that moved into a less severe functional level was higher than those that moved into a more severe functional level. As a factor influencing the change to a less severe functional level, the effect of child maturity and intervention is expected. It is necessary to also consider the development of communication skills through maturity as a cause that may affect the change in the level of CFCS in children. If the child received AAC-based interventions or other effective speech and language interventions, this would have affected the less severe functional changes in CFCS levels. As a factor influencing the change to a more severe functional level, post-seizures, other co-morbidities and losing access to AAC could be a possibility. Hidecker et al. [22] reported that seizures and other co-morbidities have a negative relation with communication function in children with CP. The number of reclassified children, especially those below 4 years, indicates that children with CP do not always maintain the same level of function. Although a 3-year to 5-year period was recommended for children and young people aged 4 to 17 with regards to the GMFCS re-evaluation period, the change rate of the CFCS found between the first and third ratings in this study may suggest a need to re-rate the participants every two years. Especially, short period re-rate of the CFCS for children below 4 years and with CP might be needed for monitoring their communication ability.

Although this study provided information on the stability of the CFCS through observations at intervals of one and two years, from the first rating, there are some limitations. First, the pilot study about the inter-rater reliability or test-retest reliability of the CFCS of this study was not completed and demographic characteristics of the assessors of the CFCS were not described. Second, there was a possibility that the occupational therapists could be misclassifying CFCS levels for children below 4 years. Third, the number of children below 4 years was relatively small and there was a high proportion of children with GMFCS level 5 observed and this proportion was higher than in a previous study [23]. Since children with severe CP showed that the stability of the functional classification might be better, the results of this study should be interpreted in consideration of the severity. Fourth, there were cases of the increase and decrease in GMFCS level, however, the results lack specificity. In future studies, it will be necessary to investigate variables that affect large functional changes.

5. Conclusions

Although the results of this study showed overall substantial agreement of the CFCS, regular re-evaluation of the CFCS levels is necessary. The differences in each research periods between the first and third ratings, with one-year intervals, suggested that there were some differences in the stability of the CFCS according to the children's ages. In future research, systematic and periodic evaluation of the CFCS levels is warranted for verifying the differences in the change rate according to age. In addition to the periodical evaluation, it is considered necessary to include changes in communication methods and comorbid diseases such as seizures after communication intervention. The results showed that the CFCS levels in children with CP increased and decreased in this study, but the factors that influenced these changes should be confirmed in further studies. Understanding why children's CFCS levels change can help with their prognosis. In addition, information on how the communication function of children with CP develops over time will help the clinician plan treatment strategies accordingly. Finally, insight into the aging-related impact on communication function in children with CP can be used to develop policies and programs that can help prepare such children for adulthood.

Funding: The author received no funding for this research.

Institutional Review Board Statement: The present study was approved by the Research Ethics Board of Jeonju University (Jeonju University IRB-1041042-2013-1).

Informed Consent Statement: Informed consent was obtained from the parents of all participants involved in the study.

Acknowledgments: Thank you to the respondents of this assessment.

Conflicts of Interest: The author declares no conflict of interest.

References

1. Linder, T.W. *Transdisciplinary Play-Based Assessment: A Functional Approach to Working with Young Children*; Raul H Brookes Publishing: Baltimore, MD, USA, 1993.
2. WHO (World Health Organization). *International Classification of Functioning Disability and Health*; World Health Organization: Geneva, Switzerland, 2001.
3. Schiariti, V.; Selb, M.; Cieza, A.; O'Donnell, M. International Classification of Functioning, Disability and Health Core Sets for Children and Youth with Cerebral Palsy: A Consensus Meeting. *Dev. Med. Child Neurol.* **2015**, *57*, 149–158. [CrossRef] [PubMed]
4. Hidecker, M.J.C.; Paneth, N.; Rosenbaum, P.L.; Kent, R.D.; Lillie, J.; Eulenberg, J.B.; Chester, K., Jr.; Johnson, B.; Michalsen, L.; Evatt, M.; et al. Developing and validating the Communication Function Classification System for individuals with cerebral palsy. *Dev. Med. Child Neurol.* **2011**, *53*, 704–710. [CrossRef] [PubMed]
5. Palisano, R.; Rosenbaum, P.; Walter, S.; Russell, D.; Wood, E.; Galuppi, B. Development and reliability of a system to classify gross motor function in children with cerebral palsy. *Dev. Med. Child Neurol.* **1997**, *39*, 214–223. [CrossRef] [PubMed]
6. Eliasson, A.C.; Krumlinde-Sundholm, L.; Rösblad, B.; Beckung, E.; Arner, M.; Öhrvall, A.M.; Rosenbaum, P. The Manual Ability Classification System (MACS) for children with cerebral palsy: Scale development and evidence of validity and reliability. *Dev. Med. Child Neurol.* **2006**, *48*, 549–554. [CrossRef] [PubMed]
7. Park, E.Y.; Kim, W.H.; Chae, S. Reliability and validity on Korean version of communication function classification system (CFCS) for individuals with cerebral palsy. *Edu. J. Phys. Multipl. Health Disabil.* **2014**, *57*, 185–203.
8. Palisano, R.J.; Cameron, D.; Rosenbaum, P.L.; Walter, S.D.; Russell, D. Stability of the gross motor function classification system. *Dev. Med. Child Neurol.* **2006**, *48*, 424–428. [CrossRef] [PubMed]
9. Öhrvall, A.M.; Krumlinde-Sundholm, L.; Eliasson, A.C. The stability of the Manual Ability Classification System over time. *Dev. Med. Child Neurol.* **2014**, *56*, 185–189. [CrossRef] [PubMed]
10. Alriksson-Schmidt, A.; Nordmark, E.; Czuba, T.; Westbom, L. Stability of the Gross Motor Function Classification System in children and adolescents with cerebral palsy: A retrospective cohort registry study. *Dev. Med. Child Neurol.* **2017**, *59*, 641–646. [CrossRef] [PubMed]
11. McCormick, A.; Brien, M.; Plourde, J.; Wood, E.; Rosenbaum, P.; McLean, J. Stability of the Gross Motor Function Classification System in adults with cerebral palsy. *Dev. Med. Child Neurol.* **2007**, *49*, 265–269. [CrossRef] [PubMed]
12. Palisano, R.J.; Avery, L.; Gorter, J.W.; Galuppi, B.; McCoy, S.W. Stability of the Gross Motor Function Classification System, Manual Ability Classification System, and Communication Function Classification System. *Dev. Med. Child Neurol.* **2018**, *60*, 1026–1032. [CrossRef] [PubMed]
13. Hidecker, M.J.C. Communication activity and participation research. *Dev. Med. Child Neurol.* **2010**, *52*, 408–409. [CrossRef] [PubMed]
14. Randall, M.; Harvey, A.; Imms, C.; Reid, S.; Lee, K.J.; Reddihough, D. Reliable classification of functional profiles and movement disorders of children with cerebral palsy. *Phys. Occup. Ther. Pediatr.* **2013**, *33*, 342–352. [CrossRef] [PubMed]
15. Hidecker, M.J.C.; Cunningham, B.J.; Thomas-Stonell, N.; Oddson, B.; Rosenbaum, P. Validity of the Communication Function Classification System for use with preschool children with communication disorders. *Dev. Med. Child Neurol.* **2017**, *59*, 526–530. [CrossRef] [PubMed]
16. Landis, J.R.; Koch, G.G. An application of hierarchical kappa-type statistics in the assessment of majority agreement among multiple observers. *Biometrics* **1977**, *33*, 363–374. [CrossRef]
17. Baer, D.M. Reviewer's comment: Just because it's reliable doesn't mean that you can use it. *J. Appl. Behav. Anal.* **1977**, *10*, 117–119. [CrossRef]
18. World Health Organization. *World Report on Disability 2011*; World Health Organization: Geneva, Switzerland, 2011.
19. Donkervoort, M.; Roebroeck, M.; Wiegerink, D.; Van der Heijden-Maessen, H.; Stam, H.; Transition Research Group South West Netherlands. Determinants of functioning of adolescents and young adults with cerebral palsy. *Disabil. Rehabil.* **2007**, *29*, 453–463. [CrossRef] [PubMed]

20. Barty, E.; Caynes, K.; Johnston, L.M. Development and reliability of the Functional Communication Classification System for children with cerebral palsy. *Dev. Med. Child Neurol.* **2016**, *58*, 1036–1041. [CrossRef] [PubMed]
21. Potter, N.L. Not there yet: The classification of communication in cerebral palsy. *Dev. Med. Child Neurol.* **2016**, *58*, 224–225. [CrossRef] [PubMed]
22. Hidecker, M.J.C.; Slaughter, J.; Abeysekara, P.; Ho, N.T.; Dodge, N.; Hurvitz, E.A.; Workinger, M.S.; Kent, R.D.; Rosenbaum, P.; Lenski, M.; et al. Early predictors and correlates of communication function in children with cerebral palsy. *J. Child Neurol.* **2018**, *33*, 275–285. [CrossRef] [PubMed]
23. Himmelmann, K.; Lindh, K.; Hidecker, M.J.C. Communication ability in cerebral palsy: A study from the CP register of western Sweden. *Eur. J. Paediatr. Neurol.* **2013**, *17*, 568–574. [CrossRef] [PubMed]

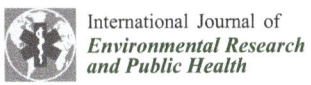

Article

Developing a Culturally Sensitive ICF-Based Tool to Describe Functioning of Children with Autism Spectrum Disorder: TEA-CIFunciona Version 1.0 Pilot Study

Silvana B. Napoli [1,*], María Paula Vitale [1], Pablo J. Cafiero [1], María Belén Micheletti [1], Paula Pedernera Bradichansky [1], Celina Lejarraga [1], Maria Gabriela Urinovsky [1], Anabella Escalante [1], Estela Rodriguez [1] and Verónica Schiariti [2]

[1] Division of Interdisciplinary Clinics, Child Developmental Pediatric Unit, Children Hospital JP Garrahan, Buenos Aires C 1245 AAM C.A.B.A, Argentina; mpauvitale@gmail.com (M.P.V.); pcafi67@gmail.com (P.J.C.); belenmicheletti@gmail.com (M.B.M.); paupeder1@gmail.com (P.P.B.); celileja@gmail.com (C.L.); gabrielaurinovsky@gmail.com (M.G.U.); ase.escalante@gmail.com (A.E.); rodriguez.estela15@gmail.com (E.R.)
[2] Division of Medical Sciences, University of Victoria, Victoria, BC V8W 2Y2, Canada; vschiariti@uvic.ca
* Correspondence: sil8napoli@gmail.com; Tel.: +54-11-4122-6000

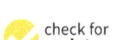

Citation: Napoli, S.B.; Vitale, M.P.; Cafiero, P.J.; Micheletti, M.B.; Bradichansky, P.P.; Lejarraga, C.; Urinovsky, M.G.; Escalante, A.; Rodriguez, E.; Schiariti, V. Developing a Culturally Sensitive ICF-Based Tool to Describe Functioning of Children with Autism Spectrum Disorder: TEA-CIFunciona Version 1.0 Pilot Study. *Int. J. Environ. Res. Public Health* **2021**, *18*, 3720. https://doi.org/10.3390/ijerph18073720

Academic Editors: Pasquale Caponnetto and Paul Tchounwou

Received: 9 January 2021
Accepted: 23 March 2021
Published: 2 April 2021

Publisher's Note: MDPI stays neutral with regard to jurisdictional claims in published maps and institutional affiliations.

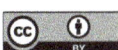

Copyright: © 2021 by the authors. Licensee MDPI, Basel, Switzerland. This article is an open access article distributed under the terms and conditions of the Creative Commons Attribution (CC BY) license (https://creativecommons.org/licenses/by/4.0/).

Abstract: Background: Autism spectrum disorder (ASD) affects the daily functioning of children and their families; however, in Argentina, there are no standardized tools to guide the description, evaluation, and follow-up of functioning and disability of children with ASD. To fill this gap, the overarching purpose of this study was to create a novel tool guided by the International Classification of Functioning, Disability, and Health (ICF) Core Sets for ASD for clinical practice. Methods: A multistep methodology was used to identify the most relevant ICF categories for an Argentinian clinical setting. The content of this ICF-based shortlist was piloted and revised according to the results. Subsequently, a toolbox of measures was proposed to operationalize each ICF category. Finally, profiles of the functioning of 100 children with ASD were created. Results: An ICF-based tool called TEA-CIFunciona was created, consisting of 32 ICF categories (10 body functions, 15 activities and participation, 7 environmental factors categories). The application of TEA-CIFunciona incorporated a family-centered approach in ASD evaluations and helped identify functional needs. Conclusions: TEA-CIFunciona is the first ICF-based instrument that guides the description of functioning of children with ASD in Argentina. TEA-CIFunciona standardizes collaborative assessments in pediatric ASD populations in Latin American contexts.

Keywords: ICF; autism spectrum disorder; functioning; child; measure; assessment

1. Introduction

Autism spectrum disorder (ASD) is a developmental disorder with a variable phenotypic expression characterized by communication and socialization difficulties and repetitive and stereotyped patterns of behavior [1,2]. ASD is generally diagnosed in early childhood and is considered to be secondary to an alteration in early brain development and neural reorganization [3]. The core symptoms of ASD have an early onset in childhood and tend to persist throughout the lifespan.

The global estimated prevalence of ASD is 1–2% [4]. In Argentina there is a lack of data on the overall prevalence of ASD; however, isolated studies have found similar figures to the prevalence estimates for the Americas by the World Health Organization (WHO) 0.7% [5,6].

Early diagnosis of ASD guides individualized early intervention. ASD diagnostic assessment warrants a detailed evaluation of the behavioral features described in manuals of diagnosis and classification, including the Diagnostic and Statistical Manual of Mental

Disorders (DSM-5) [7] and the International Statistical Classification of Diseases and Related Health Problems 10th revision [8]. However, a timely diagnosis of ASD should be complemented with a comprehensive assessment of functional needs performing everyday life activities, to ensure meaningful and adequate interventions.

In 2001 the WHO proposed the use of the International Classification of Functioning, Disability, and Health (ICF) [9] to describe functioning and disability from a biopsychosocial perspective. *Functioning* is an umbrella term to describe what a person with a health condition does or is able to do in everyday life at home, school, and in the community [9,10]. In 2007 a Child and Youth version of the ICF (ICF-CY) [11] was published specifically to capture functioning in developing individuals by adding and expanding on the descriptions of categories provided in the ICF. The ICF-CY facilitates the description of functional *abilities* and limitations in each area of development, promoting a family/child-centered approach [11]. This is important because children with neurodevelopmental disorders and their families cherish the child's functional abilities rather than the physical challenges, limitations, and participation restrictions associated with a specific diagnosis [12].

Moreover, the ICF systematically incorporates the role of environmental factors, including family, friends, therapists, societal attitudes, services, health systems and policies, and products and technology, as essential elements that facilitate or hinder participation and social inclusion [9,11]. Additionally, all content in the ICF is in conformity with international conventions and declarations on the rights of children and persons with disabilities, encouraging a human rights-based approach [9,11].

The ICF structures health and health-related domains into a hierarchy starting with components, then chapters, followed by categories. An ICF category is represented by an alphanumeric code. This code contains a letter that denotes one of the components of the ICF: body functions (b), body structures (s), activities and participation (d), and environmental factors (e) [9,11]. The component index letters are followed by a numeric code starting with the chapter number adding one digit (e.g., b1 mental functions), followed by a second-level category code adding two digits (e.g., b167 mental functions of language), and third and fourth level code by adding one digit respectively (e.g., b1670 reception of language and b16700 reception of spoken language). The categories with their corresponding codes must be completed with a qualifier: one, or more numbers after a point which denotes the severity of the problem or the extent to which a factor is a facilitator or barrier [9].

A key contribution of the ICF is to provide a framework and a structure for collecting and organizing clinical information evaluated by professionals worldwide, providing a universal language [9,11]. As such, the ICF is an important contribution to the growing interest in identifying children's needs based on their profiles of functioning rather than using only diagnostic labels, including ASD [13–15].

The practical application of the ICF-CY (from here we use 'ICF' to refer to both classifications) has been a challenge in clinical practice, including in clinical assessments of children with ASD, as the entire classification is comprehensive, consisting of 1685 ICF categories, In 2018, Bölte et al. following a rigorous step-wise multiple study methodology specified by the ICF Research Branch of the WHO Collaborating Centre for the Family of International Classifications in Switzerland, developed ICF Core Sets for ASD to facilitate its use [16]. ICF Core Sets represent shortlists of ICF categories that cover the most relevant areas of functioning and disability in a specific condition, which facilitate the application of the ICF in day-to-day practice. The Comprehensive Core Set for ASD consists of 111 categories and the common abbreviated set has 60 categories; the version for children 0–5 years of age has 73 categories, the version for children 6–16 years of age 81 categories, and the version for adults 79 categories [16,17].

Even though the ICF Core Sets for ASD, developed for the international context, highlight the most relevant categories for ASD out of the entire ICF classification, the length and complexity of these ICF Core Sets make them still difficult to use in everyday clinical encounters in Argentina.

There are multiple benefits of adopting ICF-based tools in clinical practice [15,18]. The systematic use of ICF-based tools defining the minimal key areas of functioning to be measured and reported for a given condition may be helpful to guide treatment planning, to identify facilitators and environmental barriers, and to reduce disparities in services. Moreover, ICF-based tools facilitate involvement of parents as active participants in the decision-making process on treatment goals and evaluation of intervention outcomes.

In Argentina, there is consensus on the diagnosis and treatment of people with ASD [19], but there are no guidelines that standardize the assessment of daily functioning in children with ASD. This highlights the need of a tool to systematically describe functioning of children with ASD in a comprehensive way. To fill this gap, the overall purpose of this study was to create a brief ICF-based tool to standardize assessments of ASD, with the following specific aims: (1) to identify the most relevant categories from the ICF Core Sets for ASD in order to describe the daily functioning of children with ASD in our country; (2) to propose measurement scales to evaluate each ICF category identified in aim 1; (3) to assess the feasibility of using a self-developed shortlist of ICF categories in clinical encounters; and finally (4) to describe the profile of the functioning of children with ASD at our national referral center.

2. Materials and Methods

The study is a descriptive cross-sectional design with prospective data analysis conducted between January and December 2019. Study data were collected and managed using REDCap electronic data capture tools hosted at Prof. Dr. Juan P. Garrahan" Hospital (JPGH). For statistical analysis, RStudio Software was used. The study was approved by the Ethical Review Board of JPGH and a written informed consent form was signed by parents.

2.1. Setting

The Argentinian health care system is characterized by considerable fragmentation, including a public system, work-related social insurances, and private health insurances, which causes great heterogeneity in assessments and interventions of ASD. According to the latest national census data, 36% of the population depends on publicly-funded medical insurance [20], showing the essential role of public hospitals in service provision in the country. Hence, in Argentina, there is increasing demand for providers of health services for persons with ASD in the public system, but only a few exist. One of these service providers is "Prof. Dr. Juan P. Garrahan" Hospital, the largest national public pediatric referral center in Buenos Aires, Argentina. The Division of Interdisciplinary Clinics provides consultations for the evaluation, diagnosis, and management of children with neurodevelopmental disabilities. Our division receives approximately 5000 visits per year. Out of those visits, approximately 120 visits per year are related to ASD diagnosis and a similar number to ASD follow-up visits, this reflects the average over the last three years.

2.2. Study Team—Professionals and Caregivers

Our interdisciplinary team consists of developmental pediatricians ($n = 6$), speech and language therapists ($n = 4$), and special educators ($n = 6$), with more than 15 years of experience in the diagnosis and follow-up of children with ASD. In addition, the study was conducted with active collaboration from the parents and caregivers of children with ASD attending follow-up visits at our clinic.

2.3. Study Participants

Children and their caregivers who attended regular ASD follow-up visits at the Child Developmental Pediatric Unit of the Division of Interdisciplinary Clinics at JPGH, were invited to participate, those who provided consent were included in a consecutive sampling. The inclusion criteria were a child with a diagnosis of ASD made at the Division of Interdisciplinary Clinics and age of the child under 16 years old. There were no exclusion criteria.

Children's information including gender, age, comorbidities, genetic condition, or another neurodevelopmental disorder were collected from health records. Severity of ASD was categorized following the DSM-5 levels of severity [7]. An unsatisfied basics needs (UBN) [20] score, measuring structural poverty was assigned to describe sociodemographic characteristics.

2.4. Procedure

2.4.1. Interprofessional and Family-Centered Approach

The overall purpose of this study was to create a brief culturally sensitive ICF-based tool to standardize assessments of functioning of children with ASD, especially to describe functioning in terms of performance at home, at school, and in the community. In every step of the study, the interprofessional study team, along with parents and caregivers, maintained active communication and collaborated sharing their different perspectives on day-to-day functioning. Thus, a multistep methodology was used to achieve the overall and specific aims, as follows:

- Aim (1) Identify the most relevant categories from the international ICF Core Sets for ASD to describe the daily functioning of children with ASD.

During two months, we conducted weekly sessions to familiarize ourselves with the content of the ICF classification and structure. We reviewed the literature related to the development and content of the comprehensive ASD Core Set [16,17]. In addition, electronic health records were reviewed to capture the main concerns described by families of children with ASD in previous years. Using the main concerns, each team member completed a checklist linking the meaningful concepts to the ICF categories included in the comprehensive ASD Core Set. We followed the ICF linking guidelines proposed by Cieza et al. [21]. ICF categories with an agreement of 75% or greater were included in our shortlist. This ICF-based shortlist was called TEA-CIFunciona.

- Aim (2) Propose measurement scales to evaluate each ICF category included in TEA-CIFunciona.

During the following month, we conducted weekly sessions where measurement tools were sought for each category included in our shortlist. We created a toolbox of measures to assess the categories in TEA-CIFunciona. Specifically, we tried to identify a one-to-one correspondence between an item of a measure and single ICF categories, at times this was not possible. Therefore, we proposed a set of items. When we could not identify a scale or measure to cover the content of the ICF category, we developed questions to assess that category. We ensured that the content of the questions represented the ICF category, using the ICF linking guidelines proposed by Cieza et al. [21].

- Aim (3) Feasibility and psychometric properties of TEA-CIFunciona version 0.0.

TEA-CIFunciona version 0.0 was piloted to check face validity, reliability, and feasibility in 20 patients. Interviews were conducted by two members of the study team who independently applied TEA-CIFunciona. Face validity: A questionnaire was answered by both evaluators to determine if all aspects of the consultations were included in TEA-CIFunciona. In addition, a questionnaire was answered by the parents to ensure that all their concerns were addressed; each family was additionally asked to give their opinion about the interview.

Inter-rater reliability: Two evaluators participated in each interview and independently scored all ICF categories included in TEA-CIFunciona. Cohen's Kappa statistics were used to evaluate inter-rater reliability. k of 0.61–0.80 are considered as substantial agreement and $k > 0.80$ as excellent agreement. Categories with a Kappa > 0.60 were maintained on our shortlist. Feasibility: raters were asked to provide feedback on usability, clarity, and objectivity of the TEA-CIFunciona using a brief questionnaire.

- Aim (4) Describe the profile of functioning of children with ASD using TEA-CIFunciona.

Finally, using the final version of TEA-CIFunciona (version 1.0), we described the profile of functioning of a larger group of children with ASD ($n = 100$). We translated clinical information into qualifiers following a self-developed guide, see below.

2.4.2. Translating Clinical Information and Standardized Assessment into ICF Qualifiers

As there is no gold standard to guide the translation of clinical information into ICF qualifiers, we created a guide for our pediatric clinical setting. First, we identified the best content correspondence [21] between item/s from standardized measures used in our ASD clinic and the content of the ICF categories included in TEA-CIFunciona. Then, we followed the ICF generic scale for problem severity (0–4% no problem/5–24% mild problem/25–49% moderate problem/50–95% severe problem/96–100% complete problem) [9,11] and compared it to the grading system of the assessment tools included in the toolbox. Additionally, we coded clinical information directly into ICF categories and qualifiers using our clinical expertise. Some categories were evaluated directly by parents, using the visual analog scale (VAS) as reported in other studies [22], including a visual response card created by the researchers to facilitate parents' understanding when identifying the degree of difficulty experienced by the children in a category. Parents' answers were directly translated into ICF qualifiers. Supplementary Material S1 shows examples of how clinical information and scores from standardized measures were translated into the ICF qualifiers.

3. Results

The multistep process led to the creation of TEA-CIFunciona version 1.0 and subsequently its application in clinical practice (Figure 1). TEA-CIFunciona version 1.0 consists of 32 ICF categories including, 10 body functions, 15 activities and participation, and 7 environmental factors.

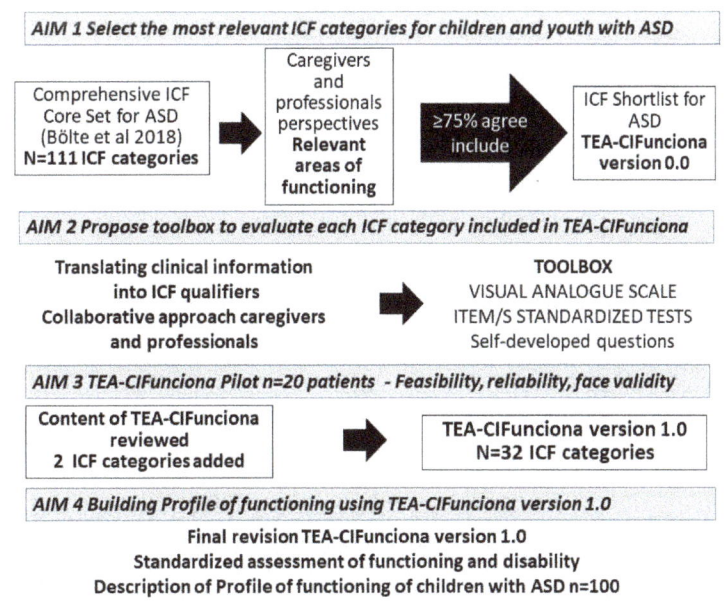

Figure 1. Multistep process for the development of TEA-CIFunciona and its clinical application.

3.1. Aim (1) Identify the Most Relevant Categories from the ICF Core Sets for ASD in Order to Describe the Daily Functioning of Children with ASD

Table 1 shows the categories included in TEA-CIFunciona version 1.0 as well as the toolbox to operationalize each category. All ICF categories were obtained from the Comprehensive Core Set for ASD, except d815 preschool education. This category was included to cover a common concern expressed by parents during clinical consultations.

Table 1. TEA-CIFunciona version 1.0 and proposed toolbox.

Content of TEA-CIFunciona (n = 32 ICF Categories)		Item/s Used to Assess Content	Alternative Item/s and Tools to Assess the Content of Each Category (Based on Availability of Tools)			
Body Functions (b)						
b117	Intellectual functions	CAT/CLAMS–Cognitive domain *	WPPSI *	S. Binet		
b125	Dispositions and intra-personal functions	VAS (parents) *				
b134	Sleep functions	VAS (parents) *				
b140	Attention functions	VAS (parents) *				
b156	Perceptual functions	VAS (parents) *				
b1670	Reception of language	VABS (Subdomain receptive) *	CELF	GARDNER	PLS	CLAMS (CD receptive)
b1671	Expression of language	VABS (Subdomain expressive) *	CELF	GARDNER	PLS	CLAMS (CD expressive)
b7602	Coordination of voluntary movements	VAS (parents) *				
b7652	Tics and mannerisms	ADI-R (item 77) *	ADOS (ítem: D2 module 2,3 ó 4)			
b7653	Stereotypies and motor perseveration	ADI-R (item 78) *				
Activities and Participation (d)						
d110	Watching	ADI-R (item 50) *				
d115	Listening	CARS (item 8) *				
d130	Copying	CARS (item 2) *				
d155	Acquiring skills	VABS * (Domain Daily Living Skills)				
d250	Managing one's own behavior	CARS (item 6) *				
d330	Speaking	Observation/Interview *				
d335	Producing nonverbal messages	ADI-R (42, 43, 44 and 45) *	ADOS 2 (module 2 A7)			
d350	Conversation	ADI-R (ítem 35) *	ADOS 2 (module 2 A5)			
d530	Toileting	VAS * (parents)				
d550	Eating	VAS * (parents)				
d720	Complex interpersonal interactions	VABS * (Subdomain Interpersonal Relationships)				
d7500	Informal relationships with friends	PEDSQL* (Social Functioning)				
d815	Preschool education	VAS * (parents)				
d820	School education	VAS * (parents)				
d920	Recreation and leisure	VABS * (subdomain Leisure Time)				

Table 1. *Cont.*

Content of TEA-CIFunciona (n = 32 ICF Categories)		Item/s Used to Assess Content	Alternative Item/s and Tools to Assess the Content of Each Category (Based on Availability of Tools)
		Environmental Factors (e)	
e125	Products and technology for communication	Self-developed question *	
e310	Immediate family	Family Apgar *	
e355	Health professionals	VAS *	
e430	Individual attitudes of people in positions of authority	VAS *	
e5502	Legal policies	Self-developed question *	
e555	Associations and organizational services, systems and policies	VAS *	
e5800	Health services, systems and policies	Self-developed question *	

* Denotes item or items used to assess the content of each category included in TEA-CIFunciona, the items were selected from standardized measurements. As shown, some categories were assessed using VAS or self-developed questions. First column describes the toolbox used in this study, the second column proposes alternative options to assess each category. **CAT/CLAMS:** Clinical Adaptive Test/Clinical Linguistic and Auditory Milestone Scale, **ADI-R:** Autism Diagnostic Interview-Revised, **ADOS-2:** Autism Diagnostic Observation Schedule-2, **WPPSI:** Wechsler Preschool and Primary Scale of Intelligence, **CARS:** Childhood Autism Rating Scale, **VABS:** Vineland Adaptive Behavior Scales 2, **CUD:** Unique Disability Certificate, **VAS:** Visual Analog Scale, **PedsQL:** Pediatric Quality of Life Inventory, **S. Binet:** Stanford-Binet Intelligence Scales, **Gardner:** Test de figura/palabra receptivo y expresivo Gardner, **PLS:** Preschool Language Scale, **CELF-4:** Clinical Evaluation of Language Fundamentals 4, **Family APGAR:** Adaptability, Partnership, Growth, Affection, and Resolve.

3.2. Aim (2) Propose Measurement Scales to Assess Each ICF Category. Development of a Toolbox

All selected scales are used regularly in assessments of ASD, and the study team is trained in their use. The selection of the tools was based on consensus. From each tool we selected the item/s that best covered the content of the ICF category (Table 1). Experts from other national and international institutions were consulted to provide feedback on the proposed toolbox.

3.3. Aim (3) Feasibility and Psychometric Properties of TEA-CIFunciona

We showed that TEA-CIFunciona was reliable, relevant, and feasible for application in our busy clinical consultations. After we piloted the first version of TEA-CIFunciona, we revised the tool based on parents' and professionals' feedback. Hence, two categories were added, as follows: Individual attitudes of people in positions of authority (e430) and Associations and organizational services, systems, and policies (e555). Two categories (b125 and b140) showed a lower level of agreement than expected; therefore, it was agreed to prioritize parents' opinion and they scored the categories using the VAS.

3.4. Aim (4) Describe the Profile of Functioning of Children with ASD Using TEA-CIFunciona; Clinical and Demographic Variables of the Sample

Table 2 shows the general characteristics of the sample using the TEA-CIFunciona version 1.0. Overall, 100 children were assessed, 81% were boys, with a mean age of 7 years and 4 months (range, 3 to 16 years), 10% had structural poverty (positive UBN score), and 20% lacked health insurance coverage. Almost 69% presented with an associated medical condition (e.g., sleep disorder, obesity, epilepsy) and 70% with associated developmental disorder (e.g., intellectual disability, developmental coordination disorder). Importantly, we included a representative sample of all severity levels for ASD proposed by the DSM-5 [7].

Table 2. Characteristics of the sample using TEA-CIFunciona version 1.0.

Characteristics of the Children with ASD	
Sample size	100
Age in months. Median (range)	89 (36; 192)
Age < 6 years	39% (39)
Age 6–16 years	61% (61)
Age of ASD diagnosis. Median (range)	42.5 (20;112)
Gender % (n)	Boys 81% (81)
	Girls 19% (19)
UBN (Unsatisfied Basic Needs)	10% (10)
Severity level (DSM-5) I Requiring support II Requiring substantial support III Requiring very substantial support	30% (30) 42% (42) 28% (28)
Language	Yes 67% (67)
	No 33% (33)
Attending school	Yes 97% (97)
	No 3% (3)
Associated medical conditions *	69% (69)
Sleep disorder	32% (22)
Obesity	20% (14)
Genetic syndrome	10% (7)
Chronic disease	5.8% (4)
Epilepsy	2.8% (2)
Associated developmental disorder **	70% (70)
Intellectual Disability/GDD	Yes 42% (30)
	No 12.8% (9)
	Not evaluated 61% (of the total sample)
Developmental Coordination Disorder	17% (12)
Anxiety	14% (10)
Language disorder	12.8% (9)
Behavioral disorder	8.5% (6)
ADHD (Attention Deficit Hyperactivity Disorder)	8.5% (6)
Hearing Impairment	5.7% (4)
Learning disorders	4.3% (3)

* Associated medical condition: The values expressed in % were calculated from the 69% (the sample with an associated medical condition). The same child may have more than one associated medical condition.
** Associated developmental disorder: The values expressed in % were calculated from the 70% (the sample with an associated developmental disorder). The same child may have more than one associated developmental disorder.

3.5. Profile of Functioning Using TEA-CIFunciona Version 1.0 (n = 100 Children with ASD)

Table 3 shows the frequency of the impairments, limitations, and restrictions in daily functioning in the corresponding components of body functions, activities and participation, and environmental factors. In the component body functions, intrapersonal functioning (b125) was considered to be a moderate or severe problem in 61% of the children. A moderate-to-complete problem was observed in reception of language (b1670) in 45% and in expression of language (b1671) in 73%.

In activities and participation, almost 20% of caregivers reported that their children had severe problems in relation to toileting (d530) and eating (d550). Education, considering school and preschool education (d815 and 820), appeared to be a problem in 40% of the sample, with different levels of severity. Speaking (d330) and conversation (d350) were considered moderate to complete problems in 33% and 79% of the children, respectively. Maintaining a relationship (d720 and d7500) and the use of leisure time (d920) were common functional challenges.

Regarding environmental factors, although the majority of parents considered attitudes of people in positions of authority (e430) a facilitator, many (24%) found it to be a barrier. Immediate family (e310) was a facilitator in 97% and health professionals (e355) in 61% of the sample.

Parents most often described problems in dispositions and intra-personal functions (b125), attention functions (b140), perceptual functions (b156), and eating (d550). Overall, support from parents' associations (for example NGOs) was seen as facilitators but appear to be an underused resource for families.

Figure 2A,B summarize the profiles of functioning of children with ASD under 6 years and ≥6 to 16 years, using TEA-CIFunciona version 1.0. As shown, there are many commonalities among the groups; however, each age-group shows unique functional characteristics and environmental factors, for example, in areas of receptive language, coordination of movements, copying skills, speaking, producing non-verbal messages, conversation, and using or accessing products and technologies for communication. Using TEA-CIFunciona, we were able to show that younger children with ASD have greater impact on functioning and less access to products and technology for communication. This information can guide interventions as well as modifications of the environment.

Table 3. Frequency (%) of impairment, limitations/restrictions, barrier or facilitator in body functions, activities and participation and environmental factors, (n = 100 children with ASD).

Category	Body Functions	Qualifier 0 (No Problem)	Qualifier 1 (Mild Problem)	Qualifier 2 (Moderate Problem)	Qualifier 3 (Severe Problem)	Qualifier 4 (Complete Problem)	Qualifier 8 (No Specified)	Qualifier 9 (Not Applicable)
b117	Intellectual functions	9	12	10	7	1	61	-
b125	Dispositions and intra-personal functions	5	34	52	8	1	-	-
b134	Sleep functions	66	12	13	9	-	-	-
b140	Attention functions	20	49	19	12	-	-	-
b156	Perceptual functions	33	35	17	10	5	-	-
b1670	Reception of language	16	39	32	11	2	-	-
b1671	Expression of language	6	21	56	11	3	-	-
b7602	Coordination of voluntary movements	58	22	16	14	1	-	-
b7652	Tics and mannerisms	37	29	27	3	-	-	-
b7653	Stereotypies and motor perseveration	19	38	35	7	-	-	-

Category	Activities and Participation	Qualifier 0	Qualifier 1	Qualifier 2	Qualifier 3	Qualifier 4	Qualifier 8	Qualifier 9
d110	Watching	13	51	31	5	-	-	-
d115	Listening	19	45	29	7	-	-	-
d130	Copying	33	43	20	4	-	-	-
d155	Acquiring skills	10	46	36	7	1	-	-
d250	Managing one's own behavior	10	31	52	5	2	-	-
d330	Speaking	41	26	16	11	6	-	-
d335	Producing nonverbal messages	27	36	24	11	2	-	-
d350	Conversation	3	18	34	38	7	-	-
d530	Toileting	56	12	13	11	8	-	-
d550	Eating	31	22	28	11	8	-	-
d720	Complex interpersonal interactions	4	20	65	10	1	-	-
d7500	Informal relationships with friends	3	19	43	20	3	12	-
d815	Preschool education	24	8	4	2	4	-	58
d820	School education	36	6	4	5	7	-	42
d920	Recreation and leisure	1	29	53	14	3	-	-

Category	Environmental Factors	Mild barrier (1)	Moderate barrier (2)	Severe barrier (3)	Total barrier (4)	No barrier/Facilitator (0)	Mild facilitator (+1)	Moderate facilitator (+2)	Severe facilitator (+3)	Total facilitator (+4)	No specified	Not applicable
e125	Products and technology for communication	16	19	19	3	19	3	8	11	2	-	-
e310	Immediate family	-	1	-	-	3	13	32	44	7	-	-
e355	Health professionals (pediatrician)	-	5	8	1	18	15	24	22	-	7	-
e430	Individual attitudes of people in positions of authority (school authorities)	6	3	12	3	3	8	36	23	1	1	4
e550	Legal policies	-	-	3	-	-	-	-	97	-	-	-
e555	Associations and organizational services, systems and policies	2	2	-	-	49	8	11	13	1	14	-
e5800	Health services, systems and policies	2	1	13	8	-	15	19	42	-	-	-

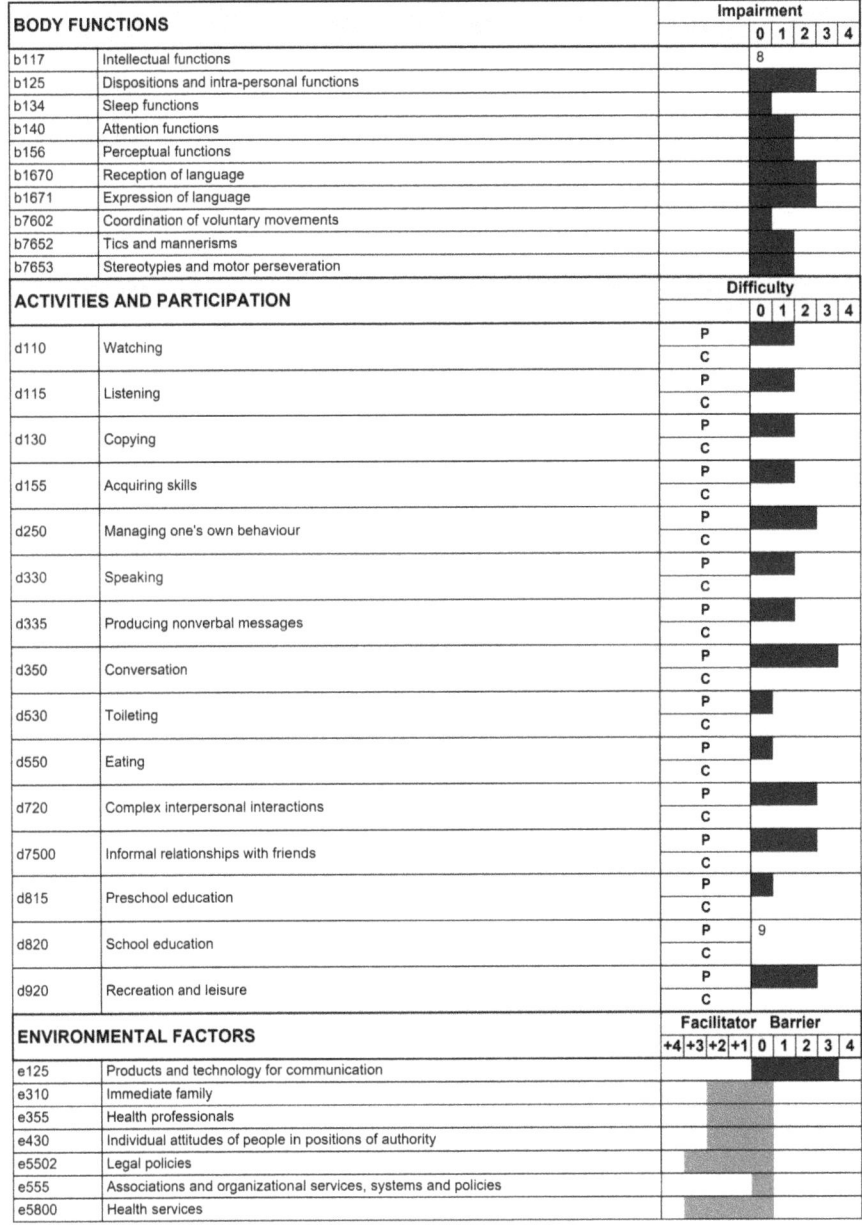

(A)

Figure 2. *Cont.*

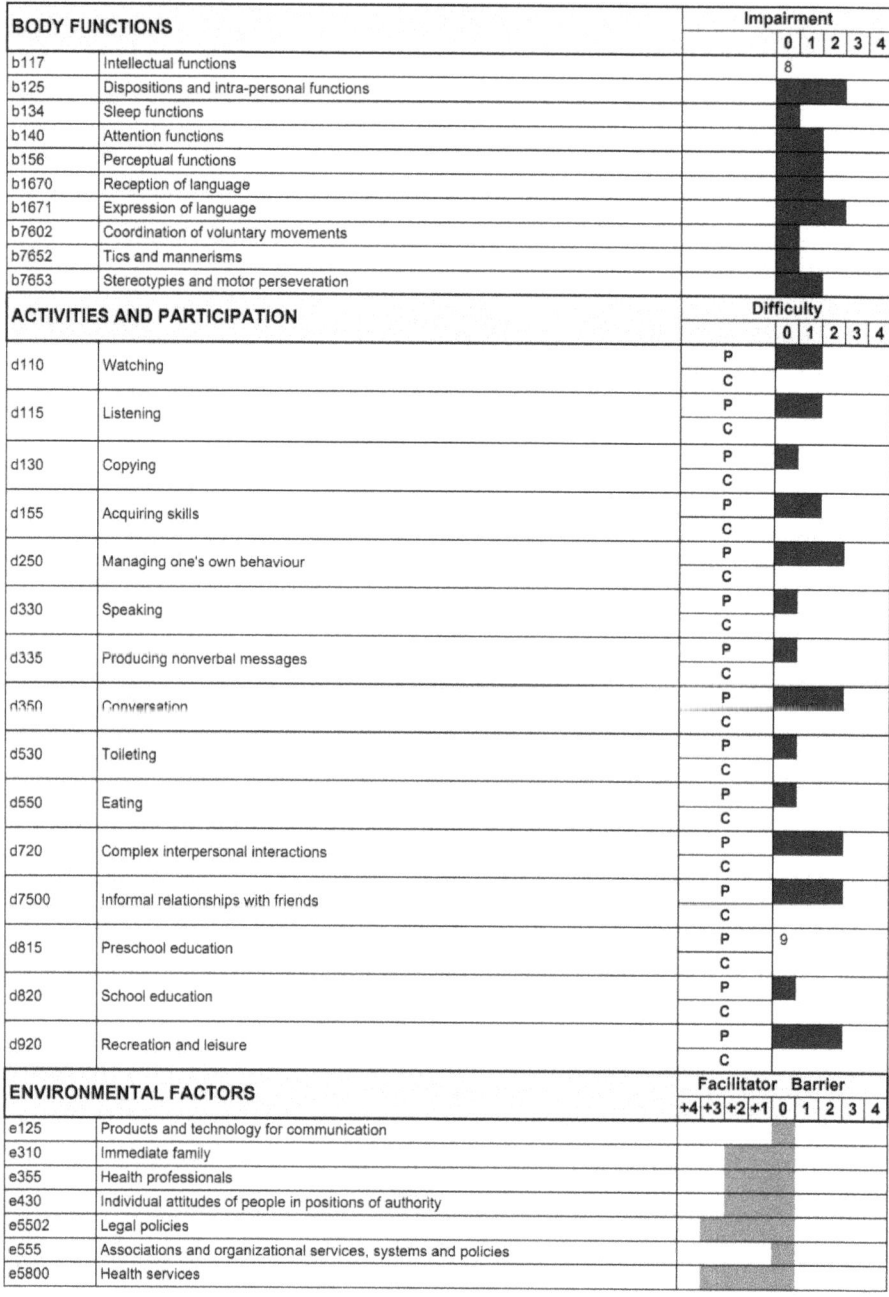

(B)

Figure 2. (**A**) Profile of functioning of children with ASD (autism spectrum disorder) < 6 years of age using TEA-CIFunciona version 1.0. (**B**) Profile of functioning of children with ASD 6 to 16 years of age using TEA-CIFunciona version 1.0.

ICF Qualifiers in body functions, body structures and activities and participation: 0 = no problem; 1 = mild problem; 2 = moderate problem; 3 = severe problem; and, 4 = complete problem. ICF Qualifiers in environmental factors: 0 = no barrier/facilitator; +1 = mild facilitator; +2 = moderate facilitator; +3 = substantial facilitator; +4 = complete facilitator; 1 = mild barrier; 2 = moderate barrier; 3 = substantial barrier; and 4 = complete barrier. The component personal factors (pf) does not have ICF categories assigned, therefore it is recommended to add themes representing personal factors to complement the profile of functioning.

The ICF qualifiers used to create the profile of functioning of this study sample represent the qualifiers that have the highest percentage within each ICF category. This profile of functioning was built using the ICF-based documentation form on this web page https://icf-core-sets.org/es/page0.php (accessed on 1 April 2019), courtesy ICF Research Branch. P (performance): describes what an individual does in his or her current environment. C (capacity): describes an individual's ability to execute a task or an action, meaning the highest probable level of functioning that a person may reach in a "standardized" environment.

4. Discussion

This study describes the creation of a novel ICF-based instrument called TEA-CIFunciona version 1.0. This is the first study conducted in Latin America that describes functioning in children with ASD. The contributions of this study are multiple, as follows: (1) identification of the most relevant areas of functioning and disability to standardize assessments of children with ASD in Argentina; (2) proposing a toolbox with standardized scales and questionnaires to operationalize the categories selected; (3) description of the profile of functioning of a large sample of children with ASD (n = 100) in the region using the ICF universal language.

4.1. Benefits of Using TEA-CIFunciona Version 1.0

TEA-CIFunciona incorporates the most relevant ICF categories for our cultural and pediatric setting. The application of TEA-CIFunciona helped us to incorporate a family-centered approach in the clinic. Consideration of parental views shifted the focus of follow-up visits towards the aspects of daily living significant to them. This modified the team's perspective; thus, parents' point of view and concerns were prioritized while taking into account the available resources.

In addition, the recognition of children's strengths and abilities was highly appreciated by the parents. For example, use of eating utensils may not be important to the practitioner, but may be essential to them. Generally, these skills can only be appreciated by the professional after a thorough investigation of everyday activities [23].

The systematic consideration of environmental characteristics allows us to draw some general conclusions regarding the difficulties these children and their families must overcome, and which support they considered most important. In most cases, the immediate family was identified as a substantial or complete facilitator, and its absence as an important barrier. This confirms once again not only the importance of a strong family structure, but also the need for support networks in the community and the notion that clinical interventions are successful when the uniqueness and diversity of families are recognized [24].

Another finding was that the pediatrician was identified as a facilitator in only 61% of the cases. The reasons given for this rating were lack of knowledge on ASD, or negative attitude. Often children with ASD do not have a primary care pediatrician and parents navigate a fragmented health care system without guidance. Sometimes the pediatrician is unaware of the family's priorities, and whether treatments or supports are working. Hence, the application of TEA-CIFunciona can improve service provision for ASD, as it explicitly examines the components of functioning that are often left out of traditional health care provision. TEA-CIFunciona could help communicate functional information in a simple way (for example using an illustration shown in Figure 2), and therefore may encourage the pediatrician to collaborate in teamwork and adopt a social model to evaluate disability.

TEA-CIFunciona showed extremely varied school experiences, being very positive for some children and extremely negative for others. The latter was associated with negative attitudes of the teachers and problems in adopting effective individual educational strategies, such as anticipation pictures, calendars, or communication devices.

Again, TEA-CIFunciona helped us identify the main environmental barrier in our national context. We found that augmentative communication technology was not commonly used. The devices were unknown to many of the parents and therapists but highly valued by those who did use them. Although evidence is limited, different studies have reported on the possible benefits of augmentative communication devices for children with autism. Therefore, the lack of use or restricted use was considered as a barrier, mainly in children with important verbal language impairment [25].

4.2. User Instructions TEA-CIFunciona

To facilitate adoption and implementation of TEA-CIFunciona in clinical practice, we propose simple user instructions (Figure 3). Briefly, (1) to apply TEA-CIFunciona children and youth have to have a confirmed diagnosis of ASD, using validated diagnostic tools; (2) a multi-disciplinary team with active collaboration with parents and/or caregivers and children with ASD—when possible should participate in the assessment process, a proposed toolbox of items is suggested to address each ICF category contained in TEA-CIFunciona version 1.0; then (3) build a profile of functioning to summarize the findings of the assessment and highlights functional strengths and needs, along with environmental barriers and facilitators; finally (4) develop a functional comprehensive collaborative plan of intervention.

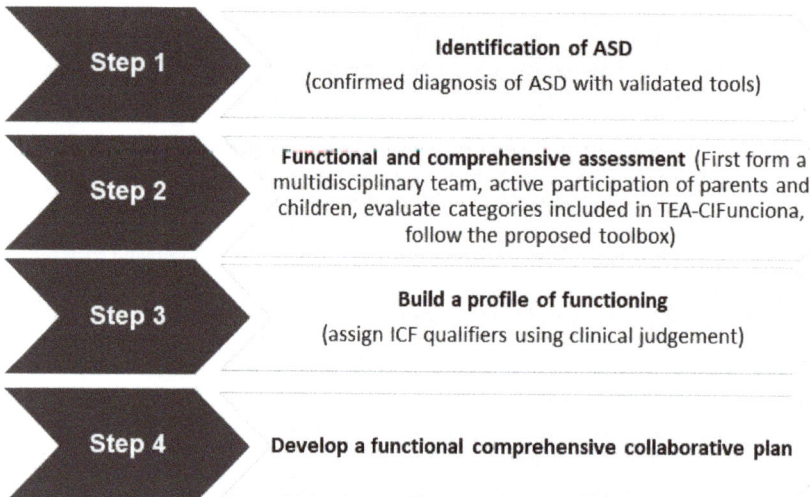

Figure 3. User instructions TEA-CIFunciona version 1.0.

4.3. Contributions of TEA-CIFunciona to Clinical Settings

This study proposes a new culturally sensitive ICF-based tool for clinicians working in the field of childhood-onset disabilities, contributing to the few pediatric ICF tools available today [13]. The application of TEA-CIFunciona could facilitate comparison of outcomes and results of intervention across the country and hopefully in other countries in Latin-America. However, clinical experience as well as training in the use and the ICF language, are needed.

4.4. Additional Considerations and Contributions to the International Community

Asking about parents' concerns and opinions also forces us to reconsider what the goals of treatment should be, who should set the priorities for a child, how to assess quality of care and support services, and even when to discontinue treatments. As described by Campos et al. in a recent qualitative study applying the ICF in a pediatric Latin American setting, it is crucial to incorporate parents' perspective when describing functional needs and setting goals for interventions, as parents are the ones who live and experience the main functional limitations of their children [26].

To our knowledge, this study describes the first attempt to operationalize the content of the ICF Core Sets for ASD in a pediatric clinical setting, as such; the multi-step methodology applied for developing TEA-CIFunciona may encourage the international community to replicate our effort in different cultural settings around the globe, and identify the most relevant items or tools to assess the content of the ICF Core Sets for ASD in their countries.

In addition, by providing evidence of functional needs and environmental barriers TEA-CIFunciona has the potential to guide health policies and may be useful guiding data collection at a regional or global level, facilitating comparisons across settings, guiding resource allocation, professional training, and capacitation. Overall, TEA-CIFunciona proved to be a practical framework and guideline for comprehensive assessments of ASD, although the time necessary for the interview may be a limiting factor.

4.5. Limitations

The translation of the scores of different grading scales into the ICF qualifiers posed several challenges. It is important to note that there is no gold standard that we could follow, currently, there are no rules guiding how to translate clinical information into ICF qualifiers in pediatric populations. Other studies applying the ICF in pediatric populations have used clinical judgement [10,22]. Our process required adjustments and modifications until the final guidelines for assigning the qualifiers were proposed. The lack of standardized tools to evaluate some of the categories, mostly those related to environmental factors, may be an additional limitation.

Finally, the selection of categories from the comprehensive ASD Core Set may have left out specific aspects that would be important in the evaluation of some children with ASD. Further revisions and larger studies across the country are needed.

5. Conclusions

In conclusion, implementation of TEA-CIFunciona version 1.0 is feasible and standardizes the assessment of children with ASD in our country. The toolbox operationalizes the content of TEA-CIFunciona and facilitates building a profile of functioning of children with ASD. This study may encourage colleagues to adopt TEA-CIFunciona, systematize the evaluations of patients with ASD using a biopsychosocial approach, benefitting both the children and their families. Although these findings describe a specific population, they may shed light on issues that are common to other children with ASD, regardless of where they live [23].

Future Steps

Regarding the next steps, it will be necessary to expand the use of this tool in other contexts, starting with community centers in Argentina and then in other Latin American countries with similar cultural background to identify common barriers and facilitators, to obtain a more representative functional data of this population. This could help to optimize delivery of health and rehabilitation services, to contribute to evidence-based policies, and to respond most adequately to children's and family's needs. Finally, we expect that after ongoing clinical application of TEA-CIFunciona version 1.0 in different settings, and based on feedback and lessons learned, future revisions will be required to include updates and recommendations not only from the professionals and caregivers' perspectives on daily functioning but from the children and youth with ASD perspectives as well.

Supplementary Materials: The following are available online at https://www.mdpi.com/article/10.3390/ijerph18073720/s1. Examples of translation strategies for ICF categories included in TEA-CIFfunciona version 1.0 for the components body functions, activities and participation and environmental factors.

Author Contributions: Conceptualization, S.B.N. and M.P.V. and V.S.; Methodology S.B.N., M.P.V. and V.S.; Software S.B.N. and M.P.V.; Formal Analysis S.B.N. and M.P.V.; Investigation S.B.N., M.P.V., P.J.C., M.B.M., P.P.B., C.L., M.G.U., A.E., Writing—Original Draft Preparation, S.B.N., M.P.V., P.J.C., M.B.M. and V.S.; Review, S.B.N., M.P.V., E.R. and V.S.; Writing & Editing, S.B.N., M.P.V. and V.S. All authors have read and agreed to the published version of the manuscript.

Funding: Maria Paula Vitale was funded by a Foundation Garrahan research fellow grant.

Institutional Review Board Statement: The study was approved by the Ethical Review Board of JPGH.

Informed Consent Statement: Informed consents were granted by all participants of this study.

Data Availability Statement: Due to privacy and confidentiality issues, we only share aggregated data in this study.

Acknowledgments: We express our thanks to all the children and their caregivers who participated in this study for their invaluable contribution.

Conflicts of Interest: The authors declare no conflict of interest.

References

1. Tuchman, R.; Rapin, I. *Autism: A Neurological Disorder of Early Brain Development*, 1st ed.; Mac Keith Press: London, UK, 2006; pp. 1–18.
2. Lord, C.; Elsabbagh, M.; Baird, G.; Veenstra-Vanderweele, J. Autism spectrum disorder. *Lancet* **2018**, *392*, 508–520. [CrossRef]
3. O'Reilly, C.; Lewis, J.D.; Elsabbagh, M. Is functional brain connectivity atypical in autism? A systematic review of EEG and MEG studies. *PLoS ONE* **2017**, *12*, e0175870. [CrossRef]
4. Myers, J.; Chavez, A.; Hill, A.P.; Zuckerman, K.; Fombonne, E. Epidemiological Surveys of Autism Spectrum Disorders. *Autism Pervasive Dev. Disord.* **2019**, 25–60. [CrossRef]
5. Contini, L.E.; Astorino, F.; Manni, D.C. Estimación de la prevalencia temprana de Trastornos del Espectro Autista. *Santa Fe-Argentina. Boletín Técnico.* **2017**, *13*, 12–13.
6. Elsabbagh, M.; Divan, G.; Koh, Y.-J.; Kim, Y.S.; Kauchali, S.; Marcín, C.; Montiel-Nava, C.; Patel, V.; Paula, C.S.; Wang, C.; et al. Global Prevalence of Autism and Other Pervasive Developmental Disorders. *Autism Res.* **2012**, *5*, 160–179. [CrossRef] [PubMed]
7. American Psychiatric Association. *Diagnostic and Statistical Manual of Mental Disorders*, 5th ed.; (DSM-5); American Psychiatric Association: Washington, DC, USA, 2013.
8. World Health Organization. *International Statistical Classification of Disease and Related Health Problems*, 10th ed.; World Health Organization: Geneva, Switzerland, 2010.
9. World Health Organization. *International Classification of Functioning, Disability and Health*; WHO: Geneva, Switzerland, 2001.
10. Schiariti, V.; Longo, E.; Shoshmin, A.; Kozhushko, L.; Besstrashnova, Y.; Król, M.; Campos, T.N.C.; Ferreira, H.N.C.; Verissimo, C.; Shaba, D.; et al. Implementation of the International Classification of Functioning, Disability, and Health (ICF) Core Sets for Children and Youth with Cerebral Palsy: Global Initiatives Promoting Optimal Functioning. *Int. J. Environ. Res. Public Health* **2018**, *15*, 1899. [CrossRef] [PubMed]
11. World Health Organization. *International Classification of Functioning, Disability and Health: Children & Youth Version*; World Health Organization: Geneva, Switzerland, 2007.
12. Schiariti, V.; Sauve, K.; Klassen, A.F.; O'Donnell, M.; Cieza, A.; Mâsse, L.C. 'He does not see himself as being different': The perspectives of children and caregivers on relevant areas of functioning in cerebral palsy. *Dev. Med. Child Neurol.* **2014**, *56*, 853–861. [CrossRef] [PubMed]

13. Schiariti, V.; Mahdi, S.; Bölte, S. International Classification of Functioning, Disability and Health Core Sets for cerebral palsy, autism spectrum disorder, and attention-deficit-hyperactivity disorder. *Dev. Med. Child Neurol.* **2018**, *60*, 933–941. [CrossRef] [PubMed]
14. Castro, S.; Ferreira, T.; Dababnah, S.; Pinto, A.I. Linking autism measures with the ICF-CY: Functionality beyond the borders of diagnosis and interrater agreement issues. *Dev. Neurorehabilit.* **2013**, *16*, 321–331. [CrossRef] [PubMed]
15. De Schipper, E.; Lundequist, A.; Coghill, D.; De Vries, P.J.; Granlund, M.; Holtmann, M.; Jonsson, U.; Karande, S.; Robison, J.E.; Shulman, C.; et al. Ability and Disability in Autism Spectrum Disorder: A Systematic Literature Review Employing the International Classification of Functioning, Disability and Health-Children and Youth Version. *Autism Res.* **2015**, *8*, 782–794. [CrossRef] [PubMed]
16. Bölte, S.; Mahdi, S.; De Vries, P.J.; Granlund, M.; Robison, J.E.; Shulman, C.; Swedo, S.; Tonge, B.; Wong, V.; Zwaigenbaum, L.; et al. The Gestalt of functioning in autism spectrum disorder: Results of the international conference to develop final consensus International Classification of Functioning, Disability and Health core sets. *Autism* **2018**, *23*, 449–467. [CrossRef] [PubMed]
17. Bölte, S.; de Schipper, E.; Robison, J.E.; Wong, V.C.; Selb, M.; Singhal, N.; De Vries, P.J.; Zwaigenbaum, L. Classification of Functioning and Impairment: The Development of ICF Core Sets for Autism Spectrum Disorder. *Autism Res.* **2014**, *7*, 167–172. [CrossRef] [PubMed]
18. Schiariti, V.; Selb, M.; Cieza, A.; O'Donnell, M. International Classification of Functioning, Disability and Health Core Sets for children and youth with CP: Contributions to clinical practice. *Dev. Med. Child Neurol.* **2015**, *57*, 203–204. [CrossRef] [PubMed]
19. Ministry of Health, Argentina. Consenso Sobre Diagnóstico y Tratamiento de Personas con Trastorno del Espectro Autista. Available online: https://www.argentina.gob.ar/sites/default/files/consenso-tea.pdf. (accessed on 5 August 2019).
20. INDEC. Censo Nacional de Población, Hogares y Viviendas. Available online: https://www.indec.gob.ar/indec/web/Nivel4-CensoNacional-3-3-Censo-2010 (accessed on 5 January 2019).
21. Cieza, A.; Fayed, N.; Bickenbach, J.; Prodinger, B. Refinements of the ICF Linking Rules to strengthen their potential for establishing comparability of health information. *Disabil. Rehabil.* **2016**, *41*, 574–583. [CrossRef] [PubMed]
22. Ferreira, H.N.C.; Schiariti, V.; Regalado, I.C.R.; Sousa, K.G.; Pereira, S.A.; Fechine, C.P.N.D.S.; Longo, E. Functioning and Disability Profile of Children with Microcephaly Associated with Congenital Zika Virus Infection. *Int. J. Environ. Res. Public Heal.* **2018**, *15*, 1107. [CrossRef] [PubMed]
23. Ketelaar, M.; Bogossian, A.; Saini, M.; Visser-Meily, A.; Lach, L. Assessment of the family environment in pediatric neurodisability: A state-of-the-art review. *Dev. Med. Child. Neurol.* **2017**, *59*, 259–269. [CrossRef] [PubMed]
24. Mahdi, S.; Albertowski, K.; Almodayfer, O.; Arsenopoulou, V.; Carucci, S.; Dias, J.C.; Khalil, M.; Knüppel, A.; Langmann, A.; Lauritsen, M.B.; et al. An International Clinical Study of Ability and Disability in Autism Spectrum Disorder Using the WHO-ICF Framework. *J. Autism Dev. Disord.* **2018**, *48*, 2148–2163. [CrossRef] [PubMed]
25. Brignell, A.; Song, H.; Zhu, J.; Suo, C.; Lu, D.; Morgan, A.T. Communication intervention for autism spectrum disorders in minimally verbal children. *Cochrane Database Syst. Rev.* **2016**, *2016*. [CrossRef]
26. Campos, T.N.C.; Schiariti, V.; Gladstone, M.; Melo, A.; Tavares, J.S.; Magalhães, A.G.; Longo, E. How congenital Zika virus impacted my child's functioning and disability: A Brazilian qualitative study guided by the ICF. *BMJ Open* **2020**, *10*, e038228. [CrossRef] [PubMed]

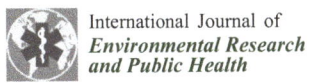

Article

Cross-Cultural Adaptation and Validation of the Brazilian Portuguese Version of an Observational Measure for Parent–Child Responsive Caregiving

Alessandra Schneider [1], Michelle Rodrigues [1], Olesya Falenchuk [2], Tiago N. Munhoz [3,4], Aluisio J. D. Barros [4], Joseph Murray [4,5], Marlos R. Domingues [6] and Jennifer M. Jenkins [1,*]

1. Department of Applied Psychology and Human Development, University of Toronto, Toronto, ON M5S, Canada; alessandra.schneider@mail.utoronto.ca (A.S.); michelle.rodrigues@mail.utoronto.ca (M.R.)
2. Ontario Institute for Studies in Education, University of Toronto, Toronto, ON M5S, Canada; olesya.falenchuk@utoronto.ca
3. Faculty of Psychology, Federal University of Pelotas, Pelotas 96010900, Brazil; tyagomunhoz@hotmail.com
4. Postgraduate Program in Epidemiology, Federal University of Pelotas, Pelotas 96010900, Brazil; abarros.epi@gmail.com (A.J.D.B.); j.murray@doveresearch.org (J.M.)
5. Human Development and Violence Research Centre, Federal University of Pelotas, Pelotas 96010900, Brazil
6. Postgraduate Program in Physical Education, Federal University of Pelotas, Pelotas 96010900, Brazil; marlosufpel@gmail.com
* Correspondence: jenny.jenkins@utoronto.ca

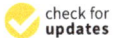

Citation: Schneider, A.; Rodrigues, M.; Falenchuk, O.; Munhoz, T.N.; Barros, A.J.D.; Murray, J.; Domingues, M.R.; Jenkins, J.M. Cross-Cultural Adaptation and Validation of the Brazilian Portuguese Version of an Observational Measure for Parent–Child Responsive Caregiving. *Int. J. Environ. Res. Public Health* **2021**, *18*, 1246. https://doi.org/10.3390/ijerph18031246

Academic Editor: Verónica Schiariti
Received: 23 December 2020
Accepted: 25 January 2021
Published: 30 January 2021

Publisher's Note: MDPI stays neutral with regard to jurisdictional claims in published maps and institutional affiliations.

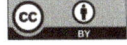

Copyright: © 2021 by the authors. Licensee MDPI, Basel, Switzerland. This article is an open access article distributed under the terms and conditions of the Creative Commons Attribution (CC BY) license (https:// creativecommons.org/licenses/by/ 4.0/).

Abstract: Responsive caregiving is the dimension of parenting most consistently related to later child functioning in both developing and developed countries. There is a growing need for efficient, psychometrically sound and culturally appropriate measurement of this construct. This study describes the cross-cultural validation in Brazil of the Responsive Interactions for Learning (RIFL-P) measure, requiring only eight minutes for assessment and coding. The cross-cultural adaptation used a recognized seven-step procedure. The adapted version was applied to a stratified sample of 153 Brazilian mother–child (18 months) dyads. Videos of mother–child interaction were coded using the RIFL-P and a longer gold standard parenting assessment. Mothers completed a survey on child stimulation (18 months) and child outcomes were measured at 24 months. Internal consistency ($\alpha = 0.94$), inter-rater reliability ($r = 0.83$), and intra-rater reliability ($r = 0.94$) were all satisfactory to high. RIFL-P scores were significantly correlated with another measurement of parenting (r's ranged from 0.32 to 0.47, $p < 0.001$), stimulation markers ($r = 0.34$, $p < 0.01$), and children's cognition ($r = 0.29$, $p < 0.001$), language ($r = 0.28$, $p < 0.001$), and positive behavior ($r = 0.17$, $p < 0.05$). The Brazilian Portuguese version is a valid and reliable instrument for a brief assessment of responsive caregiving.

Keywords: responsive caregiving; parent–child interaction; observational measurement; thin slice methodology; low- and middle-income countries; Brazil

1. Introduction

Responsive caregiving is a key element in fostering young children's developmental potential [1–4]. This special type of caregiving integrates sensitivity (defined as the caregiver´s ability to notice, interpret, and respond appropriately to an infant´s signals, needs, and internal state [5]) and stimulation (described as expanding and building on a child's interest by talking, pointing and demonstrating in a developmentally appropriate way that supports early learning [6]). These attuned and reciprocal interactions—previously operationalized as cognitive sensitivity [7] or responsive stimulation [3]—have been found to predict cognitive [4,8,9], socioemotional [10,11], and brain development in young children [12]. This aspect of parenting is best assessed observationally as caregivers can only report on responses to signals that they notice and not those they miss or misinterpret [13,14].

The Responsive Interactions for Learning (RIFL) measure combines the well-understood concepts of sensitivity and stimulation in a brief, observational tool that can be used to assess responsive caregiving at the population level. It has been shown to have good reliability and validity in mothers, fathers, and siblings and is referred to as RIFL-P for parents [15] and RIFL-S for siblings [7,16]. The coding scheme for this instrument uses a thin-slice methodology proposed by Ambady [17], who argued that when a construct is well articulated, it can be accurately, intuitively, and rapidly rated. Thin-slice ratings have been shown to have similar psychometric properties to labor-intensive coding schemes [7,15].

Considering that most instruments measuring parental responsivity have been developed in Western countries based on middle-class samples [18], one cannot presume that specific behaviors observed for those families and assessed by those instruments are generalizable across cultures. To overcome this, the field recommends adaptation of instruments with documented validity rather than the development of new ones since cross-cultural adaptation is faster, easier, and less expensive [19,20]. Experimental and correlational studies performed in Brazil have shown cultural evidence of the importance of the construct of responsivity/sensitivity in the Brazilian society [21–23].

Given the public health importance of early responsivity to child development, and considering that responsive caregiving is the cornerstone of successful early childhood development (ECD) interventions [24,25], there is an urgent need for valid and reliable measures appropriate for use in large-scale studies. Screening of parental responsivity at the level of population groups could aid in identifying those caregivers who may benefit from parenting programs. There is also growing recognition of the need to integrate behavioral services into primary care [26] to strengthen early identification and access to appropriate interventions [27]. This is especially relevant in Brazil, as this country has been implementing massive ECD home visiting programs among disadvantaged families [28,29] and parent training programs to coach caregivers on positive parent–child interactions [30].

The aim of the study was to describe the cross-cultural adaptation process and validation of the Brazilian Portuguese RIFL-P, thus providing a culturally adapted, validated, and appropriate observational instrument to assess responsive caregiving in Brazilian parent–child dyads.

2. Materials and Methods

The University of Toronto Research Ethics Board, as well as the Ethics Committee of the Medical School of the Federal University of Pelotas approved the study. All participants signed an informed consent form before being enrolled in this study.

2.1. Participants

Participants of phase 1 (cross-cultural adaptation) and phase 2 (testing the new measure) were different. For phase 1, nineteen participants took part, including supervisors and home visitors from the *Primeira Infância Melhor* program ($N = 17$) and two child health university professors.

The phase 2 study was based on a subsample of the 2015 Pelotas Birth Cohort Study [31] when the children were 18 months old. The target sample size was $N = 155$, based on budgetary constraints and practice in the field [32,33]. The Pelotas cohort used demographic data collected within two days of the child's birth to identify a subpopulation of children eligible for the current parenting study. Three hundred and ninety-five families satisfied the selection criteria (full-term, singleton, normal birth weight, and aged between 17 and 18 months during a six-week data collection period). Families were stratified by wealth quintiles according to household assets assessed at the child's birth and recruited until the target sample size was achieved. Recruiting stopped after 178 families were contacted, 23 families refused (13%) and the target sample of $N = 155$ was achieved. Observational data were collected for 155 mother–child dyads. Two film clips were excluded for technical reasons (duration of less than 5 min and third-party interference in the task). The final sample of 153 dyads was determined to be optimal based on the proposed analyses and expected results [34]. Mean child age was 17.9 months (SD = 0.27), mean gestational age was 39.4 weeks (SD = 1.23; range = 37–41.9 weeks). Females outnumbered males (females = 55.5%, males = 44.5%). The participating families' socioeconomic levels were represented equally in the upper four quintiles with about 22% each, while the first quintile (the poorest) accounted for about 12% of the children. Children in the 2015 Pelotas Birth Cohort were followed up at 24 months of age, and developmental outcomes were collected [35]. The relationship between our new parental responsivity measure and children's developmental outcomes could therefore be examined in the 153 families of our sample.

2.2. The Responsive Interactions for Learning Measure, Version for Parents

The RIFL-P (previously known as Cognitive Sensitivity) is a unidimensional 11-item observational instrument designed to provide a rapid assessment of the extent to which a parent identifies and responds, incorporating sensitivity and stimulation, to the feelings and thoughts of the child with whom they are interacting. The RIFL-P measures three interconnected skills of the caregiver—(i) communicative clarity (providing meaningful verbal/nonverbal inputs to the child and fostering of shared understanding of the goals of the task); (ii) mind-reading (thinking about what the child knows and understands); and (iii) mutuality building (promoting reciprocity)—through a challenging task that elicits cooperation. Assessment uses a thin slice methodology and takes around eight minutes to administer and code (five minutes of observation of interaction, three minutes to code). After watching a 5-min video recording just once, raters apply codes to each of the 11 items using a five-point Likert scale, ranging from 1 ("Not at all true") to 5 ("Very true"). A mean of the 11 items is calculated, yielding a composite score of responsivity that can range from 1 to 5. Currently, the training of RIFL-P raters is completed in less than eight hours through a password-protected, open-source online asynchronous course offered by the University of Toronto, which is available in English, Portuguese, and Spanish. Psychometric properties of the original instrument were found to be strong (inter-rater reliability (IRR) was $\alpha = 0.84$; internal consistency of the scale was $\alpha = 0.92$) [15]. RIFL scores assessed both for parents and siblings have been found to be associated with contextual risk (inversely), traditional measures of maternal sensitivity, and a range of child outcomes, including receptive vocabulary, executive functioning, theory of mind, and academic achievement [7,15,36].

2.3. Phase 1: Cross-Cultural Adaptation of the RIFL-P

Phase 1 was the cross-cultural adaptation of the RIFL-P from the source to the target language. Prior to conducting this phase, written permission from the developers of the original measure was obtained. A well-established method [19,37] was used for this phase, based on six steps (see Figure 1) that maximize the level of semantic, idiomatic, conceptual, and experiential equivalence achieved between the original and adapted versions of the instrument.

At the end of each step, a written report and/or an updated version of the instrument were produced and used to guide the next step. The focus groups and the formation of an expert committee ensured conceptual and functional content validity [38]. The first author (AS) coordinated the two 2-h group sessions with nine and eight participants each. Participants were asked to read and discuss all the items in the scale, the response options, and the extent to which the wording was clear and comprehensible. They collectively rated the comprehensibility of the scale on a three-point scale. They were asked to consider whether the items were representative of the parenting of Brazilian parents and to raise any other important aspects of parenting that came to mind. Back translation was elaborated with a double purpose, i.e., highlighting translation deficiencies and allowing for review of possible cultural differences by the original developers. Back translation is viewed as an additional quality control check [19,39]. It is also essential in a cross-cultural adaptation of an observational measure to contextualize the coding in the new culture [32], as described below.

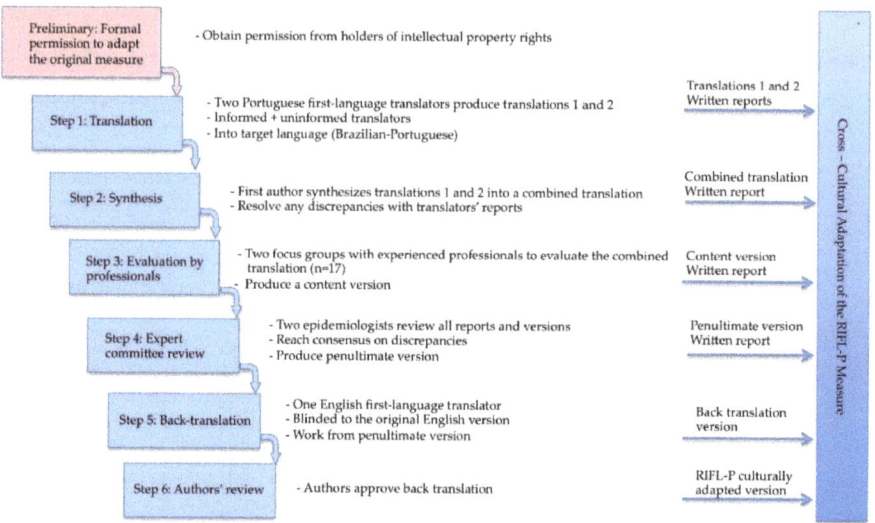

Figure 1. Step sequence for the cross-cultural adaptation process—the Brazilian Portuguese version of the RIFL-P measure (adapted from Beaton et al. [19]).

2.4. Phase 2: Testing the New Measure

This phase included the collection and analysis of 155 videos of mother–child interaction. This phase had two components: Coder Training and Full Psychometrics. The purpose of Coder Training was to train the second coder in the reliability criteria and to elaborate the coder manual (for future training of coders) with specific information about the Brazilian context and parenting. This was done with the first 39 dyads from the full sample. The purpose of the Full Psychometrics component was to establish the reliability and validity of the Brazilian Portuguese RIFL-P measure (namely, *Interações Responsivas para a Aprendizagem*).

2.4.1. Measures

The RIFL-P (Brazilian Portuguese Version)

Mothers were given a task to do with their children. The mother sat on a yoga mat and played with her child for five minutes. She was shown pictures of patterns on the shape and color sorter of varying degrees of difficulty and asked to encourage the child to make the patterns with her. The goal was to elicit maternal behaviors and speech related to helping and teaching when the task was slightly too developmentally challenging for the child. Following training on the scale, and after watching the recording once, raters applied codes to each of the 11 items using a five-point Likert scale, ranging from 1 ("Not at all true") to 5 ("Very true"). The task plus coding took around eight minutes.

Parenting Interactions with Children: Checklist of Observations Linked to Outcomes, PICCOLO (Brazilian Portuguese Version)

PICCOLO is a strengths-based checklist of 29 observable behaviors used to assess positive parenting interactions with children aged 10 to 47 months [40]. PICCOLO items are clustered in four domains with seven to eight items per domain: (a) affection (warmth, physical closeness, and positive expressions toward the child); (b) responsiveness (responding sensitively to a child's cues, needs, interests, and behaviors); (c) encouragement (active support of play, exploration, curiosity, skills, and creativity); and (d) teaching (shared conversations and play, cognitive stimulation, explanations, and questions). After watching a 10-min film clip once, raters coded items on a three-point ordinal scale from "Absent", or not seen, to "Clearly" seen. The task plus coding took around 45 min. Psychometric properties of the original instrument have been found to be strong (IRR ranged between $r = 0.74$ for the responsiveness domain and $r = 0.80$ for the affection domain; Cronbach's α coefficient = 0.91 for the total PICCOLO score (ranging from α's of 0.75 for the responsiveness domain to 0.80 for the teaching domain)) [40], as have those of the PICCOLO Brazilian Portuguese version (IRR ranged between $r = 0.63$ for the encouragement domain and $r = 0.77$ for the affection domain; Cronbach's α coefficient = 0.94 for the total PICCOLO score (ranging from α's of 0.79 for the affection and teaching domains to 0.86 for the responsiveness and encouragement domains)) [41].

INTERGROWTH-21st Neurodevelopment Assessment

The INTERGROWTH-21st Neurodevelopment Assessment (INTER-NDA) is a valid and reliable international standardized screening assessment of early child development at 2 years of age [42]. This multidimensional measure provides a comprehensive, rapid assessment of cognition, fine and gross motor skills, language, and positive and negative behavior for children aged 22–30 months. Its 37 items are administered in approximately 15 min using a combination of psychometric techniques, such as direct administration, concurrent observation, and caregiver reports. For all INTER-NDA domains, except for negative behavior, higher scores reflect better outcomes. The INTER-NDA has demonstrated good to acceptable agreement with the Bayley Scales of Infant and Toddler Development, Third Edition [43]. The INTER-NDA is designed to be applied by nonspecialists to high-, middle-, and low-income populations. The INTER-NDA instrument was used to evaluate the development of 3776 children aged 24 months from the 2015 Pelotas Birth Cohort Study in Southern Brazil [35].

Five Stimulation Markers

This scale was developed by Barros and colleagues [44] to examine the extent to which children experienced a cognitively stimulating environment. Mothers answered no/yes (no = 0, yes = 1) to the following questions about their children's activities in the past week: whether someone read or told a story to the child; whether the child went to a park or playground; whether the child had a story book; whether the child watched TV; whether the child visited anyone's house. The responses for the five items were summed, resulting in a scale from 0 to 5 points. The scale has been found to be related to child development outcomes in Brazil, particularly amongst children whose mothers are low in education [44].

2.4.2. Procedures

Data collection for phase 2 included a home visit to film mother–child interactions (10 min PICCOLO task followed by the 5 min RIFL-P task) when children were around 18 months old. The mothers answered a one-page questionnaire about the five stimulation markers before the home visit was terminated. The filmed interactions (collected at 18 months) were coded and analyzed in relation to demographic data (collected up to two days after delivery, in the perinatal period) of the 2015 Pelotas Birth Cohort Study and developmental data collected when children reached 24 months of age.

2.4.3. Data Coding Procedures

The first (AS) and fourth (TNM) authors, trained by expert coders, scored the RIFL-P videos. Raters were trained until the inter-rater reliability of $r > 0.80$ was reached and then coded the remaining videos independently. Reliability testing was conducted using every fourth film throughout data coding. Following the submission of reliability scores, discrepancies were discussed to minimize rater drift. Scale developers were consulted on three occasions.

2.5. Data Analysis

Investigation of psychometric properties of the adapted RIFL-P instrument included inter- and intra-rater reliability (Pearson correlation coefficient), item-level descriptive statistics, and confirmatory factor analysis (CFA). The internal consistency of the adapted version was computed using Cronbach's alpha.

To examine convergent validity, the composite score of RIFL-P was correlated with the scores of the PICCOLO Brazilian Portuguese version, Five Stimulation Markers, and INTER-NDA scales. Discriminant validity was tested by examining the relationship between gender and the RIFL-P scores and no significant association was expected. Different types of correlation were used dependent on variable type (Pearson product-moment correlation for continuous variables, point-biserial correlation for binary and continuous variables, and Spearman's correlation for ordinal variables). Statistical analyses were conducted using the Statistical Package for Social Sciences (SPSS, Inc., Chicago, IL, USA) for Windows (version 21.0; Microsoft Corporation, Redmond, WA, USA), and the Stata® version 13.0 software.

3. Results

3.1. Phase 1: Cross-Cultural Adaptation of the RIFL-P

Three key adaptations were made during development of the Brazilian Portuguese RIFL-P version. First, the term "parent" was replaced by "caregiver". Second, in Portuguese, "mind reading" was translated as "thought reading" (*leitura do pensamento*) in order to preserve conceptual equivalence. Third, definitions of the scoring rubrics of the adapted RIFL-P version were expanded to include a specific rubric for score 3 ("Sometimes true/I partially agree") and descriptions of scores 1 and 5 of the Likert scale gained one more expression (i.e., 1 = "Not at all true/I totally disagree"; 5 = "Very true/I totally agree"). The adapted RIFL-P coding sheet and manual, in Brazilian Portuguese, are presented as Appendices A and B respectively.

3.2. Phase 2: Testing the New Measure

3.2.1. Coder Training

Additional guidelines for Brazilian coders (i.e., examples of culture-specific behaviors) were elaborated for five of the 11 items to adapt the measure, both culturally and psychometrically, for use with the local population. Three items were coded infrequently (1, 3, and 8), meaning that what was average for those behaviors for Canadian mothers was not average for Brazilian mothers. In order to ensure the underlying normal distribution on all items in the adapted RIFL-P measure, the scoring rubrics for those three items were softened in the Portuguese Brazilian version.

3.2.2. Full Psychometrics

Descriptive statistics for the RIFL-P items in the Brazilian sample are presented in Table 1. The table shows that the least frequently observed item in the Brazilian sample was item 8, namely "This parent is good at rephrasing what the child does not understand" and the most frequently observed behavior was item 1 "This parent gives clear and specific verbal directions".

Table 1. Descriptive statistics of responsive interactions for learning items (English and Portuguese versions) in the Brazilian sample.

Item (English)	Item (Portuguese)	Brazilian Sample (n = 153)	
		M	SD
1. This parent gives clear and specific verbal directions.	1. Este cuidador dá instruções verbais claras e específicas.	3.27	1.5
2. This parent gives positive nonverbal directions.	2. Este cuidador dá instruções não verbais positivas.	2.87	0.85
3. This parent reminds the child about goals/rules of the task.	3. Este cuidador lembra a criança dos objetivos/regras da tarefa.	2.65	0.84
4. This parent will try to complete the task in a way that is sensitive to the child's needs and desires.	4. Este cuidador procura completar a tarefa de maneira sensível às necessidades e aos desejos da criança.	2.71	0.88
5. This parent will try to follow the rules in a way that is sensitive to the child's needs and desires.	5. Este cuidador procura seguir as regras de maneira sensível às necessidades e aos desejos da criança.	2.35	1.01
6. This parent is clear in his/her requests for help.	6. Este cuidador pede ajuda de maneira clara.	2.75	0.91
7. This parent is *sensitively* responsive to the child's requests for help, even those that are subtle/nonverbal.	7. Este cuidador responde *sensivelmente* aos pedidos de ajuda da criança, mesmo os sutis e/ou não verbais.	2.44	0.9
8. This parent is good at rephrasing what the child does not understand.	8. Este cuidador consegue reformular instruções que a criança não entende.	1.98	1.06
9. This parent is sensitive to what the child knows and/or understands.	9. Este cuidador é sensível ao que a criança sabe e/ou compreende.	2.43	0.86
10. This parent gives positive feedback to reinforce the child.	10. Este cuidador oferece *feedback* positivo para reforçar o comportamento da criança.	2.96	1.37
11. This parent promotes turn taking between himself/herself and the child.	11. Este cuidador incentiva a alternância na interação com a criança.	2.41	0.88

Note: M = mean; SD = standard deviation.

Reliability

Inter-rater reliability of the total scale score was high ($r = 0.83$), well above the acceptable minimum of 0.70 [45]. Intra-rater reliability, or rating consistency by the same rater two weeks apart, was also high ($r = 0.94$).

Factorial Structure

Confirmatory factor analysis was conducted to investigate whether the unidimensional structure of the original RIFL-P instrument applied to the Portuguese version. Model fit for the one-dimensional CFA model was less than optimal (RMSEA = 0.12; CFI = 0.93; TLI = 0.92; cut-off recommendations for acceptable fit require RMSEA < 0.06; CFI > 0.95; TLI > 0.95) [46]. A likelihood ratio test comparing the CFA model to the saturated model was significant, $\chi^2(44) = 143.55$, $p < 0.001$. Investigation of the modification indices showed very high correlations across three pairs of items (3 and 8, 1 and 6, and 8 and 10; modification indices were 31.95, 16.88, and 13.52, respectively). Consequently, the insufficient model fit in the CFA analysis was not due to deficient relationships among the items but rather to potential redundancies among some of them. Once the CFA model was modified to take these correlations into account, the model fit indices were high (RMSEA = 0.05; CFI = 0.97; TLI = 0.96). All 11 items had high standardized factor loadings on a single factor (ranging from 0.61 to 0.90, shown in Table 2). The percentage of variance explained by the latent factor in each item (R^2) ranged between 0.37 and 0.81. This unidimensional structure was further confirmed with the internal consistency analysis. The Cronbach's alpha was 0.94, with item-total correlations ranging between 0.61 and 0.88.

Table 2. Item loadings for the Responsive Interactions for Learning measure in the Brazilian sample.

Scale/Item	Standardized Factor Loadings	R^2
1. This parent gives clear and specific verbal directions.	0.61	0.37
2. This parent gives positive nonverbal directions.	0.76	0.57
3. This parent reminds the child about goals/rules of the task.	0.79	0.62
4. This parent will try to complete the task in a way that is sensitive to the child's needs and desires.	0.89	0.80
5. This parent will try to follow the rules in a way that is sensitive to the child's needs and desires.	0.90	0.81
6. This parent is clear in his/her requests for help.	0.89	0.79
7. This parent is *sensitively* responsive to the child's requests for help, even those that are subtle/nonverbal.	0.87	0.75
8. This parent is good at rephrasing what the child does not understand.	0.83	0.68
9. This parent is sensitive to what the child knows and/or understands.	0.85	0.73
10. This parent gives positive feedback to reinforce the child.	0.65	0.42
11. This parent promotes turn taking between himself/herself and the child.	0.69	0.48

Note: All standardized factor loadings are significant at the 0.001 level. R^2 = coefficient of determination.

Based on the results of psychometric analyses, composite RIFL-P scores were computed as the mean of the 11 items. The mean Brazilian Portuguese RIFL-P score was 2.62 (SD = 0.81), ranging between 1.09 and 4.82. Comparable scores for the original measure, in a sample of Canadian mother–child dyads, had a mean of 3.24 (SD = 0.70), with a minimum score of 1.18 and a maximum score of 4.91 [15]. The differences between the average RIFL-P scores in the Brazilian Portuguese and Canadian samples was statistically significant, t(437) = 8.36, $p < 0.001$, with a large effect size (Cohen's d = 0.82). RIFL-P composite scores were positively correlated with family socioeconomic status (Spearman's $\rho = 0.46, p < 0.001$).

Convergent and Discriminant Validity

The convergent validity analyses showed that the adapted RIFL-P was significantly associated with all four Brazilian Portuguese PICCOLO domains ($r = 0.32$ for affection; $r = 0.37$ for responsiveness; $r = 0.41$ for encouragement; and $r = 0.47$ for teaching, $p < 0.001$) and the PICCOLO total score ($r = 0.44, p < 0.001$). In addition, the adapted RIFL-P was significantly associated with the Five Stimulation Markers ($r = 0.34, p < 0.01$) and a range of child outcomes assessed by the INTER-NDA, including cognition ($r = 0.29, p < 0.001$), language ($r = 0.28, p < 0.001$), and positive behavior ($r = 0.17, p < 0.05$). Its association with fine motor skills ($r = 0.16, p = 0.055$) was borderline significant and it was not significantly associated with gross motor skills ($r = 0.13, p = 0.110$) or negative behavior scores ($r = -0.001, p = 0.992$). With respect to discriminant validity, RIFL-P was not expected to correlate with gender ($r = -0.22, p < 0.01$) but it did. The RIFL-P scores for boys were lower than for girls.

4. Discussion

Responsive caregiving is a dimension of parenting in the early childhood years that is consistently related to subsequent cognitive and socioemotional aspects of functioning [2,47,48]. This aspect of caregiving is modifiable. Results from randomized controlled trials in developed and developing countries show that it is possible to improve this aspect of parenting, that doing so improves children's developmental outcomes, and that it may be the modifiable risk factor with the strongest effect on later brain development [3,49,50]. Although marked improvements to long-term child outcomes have now been demonstrated for parental responsivity interventions [4], moving from efficacy to effectiveness has proven to be a substantial challenge. If scalability is to be achieved, it is essential to have an instrument that can measure parental responsivity. Unfortunately, however, observational measures are the only ones that show good validity and most previous measures take a long time to administer and code. On the other hand, the literature suggests that adaptation of instruments that have shown reliability and validity evidence is more advantageous in LMIC than novel instrument development [19].

The cross-cultural adaptation of RIFL-P involved gold standard methodology to avoid cultural bias and the measure was successfully adapted to Portuguese and the Brazilian context. The adapted RIFL-P measure showed strong psychometric properties, mirroring the findings from the original instrument. As it is efficient, only taking eight minutes to assess and code, it is a measure that can be used at the population level. Since the sample was based on a stratified sample from a population cohort in one city of Brazil and refusal rates from the cohort were low, a high level of representativeness was achieved. A recent global effort led by the World Health Organization and UNICEF to monitor the Nurturing Care Framework's responsive caregiving component only provided proxy indicators (e.g., parental mental health, childcare availability, parental support) [51]. To make real progress in this realm, it is imperative to assess responsive interactions at the population level with measures, such as RIFL-P, that are psychometrically strong and quick to train, administer, and code. An online course in three languages is available to researchers or parenting professionals free of charge by contacting the first or last authors.

Four findings are worthy of further comment. First, the mean score for responsive interactions in Brazil was lower than that found in Canada. This was expected given the results of earlier studies in which the parenting of Latino mothers has been found to be more directive and controlling [52], with a lack of emphasis on understanding the child's internal goals and need for autonomy [53]. Of course, cultures differ in their values, customs, and beliefs [54], with the result that some parental behaviors receive less attention than others [55]. Regarding childrearing practices, Latino mothers tend to value obedience and politeness, physically guide their toddler's actions, attribute less importance to children's autonomy, and report greater use of discipline as a teaching method when compared to European American mothers of the same socioeconomic status [56]. Given that parental responsivity (although lower in Brazil) was found to relate to children's developmental outcomes, this does suggest that improving parental responsivity should be an important policy goal in Brazil. Second, in this study, Brazilian mothers were more responsive to girls than to boys, according to the RIFL-P scores. This finding should be cautiously interpreted as the same gender difference was not observed based on PICCOLO scores and a meta-analysis of parenting as a function of gender reported no significant differences [57]. An examination of this in future studies in Brazil is encouraged. Third, for purposes of criterion validity, we examined relationships with child outcomes, as well as other indices of parenting and contextual risk. Findings showed that both parenting measures were significantly related (i.e., RIFL-P and PICCOLO scores), as well as RIFL-P scores and a measure of parenting stimulation [44], and the strongest relationships with child outcomes were observed for the cognitive and language domains, which is in line with previous findings for the RIFL-P in a Canadian sample [15]. RIFL-P scores, both in Brazil and Canada, have been found to be associated with contextual risk (inversely). Fourth, as in previous work, low socioeconomic status (SES) was found in the current study to be associated with lower levels of parental responsivity. The association between socioeconomics and parenting has been widely reported [58] with evidence that economic hardship leads to parental emotional distress which impairs parenting [59]. It is also notable that economic hardship does not operate on its own. SES clusters risk [60] such that children are exposed to multiple challenges that compromise development (e.g., maternal depression, unemployment, domestic violence, poor neighborhoods) and parenting [61].

Limitations and Future Directions

This research has limitations that should be considered when interpreting the results. Although the study tested the instrument using an adequate sample in terms of size (n = 153) and socioeconomic variability, thus ensuring its statistical power, the numbers were not sufficient to provide normative data, and the age range of the children was limited to 18-month-old toddlers. A large study would be necessary for RIFL-P standardization and, therefore, for its clinical use.

The significance and novelty of this study was the development of a Brazilian Portuguese version of a psychometrically sound measure of responsive caregiving that requires little training (free, online), uses a short video clip of caregiver–child interaction (5 min), and takes little time to code (approximately 3 min per interaction). Thus, the adapted RIFL-P instrument represents a suitable measure for application in large-scale studies in Brazil to potentially impact policy, practice, and research.

5. Conclusions

The culturally adapted Brazilian Portuguese version of the RIFL-P measure proved to be a valid and reliable instrument for a brief assessment of responsive caregiving in parent–child interactions in Brazil. Efficient and valid measuring instruments of responsive caregiving appropriate to primary care settings are essential tools to advance ECD policies and programs. This study is one of the first of its kind, designed to provide a culturally adapted, reliable, and valid strengths-based measure of responsive parenting interactions with children under two years of age in Brazil.

Author Contributions: Conceptualization: A.S., A.J.D.B., J.M.J., M.R.; methodology: A.S., O.F., J.M.J.; sample: T.N.M., A.J.D.B., J.M., M.R.D.; software: A.S., O.F.; formal analysis: A.S., O.F.; resources: O.F., T.N.M., A.J.D.B., J.M., M.R.D.; data curation: A.S.; writing—original draft preparation: A.S., A.J.D.B., J.M.J., M.R., T.N.M., J.M., M.R.D.; supervision: A.J.D.B., O.F., J.M.J.; funding acquisition: A.S. All authors have read and agreed to the published version of the manuscript.

Funding: This study was financed in part by the Coordenação de Aperfeiçoamento de Pessoal de Nível Superior–Brasil (CAPES)–Finance Code 001.

Institutional Review Board Statement: The study was conducted according to the guidelines of the Declaration of Helsinki, and approved by the Research Ethics Board of the UNIVERSITY OF TORONTO (protocol code 33024 of June 27, 2016) and the Ethics Committee of the Medical School of the FEDERAL UNIVERSITY OF PELOTAS (protocol code 1.717.977 of 8 September 2016).

Informed Consent Statement: Informed consent was obtained from all subjects involved in the study.

Data Availability Statement: The data that support the findings of this study are available from the corresponding author, upon reasonable request.

Acknowledgments: We are grateful to the families who gave their time so generously and have contributed to knowledge of parental interactions in Brazil. We thank the Postgraduate Program in Epidemiology at the Federal University of Pelotas, Brazil for the partnership.

Conflicts of Interest: The authors declare no conflict of interest.

Appendix A. RIFL-P Coding Sheet (Brazilian Portuguese Version)

ID:_____Codificador:_____Hora/início:_____Hora/fim:_____Data/codificação:____/_

Interações Responsivas para a Aprendizagem
Codificação de Interações Breves em Duplas Cuidador-Criança

- Responda às perguntas abaixo com base na interação deste cuidador especificamente com esta criança.
- Pontue rapidamente, de acordo com suas reações iniciais e impressões gerais; não se detenha demais em nenhum item.
- Use todas as informações disponíveis, incluindo as não verbais, para formar sua reação e impressões.
- Tente usar toda escala de 5 pontos, não deixe itens em branco (dê a cada item seu melhor palpite/avaliação).
- Observe somente por 5 min. Se ultrapassar 5 min, interrompa.

Dê sua impressão de como este cuidador interage com a criança no dia-a-dia, com base no que você observou:	(Nada verdadeiro/Discordo totalmente)		(Algumas vezes verdadeiro/Concordo parcialmente)		(Muito verdadeiro/ Concordo totalmente)
Clareza na Comunicação					
1. Este cuidador dá instruções verbais claras e específicas.	1	2	3	4	5
2. Este cuidador dá instruções não verbais positivas.	1	2	3	4	5
3. Este cuidador lembra a criança dos objetivos/regras da tarefa.	1	2	3	4	5
4. Este cuidador procura completar a tarefa de maneira sensível às necessidades e aos desejos da criança.	1	2	3	4	5
5. Este cuidador procura seguir as regras de maneira sensível às necessidades e aos desejos da criança.	1	2	3	4	5
6. Este cuidador pede ajuda de maneira clara.	1	2	3	4	5
Leitura do Pensamento					
7. Este cuidador responde *sensivelmente* aos pedidos de ajuda da criança, mesmo os sutis e/ou não verbais.	1	2	3	4	5
8. Este cuidador consegue reformular instruções que a criança não entende.	1	2	3	4	5
9. Este cuidador é sensível ao que a criança sabe e/ou compreende.	1	2	3	4	5
Desenvolvimento da Mutualidade					
10. Este cuidador oferece *feedback* positivo para reforçar o comportamento da criança.	1	2	3	4	5
11. Este cuidador incentiva a alternância na interação com a criança.	1	2	3	4	5

Appendix B. RIFL-P Manual (Brazilian Portuguese Version)

Interações Responsivas para a Aprendizagem
Codificação de Interações Breves em Duplas Cuidador-Criança

- Responda às perguntas abaixo com base na interação do cuidador especificamente com esta criança.
- Pontue rapidamente, de acordo com suas reações iniciais e impressões gerais; não se detenha demais em nenhum item.
- Use todas as informações disponíveis, incluindo as não verbais, para formar sua reação e impressões.
- Tente usar toda a escala de 5 pontos, não deixe itens em branco (dê a cada item seu melhor palpite/avaliação).

	1 = Nada verdadeiro/Discordo totalmente
	2
Escala Likert de 5 pontos	3 = Pouco verdadeiro/Concordo
	4
	5 = Muito verdadeiro/Concordo totalmente

CLAREZA NA COMUNICAÇÃO

1. Este cuidador dá instruções verbais claras e específicas.

Este item se refere a comandos verbais com informações específicas e não genéricas. O cuidador dá informações suficientes para que a criança complete a tarefa, sem ser vago ou ambíguo.

Exemplos: "Coloque o bloco azul grande ao lado do bloco amarelo pequeno"; "Conte quatro círculos e depois coloque aqui"; "É o bloco verde claro"; "Vamos separar os blocos, você pega os azuis claros e eu pego os azuis escuros"; **ao invés de** "Coloque esse lá"; "Me dê aquele"; "Separe os blocos."

2. Este cuidador dá instruções não verbais positivas.

Este item se refere ao uso de ações físicas para comunicar o que a criança deve fazer a seguir, incluindo também a modelagem. As ações são consideradas "positivas" na medida em que promovem a realização da tarefa de forma colaborativa, não agressiva e não hostil.

Exemplos: "Guiar a mão da criança, apontar para o lugar correto, apontar para a figura, apontar para um objeto e sugerir que a criança o pegue, servir de modelo, modelar ("Olha o que a mamãe vai fazer" ou "Olha só [e mostra como a criança deve fazer]").

3. Este cuidador lembra a criança dos objetivos/regras da tarefa.

O cuidador cria um contexto para a atividade, comunicando à criança a ideia geral da tarefa, os objetivos e os passos a seguir.

Exemplos: "Lembra que nós estamos tentando copiar essa figura"; "A gente quer construir uma casa"; "Nós queremos colocar todos os blocos azuis para baixo"; "Agora vamos montar o braço"; "Não esqueça que só temos 5 min".

4. Este cuidador procura completar a tarefa de maneira sensível às necessidades e aos desejos da criança.

Este item descreve a clareza com que o cuidador comunica à criança que há uma tarefa a ser feita na qual ele está engajado, estimulando assim a participação da criança. O cuidador demonstra envolvimento na atividade e esforço em completá-la. Se a criança parece não estar muito interessada na tarefa ou demonstra dificuldade, o cuidador procura contemplar com sensibilidade tanto os desejos/necessidades da criança quanto o objetivo da tarefa. Não é necessário que a atividade seja realizada corretamente, mas o cuidador deve tentar seguir a estrutura da tarefa. Um cuidador que desconsidera as necessidades da criança para completar a tarefa terá pontuação mais baixa nesse item, assim como um cuidador que não tenta modelar a estrutura e os objetivos da atividade. Um cuidador que leva em conta as necessidades da criança e também as exigências da tarefa deverá ter pontuação mais alta.

Exemplos: Seguir o ritmo da criança, fornecer uma orientação completa e abrangente, demonstrar paciência quando a criança está tentando realizar a tarefa, reformular as instruções quando a criança não entende.

5. Este cuidador procura seguir as regras de maneira sensível às necessidades e aos desejos da criança.

O cuidador segue as instruções do entrevistador, incluindo quaisquer regras mencionadas (p. ex., tocar nas cores certas), levando em consideração as necessidades da criança. Se a criança não compreende, então o cuidador explica as regras. Se a criança não demonstra interesse em seguir as regras, o cuidador procura de maneira sensível fazer com que a criança siga as regras. Um cuidador que desconsidera as necessidades da criança para seguir rigidamente as regras terá pontuação mais baixa nesse item. Um cuidador que leva em conta as necessidades da criança e também as regras da tarefa deverá ter pontuação mais alta.

Exemplos: O cuidador segue as regras da tarefa, lembra a criança sobre as regras, o cuidador é flexível quando a criança insiste em não seguir as regras e tenta fornecer oportunidades de aprendizagem.

6. Este cuidador pede ajuda de maneira clara.

O cuidador se comunica de uma forma que a criança consegue compreender. Este item não se refere especificamente a instruções verbais ou não verbais, mas à clareza geral da comunicação.

LEITURA DO PENSAMENTO

7. Este cuidador responde *sensivelmente* aos pedidos de ajuda da criança, mesmo os sutis e/ou não verbais.

Quando a criança demonstra precisar de ajuda (de modo verbal ou não verbal), o cuidador percebe e responde adequadamente. O cuidador não ignora sinais sutis ou óbvios de que a criança precisa de ajuda. Esse item *não* inclui respostas em tom irritado, frustrado ou hostil.

Exemplos: [A criança não consegue achar o bloco] "Esse está difícil de encontrar, não é?"; [A criança não consegue achar o bloco] "Olha o bloco ali!"; [puxa para perto o bloco que a criança está procurando].

CLAREZA NA COMUNICAÇÃO
8. Este cuidador consegue reformular instruções que a criança não entende.
Quando a criança tem dificuldade em entender as instruções ou a tarefa, o cuidador percebe e ajusta a linguagem para que ela compreenda melhor.
Exemplos: O cuidador percebe que a criança não está conseguindo achar o bloco amarelo pequeno, e diz "Procure o que tem só 4 círculos"; [ao construir o robô] a criança não responde quando o cuidador diz "Vamos começar de baixo" e o cuidador reformula dizendo "De que cor são os pés do robô?".
9. Este cuidador é sensível ao que a criança sabe e/ou compreende.
O cuidador é capaz de avaliar o nível de compreensão da criança e que tipo de ajuda ela precisa em cada tarefa, identificando a zona de desenvolvimento proximal (isto é, o nível em que as instruções são mais proveitosas para a criança - nem muito fáceis, nem muito difíceis).
Exemplos: Divide a tarefa em partes menores, usa linguagem adequada para o nível de desenvolvimento da criança, dá instruções básicas e apropriadas, percebe quando a criança não compreende algo, incentiva a independência da criança quando apropriado.
DESENVOLVIMENTO DA MUTUALIDADE
10. Este cuidador oferece feedback positivo para reforçar o comportamento da criança.
O cuidador responde às ações da criança com afirmações, vocalizações e/ou comportamentos positivos.
Exemplos: "Muito bem!", "É assim mesmo!", "Beleza!", "Isso mesmo!", "Isso!", "Êee!", "Parabéns!", "Que bonito!", "Que legal!"; [bate palmas; balança a cabeça seguindo as ações da criança].
11. Este cuidador incentiva a alternância na interação com a criança.
Este item é codificado quando o cuidador incentiva a reciprocidade e a alternância na interação, verbalmente ou não, e de modo explícito (p. ex., "Agora é a sua vez") ou sutil (p. ex., "O que a gente vai fazer agora?").
Exemplos: "O próximo é você quem faz"; "Agora é a sua/minha vez"; [apontar para a criança para indicar que é a vez dela]; "Onde será que esse bloco vai... [estimulando a criança a dar sua opinião]". Outros exemplos incluem: "Agora a mãe coloca ... agora a Maria coloca"; "A mãe vai botar primeiro e depois tu tens que fazer igual"; [A criança colocou a peça na parte de cima do pino e a mãe diz] "A mãe empurra pra ti"; "Agora bota tu". Em interações altamente recíprocas, isto pode ser sutil (p. ex., o cuidador se inclina levemente para trás e/ou olha para a criança quando termina a sua vez).

References

1. Black, M.M.; Walker, S.P.; Fernald, L.C.H.; Andersen, C.T.; DiGirolamo, A.M.; Lu, C.; McCoy, D.C.; Fink, G.; Shawar, Y.R.; Shiffman, J.; et al. Early childhood development coming of age: Science through the life course. *Lancet* **2017**, *389*, 77–90. [CrossRef]
2. Madigan, S.; Prime, H.; Graham, S.A.; Rodrigues, M.; Anderson, N.; Khoury, J.; Jenkins, J.M. Parenting behavior and child language: A meta-analysis. *Pediatrics* **2019**, *144*, e20183556. [CrossRef] [PubMed]
3. Yousafzai, A.K.; Rasheed, M.A.; Rizvi, A.; Armstrong, R.; Bhutta, Z.A. Effect of integrated responsive stimulation and nutrition interventions in the Lady Health Worker programme in Pakistan on child development, growth, and health outcomes: A cluster-randomised factorial effectiveness trial. *Lancet* **2014**, *384*, 1282–1293. [CrossRef]
4. Yousafzai, A.K.; Obradović, J.; Rasheed, M.A.; Rizvi, A.; Portilla, X.A.; Tirado-Strayer, N.; Memon, U. Effects of responsive stimulation and nutrition interventions on children's development and growth at age 4 years in a disadvantaged population in Pakistan: A longitudinal follow-up of a cluster-randomised factorial effectiveness trial. *Lancet Glob. Health* **2016**, *4*, e548–e558. [CrossRef]
5. Ainsworth, M.D.S.; Blehar, M.C.; Waters, E.; Wall, S.N. *Patterns of Attachment: A Psychological Study of the Strange Situation*; Psychology Press: Hove, East Sussex, UK, 2015.
6. Vygotsky, L.S. *Mind in Society: The Development of Higher Psychological Processes*; Harvard University Press: Cambridge, MA, USA, 1980.
7. Prime, H.; Perlman, M.; Tackett, J.L.; Jenkins, J.M. Cognitive sensitivity in sibling interactions: Development of the construct and comparison of two coding methodologies. *Early Educ. Dev.* **2014**, *25*, 240–258. [CrossRef]
8. Mermelshtine, R.; Barnes, J. Maternal Responsive–didactic Caregiving in Play Interactions with 10-month-olds and Cognitive Development at 18 months. *Infant Child Dev.* **2016**, *25*, 296–316. [CrossRef]
9. Prime, H.; Wade, M.; Gonzalez, A. The link between maternal and child verbal abilities: An indirect effect through maternal responsiveness. *Dev. Sci.* **2020**, *23*, e12907. [CrossRef]
10. Bakermans-Kranenburg, M.J.; Van Ijzendoorn, M.H.; Juffer, F. Less is more: Meta-analyses of sensitivity and attachment interventions in early childhood. *Psychol. Bull.* **2003**, *129*, 195. [CrossRef]
11. Scherer, E.; Hagaman, A.; Chung, E.; Rahman, A.; O'Donnell, K.; Maselko, J. The relationship between responsive caregiving and child outcomes: Evidence from direct observations of mother-child dyads in Pakistan. *BMC Public Health* **2019**, *19*, 252. [CrossRef]

12. Bernier, A.; Calkins, S.D.; Bell, M.A. Longitudinal associations between the quality of mother–infant interactions and brain development across infancy. *Child Dev.* **2016**, *87*, 1159–1174. [CrossRef]
13. Gardner, F. Methodological Issues in the Direct Observation of Parent–Child Interaction: Do Observational Findings Reflect the Natural Behavior of Participants? *Clin. Child Fam. Psychol. Rev.* **2000**, *3*, 185–198. [CrossRef] [PubMed]
14. Lotzin, A.; Lu, X.; Kriston, L.; Schiborr, J.; Musal, T.; Romer, G.; Ramsauer, B. Observational tools for measuring parent–infant interaction: A systematic review. *Clin. Child Fam. Psychol. Rev.* **2015**, *18*, 99–132. [CrossRef] [PubMed]
15. Prime, H.; Browne, D.; Akbari, E.; Wade, M.; Madigan, S.; Jenkins, J.M. The development of a measure of maternal cognitive sensitivity appropriate for use in primary care health settings. *J. Child Psychol. Psychiatry* **2015**, *56*, 488–495. [CrossRef]
16. Sokolovic, N.; Borairi, S.; Rodrigues, M.; Perlman, M.; Jenkins, J.M. Validating an efficient measure of responsivity in father–child interactions. *Can. J. Behav. Sci.* **2021**, *53*, 84–89. [CrossRef]
17. Ambady, N. The perils of pondering: Intuition and thin slice judgments. *Psychol. Inq.* **2010**, *21*, 271–278. [CrossRef]
18. Mesman, J.; van IJzendoorn, M.H.; Bakermans-Kranenburg, M.J. Unequal in opportunity, equal in process: Parental sensitivity promotes positive child development in ethnic minority families. *Child Dev. Perspect.* **2012**, *6*, 239–250. [CrossRef]
19. Beaton, D.E.; Bombardier, C.; Guillemin, F.; Ferraz, M.B. Guidelines for the process of cross-cultural adaptation of self-report measures. *Spine* **2000**, *25*, 3186–3191. [CrossRef]
20. Epstein, J.; Santo, R.M.; Guillemin, F. A review of guidelines for cross-cultural adaptation of questionnaires could not bring out a consensus. *J. Clin. Epidemiol.* **2015**, *68*, 435–441. [CrossRef]
21. Alvarenga, P.; Cerezo, M.Á.; Wiese, E.; Piccinini, C.A. Effects of a short video feedback intervention on enhancing maternal sensitivity and infant development in low-income families. *Attach. Hum. Dev.* **2019**, *22*, 534–554. [CrossRef]
22. Ribeiro-Accioly, A.C.L.; Seidl-De-Moura, M.L.; Mendes, D.M.L.F.; Mesman, J. Maternal sensitivity in mother-infant interactions in Rio de Janeiro–Brazil. *Attach. Hum. Dev.* **2019**, *21*, 1–10. [CrossRef]
23. Wendland-Carro, J.; Piccinini, C.A.; Millar, W.S. The role of an early intervention on enhancing the quality of mother-infant interaction. *Child Dev.* **1999**, *70*, 713–721. [CrossRef] [PubMed]
24. Britto, P.R.; Lye, S.J.; Proulx, K.; Yousafzai, A.K.; Matthews, S.G.; Vaivada, T.; MacMillan, H. Nurturing care: Promoting early childhood development. *Lancet* **2017**, *389*, 91–102. [CrossRef]
25. Juffer, F.; Bakermans-Kranenburg, M.J.; van IJzendoorn, M.H. Pairing attachment theory and social learning theory in video-feedback intervention to promote positive parenting. *Curr. Opin. Psychol.* **2017**, *15*, 189–194. [CrossRef] [PubMed]
26. Stancin, T. Commentary: Integrated pediatric primary care: Moving from why to how. *J. Pediatr. Psychol.* **2016**, *41*, 1161–1164. [CrossRef]
27. Marks, K.P.; LaRosa, A.C. Understanding developmental-behavioral screening measures. *Pediatr. Rev.* **2012**, *33*, 448–457. [CrossRef] [PubMed]
28. Santos, I.; Munhoz, T.; Barcelos, R.; Blumenberg, C.; Bortolotto, C.; Matijasevich, A.; Junior, H.; Marques, L.; Correia, L.; Souza, M.; et al. *Estudo de Linha de Base da Avaliação de Impacto do Programa Criança Feliz*; Ministério da Cidadania, Secretaria de Avaliação e Gestão da Informação: Brasília, DF, Brasil, 2020.
29. Smith, J.A.; Baker-Henningham, H.; Brentani, A.; Mugweni, R.; Walker, S.P. Implementation of Reach Up early childhood parenting program: Acceptability, appropriateness, and feasibility in Brazil and Zimbabwe. *Ann. N. Y. Acad. Sci.* **2018**, *1419*, 120–140. [CrossRef] [PubMed]
30. Martins, R.C.; Machado, A.K.F.; Shenderovich, Y.; Soares, T.B.; da Cruz, S.H.; Altafim, E.R.P.; Murray, J. Parental attendance in two early-childhood training programmes to improve nurturing care: A randomized controlled trial. *Child. Youth Serv. Rev.* **2020**, *118*, 105418. [CrossRef] [PubMed]
31. Hallal, P.C.; Bertoldi, A.D.; Domingues, M.R.; Silveira, M.F.D.; Demarco, F.F.; da Silva, I.C.M.; Barros, F.C.; Victora, C.G.; Bassani, D.G. Cohort Profile: The 2015 Pelotas (Brazil) Birth Cohort Study. *Int. J. Epidemiol.* **2018**, *47*, 1048–1048h. [CrossRef]
32. Bayoğlu, B.; Unal, Ö.; Elibol, F.; Karabulut, E.; Innocenti, M.S. Turkish validation of the PICCOLO (Parenting interactions with children: Checklist of observations linked to outcomes). *Child Adolesc. Ment. Health* **2013**, *34*, 330–338. [CrossRef]
33. Vilaseca, R.; Rivero, M.; Bersabé, R.M.; Navarro-Pardo, E.; Cantero, M.J.; Ferrer, F.; Roggman, L. Spanish validation of the PICCOLO (parenting interactions with children: Checklist of observations linked to outcomes). *Front. Psychol.* **2019**, *10*, 680. [CrossRef]
34. Wolf, E.J.; Harrington, K.M.; Clark, S.L.; Miller, M.W. Sample Size Requirements for Structural Equation Models: An Evaluation of Power, Bias, and Solution Propriety. *Educ. Psychol. Meas.* **2013**, *76*, 913–934. [CrossRef] [PubMed]
35. Neves, P.A.; Gatica-Domínguez, G.; Santos, I.S.; Bertoldi, A.D.; Domingues, M.; Murray, J.; Silveira, M.F. Poor maternal nutritional status before and during pregnancy is associated with suspected child developmental delay in 2-year old Brazilian children. *Sci. Rep.* **2020**, *10*, 1–11. [CrossRef] [PubMed]
36. Prime, H.; Pauker, S.; Plamondon, A.; Perlman, M.; Jenkins, J. Sibship size, sibling cognitive sensitivity, and children's receptive vocabulary. *Pediatrics* **2014**, *133*, e394–e401. [CrossRef]
37. International Test Commission [ITC]. *The ITC Guidelines for Translating and Adapting Tests*, 2nd ed.; International Test Commission [ITC]: Luxembourg, 2017; Available online: https://www.intestcom.org/files/guideline_test_adaptation_2ed.pdf (accessed on 19 June 2020).

38. Epstein, J.; Osborne, R.H.; Elsworth, G.R.; Beaton, D.E.; Guillemin, F. Cross-cultural adaptation of the Health Education Impact Questionnaire: Experimental study showed expert committee, not back-translation, added value. *J. Clin. Epidemiol.* **2015**, *68*, 360–369. [CrossRef] [PubMed]
39. Sireci, S.G.; Yang, Y.; Harter, J.; Ehrlich, E.J. Evaluating guidelines for test adaptations: A methodological analysis of translation quality. *J. Cross-Cult. Psychol.* **2006**, *37*, 557–567. [CrossRef]
40. Roggman, L.A.; Cook, G.A.; Innocenti, M.S.; Jump Norman, V.; Christiansen, K. Parenting interactions with children: Checklist of observations linked to outcomes (PICCOLO) in diverse ethnic groups. *Infant Ment. Health J.* **2013**, *34*, 290–306. [CrossRef]
41. Schneider, A. Cross-Cultural Adaptation and Validation of Strengths-Based Parenting Measures in Brazil: PICCOLO and Cognitive Sensitivity Scale. Ph.D. Thesis, Department of Applied Psychology and Human Development, University of Toronto, Toronto, ON, Canada, 2018. Available online: https://tspace.library.utoronto.ca/bitstream/1807/89818/3/Schneider_Alessandra_201806_PhD_thesis.pdf (accessed on 15 November 2020).
42. Fernandes, M.; Villar, J.; Stein, A.; Urias, E.S.; Garza, C.; Victora, C.G.; Giuliani, F. INTERGROWTH-21st Project international INTER-NDA standards for child development at 2 years of age: An international prospective population-based study. *BMJ Open* **2020**, *10*, e035258. [CrossRef]
43. Murray, E.; Fernandes, M.; Newton, C.R.; Abubakar, A.; Kennedy, S.H.; Villar, J.; Stein, A. Evaluation of the INTERGROWTH-21st Neurodevelopment Assessment (INTER-NDA) in 2 year-old children. *PLoS ONE* **2018**, *13*, e0193406. [CrossRef]
44. Barros, A.J.; Matijasevich, A.; Santos, I.S.; Halpern, R. Child development in a birth cohort: Effect of child stimulation is stronger in less educated mothers. *Int. J. Epidemiol.* **2010**, *39*, 285–294. [CrossRef]
45. DeVellis, R.F. *Scale Development: Theory and Applications*, 3rd ed.; Sage Publications: Shazende Oaks, CA, USA, 2012.
46. Hu, L.T.; Bentler, P.M. Cutoff criteria for fit indexes in covariance structure analysis: Conventional criteria versus new alternatives. *Struct. Equ. Model. Multidiscip. J.* **1999**, *6*, 1–55. [CrossRef]
47. Browne, D.T.; Wade, M.; Prime, H.; Jenkins, J.M. School readiness amongst urban Canadian families: Risk profiles and family mediation. *J. Educ. Psychol.* **2018**, *110*, 133. [CrossRef]
48. Groh, A.M.; Fearon, R.P.; van IJzendoorn, M.H.; Bakermans-Kranenburg, M.J.; Roisman, G.I. Attachment in the early life course: Meta-analytic evidence for its role in socioemotional development. *Child Dev. Perspect.* **2017**, *11*, 70–76. [CrossRef]
49. Bick, J.; Nelson, C.A. Early experience and brain development. *WIREs Cogn. Sci.* **2017**, *8*, e1387. [CrossRef] [PubMed]
50. Landry, S.H.; Smith, K.E.; Swank, P.R.; Guttentag, C. A responsive parenting intervention: The optimal timing across early childhood for impacting maternal behaviors and child outcomes. *Dev. Psychol.* **2008**, *44*, 1335. [CrossRef]
51. United Nations Children´s Fund [UNICEF]. *Thrive Nurturing Care for Early Childhood Development. Country Profiles for Early Childhood Development*; United Nations Children´s Fund [UNICEF]: New York, NY, USA, 2020; Available online: https://nurturing-care.org/wp-content/uploads/2020/11/English.pdf (accessed on 20 December 2020).
52. Halgunseth, L.C.; Ispa, J.M.; Rudy, D. Parental control in Latino families: An integrated review of the literature. *Child Dev.* **2006**, *77*, 1282–1297. Available online: http://www.jstor.org/stable/3878432 (accessed on 12 October 2020).
53. Calzada, E.J.; Huang, K.Y.; Anicama, C.; Fernandez, Y.; Brotman, L.M. Test of a cultural framework of parenting with Latino families of young children. *Cult. Divers. Ethn. Minority Psychol.* **2012**, *18*, 285–296. [CrossRef]
54. Bornstein, M.H. *Cultural Approaches to Parenting*; Psychology Press: Hove, East Sussex, UK, 2013; 224p.
55. Bornstein, M.H.; Putnick, D.L.; Lansford, J.E.; Deater-Deckard, K.; Bradley, R.H. A developmental analysis of caregiving modalities across infancy in 38 low-and middle-income countries. *Child Dev.* **2015**, *86*, 1571–1587. [CrossRef]
56. Ispa, J.M.; Fine, M.A.; Halgunseth, L.C.; Harper, S.; Robinson, J.; Boyce, L.; Brady-Smith, C. Maternal intrusiveness, maternal warmth, and mother–toddler relationship outcomes: Variations across low-income ethnic and acculturation groups. *Child Dev.* **2004**, *75*, 1613–1631. Available online: https://www-jstor-org.myaccess.library.utoronto.ca/stable/3696666 (accessed on 12 October 2020). [CrossRef]
57. Endendijk, J.J.; Groeneveld, M.G.; Bakermans-Kranenburg, M.J.; Mesman, J. Gender-differentiated parenting revisited: Meta-analysis reveals very few differences in parental control of boys and girls. *PLoS ONE* **2016**, *11*, e0159193. [CrossRef]
58. Bradley, R.H.; Corwyn, R.F.; Burchinal, M.; McAdoo, H.P.; García Coll, C. The home environments of children in the United States Part II: Relations with behavioral development through age thirteen. *Child Dev.* **2001**, *72*, 1868–1886. [CrossRef]
59. Neppl, T.K.; Senia, J.M.; Donnellan, M.B. Effects of economic hardship: Testing the family stress model over time. *J. Fam. Psychol.* **2016**, *30*, 12–21. [CrossRef]
60. Evans, G.W.; Kim, P. Childhood poverty and young adults' allostatic load: The mediating role of childhood cumulative risk exposure. *Psychol. Sci.* **2012**, *23*, 979–983. [CrossRef] [PubMed]
61. Browne, D.T.; Leckie, G.; Prime, H.; Perlman, M.; Jenkins, J.M. Observed sensitivity during family interactions and cumulative risk: A study of multiple dyads per family. *Dev. Psychol.* **2016**, *52*, 1128–1138. [CrossRef] [PubMed]

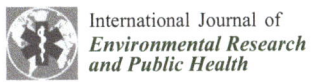

Article

Identification of Growth Patterns in Low Birth Weight Infants from Birth to 5 Years of Age: Nationwide Korean Cohort Study

So Jin Yoon, Joohee Lim, Jung Ho Han, Jeong Eun Shin, Soon Min Lee *, Ho Seon Eun, Min Soo Park and Kook In Park

Department of Pediatrics, Yonsei University College of Medicine, Seoul 06273, Korea; sojinyoon@yuhs.ac (S.J.Y.); imagine513@yuhs.ac (J.L.); feagd@yuhs.ac (J.H.H.); golden-week@yuhs.ac (J.E.S.); hseun@yuhs.ac (H.S.E.); minspark@yuhs.ac (M.S.P.); kipark@yuhs.ac (K.I.P.)
* Correspondence: smlee@yuhs.ac; Tel.: +82-2-2019-3350

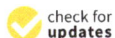

Citation: Yoon, S.J.; Lim, J.; Han, J.H.; Shin, J.E.; Lee, S.M.; Eun, H.S.; Park, M.S.; Park, K.I. Identification of Growth Patterns in Low Birth Weight Infants from Birth to 5 Years of Age: Nationwide Korean Cohort Study. *Int. J. Environ. Res. Public Health* **2021**, *18*, 1206. https://doi.org/10.3390/ijerph18031206

Academic Editor: Verónica Schiariti
Received: 7 December 2020
Accepted: 25 January 2021
Published: 29 January 2021

Publisher's Note: MDPI stays neutral with regard to jurisdictional claims in published maps and institutional affiliations.

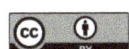

Copyright: © 2021 by the authors. Licensee MDPI, Basel, Switzerland. This article is an open access article distributed under the terms and conditions of the Creative Commons Attribution (CC BY) license (https://creativecommons.org/licenses/by/4.0/).

Abstract: This study aimed to investigate the nationwide growth pattern of infants in Korea according to the birth-weight group and to analyze the effect of growth on development. A total of 430,541 infants, born in 2013 and who received the infant health check-up regularly from 6 months to 60 months of age, were included. The weight, height, head circumferences percentiles, and neurodevelopment using screening tests results were compared among the birth-weight groups. Using longitudinal analysis, the study found a significant difference in height, weight, and head circumference, respectively, according to age at health check-up, birth weight group, and combination of age and birth weight ($p < 0.001$). The growth parameters at 60 months of age showed a significant correlation with those at 6 months of age especially in extremely low birth weight infants. The incidence of suspected developmental delay was significantly higher in infants with growth below the 10th percentiles than in those with growth above the 10th percentiles. Among 4571 (1.6%) infants with suspected developmental delay results at 60 months of age, birth weight, sex, and poor growth parameters were confirmed as associated factors. This nationwide Korean study shows that poor growth and neurodevelopment outcomes persisted among low-birth-weight infants at 60 months of age. Our findings provide guidance for developing a nationwide follow-up program for infants with perinatal risk factors in Korea.

Keywords: developmental delay; child health; birth weight; growth measurement

1. Introduction

Due to the improvement in perinatal care, the survival and major morbidity free survival of preterm infants have improved dramatically. The focus of neonatology has shifted towards improving nutrition and anthropometry [1]. Growth and nutrition in preterm infants have long-term implications for neurodevelopmental and cardiometabolic outcomes [2]; consequently, growth monitoring is a cardinal precept of pediatric practice.

A significant number of infants are discharged with their growth parameters still well below the normal range. In particular, very low birth weight (VLBW) infants and small for gestational age (SGA) preterm infants have a higher risk of growth deviations [3]. Several studies have shown an association between impaired extrauterine growth and poor long-term performance [4]. In moderate and late preterm children, poorer growth in the first seven years is associated with poorer neuropsychological functioning. Poor postnatal growth, especially head circumference, in preterm infants is associated with increased levels of motor and cognitive impairment [5].

The catch-up growth patterns of preterm infants have been a matter of debate. Approximately 80% of preterm infants after initial postnatal growth failure show catch-up growth in weight, length, and head circumference (HC), generally starting early in the first months of life and often achieving targets within the first two years of life [6]. However, late catch-up growth of preterm infants throughout childhood and even in adolescence has also been described. Catch-up growth is linked to an adverse health outcome, while rapid catch-up increases the risk of metabolic disease later in life [7].

In Korea, the total number of births in 2013 was 436,455, including 5.5% of which were low birth weight (LBW) infants and 0.7% of which were VLBW infants. The national health screening program in Korea checks anthropometric measurement and developmental progress serially until 6 years of age. However, little is known about the postnatal growth patterns of infants in Korea. Thus, it is important to use population-based nationwide data to understand of the early growth patterns of preterm infants.

This study aimed to estimate the nationwide growth patterns according to the birth-weight group and to analyze the relationship between growth and development using a population-based surveillance system. We hope that our findings will inform policymakers, medical practitioners, and public health experts, and provide guidance for developing a nationwide follow-up program for public services, especially healthcare-delivery and social welfare delivery systems.

2. Materials and Methods

2.1. Patients and Data Source

We initially identified 430,541 infants who were born in 2013 and examined their infant health check-up records for the 1st to 6th visits from the National Health Insurance Service (NHIS) database. Healthcare claims including diagnostic codes of almost all Korean residents, approximately 98% covered by NHIS and 2% by medical aid, were linked to health check databases. The data, including gestational age and birth weight, were also grouped according to the International Classification of Diseases-10 codes (ICD-10: P07.01, P07.02, P07.09-14, P07.19, P07.20, P07.23, P07.29, P07.30, P07.39) [8]. The data were entered by the hospital or obtained from self-report questionnaires used by the national health screening program. Based on the birth statistics [9], the total number of births in 2013 was 436,455, and the number of infants who lived to be at least 1 year of age was 435,150, which shows that this study population 430,541 covered 99% of national births.

The national health screening program for infants and children in Korea, launched in November 2007 is a kind of population surveillance system that consists of history taking, physical examination, anthropometric measurements, screening for visual acuity, and administration of Korean Developmental Screening Test (K-DST), oral examination, and questionnaires with anticipatory guidance [10]. The questionnaire contains the birth weight, preterm, vision, hearing, nutrition (meal, milk, snacks), multimedia, and safety education. We used only the information of birth weight and preterm status in questionnaire from family.

The period for national health screening program (1st to 6th visits) was divided and classified as follow; 6 months for 4–6 months of age, 12 months for 9–12 months of age, 24 months for 18–24 months of age, 36 months for 30–36 months of age, 48 months for 42–48 months of age, and 60 months for 54–60 months of age. The age at exam was defined as chronologic ages.

For growth assessment, the National health screening program checks anthropometric parameters including body weight, height, and HC serially at every follow-up. The percentile of growth was assessed using the Korean growth curve, which provides sex specific data. Poor growth was defined as measurements below the 10th percentile of weight, height, and head circumference individually.

The K-DST is used an effective screening tool for infants and children with neurodevelopmental disorders and has been used since 2011. It is used to verify whether infants are developmentally appropriate or neurodevelopmentally delayed in six domains: gross motor, fine motor, cognition, communication, social interaction, and self-control.

The K-DST is conducted to screen children according to their corrected age before 36 months of age as recommendation and after that age, it is allowed to take tests according to chronological age. There is no K-DST at first visit, and at 5th, 6th visit (42–48, 54–60 months of age) the participants take the test papers according to their chronological age. The participants take the tests papers at the time of their clinic visit and get the result as four categorized groups based on the standard deviation (SD) scores; the scores above 1 SD are defined as 'high-level', those between −1 and 1 SD as 'peer-level', those between −2 and −1 SD as 'follow-up test', and those below −2 SD as 'further evaluation' [11]. Additional positive questions that take into account clinically important diseases, such as cerebral palsy, language delay, and autism spectrum disorders, that should be referred for 'further evaluation' are also included in the questionnaire. To evaluate the ability of the K-DST to identify infants with developmental delay, critical cutoff scores for 6 domains were set below −1 SD [12,13]. Suspected developmental delay was defined as a K-DST result of 'further evaluation' and 'follow-up test'.

In this study, growth and developmental results were analyzed according to five stratified birth weight groups (<1000 g, 1000–1499 g, 1500–1999 g, 2000–2499 g, and 2500–4500 g). LBW infants and VLBW infants were defined as having a birth weight below 2500 g and 1500 g, respectively. Preterm infants were defined as infants born before 37 weeks of gestation.

2.2. Statistical Analyses

The cohort was stratified according to the birth weight or the age of checkup. The characteristics of the subjects were expressed as means and standard deviations for continuous variables and as percentages for categorical variables. Correlations for height, weight and HC between 6 months and 60 months of ages as time periods were computed using Pearson's correlation coefficient. Multiple logistic regression model was used to determine the independently associated factors with among infants with odds ratios (OR) and 95% confidence intervals (CI). Multivariate longitudinal data analysis was done using multivariate repeated measured model (PROC MIXED and GENMOD). All statistical analyses were performed using SAS version 9.4 (SAS Institute, Cary, NC, USA). p-values < 0.05 were considered statistically significant.

2.3. Ethics Statement

In this study, all identifiable variables, including claim-, individual-, and organizational-level identification numbers, were re-generated in random by the NHIS database to protect the patients' privacy. This study used NHIS data (NHIS-2019-1-569) maintained by the NHIS. The study protocol was approved by the Institutional Review Board of Gangnam Severance Hospital (No. 3-2019-0147). Informed consent was waived.

3. Results

3.1. Growth Outcome

Among 430,541 infants, born in 2013 and included in the study, 219,576 (51%) were male. The numbers of infants, who underwent health checks ranged from 286,331 (67%) to 347,153 (81%). The highest number of infants (n = 347,153, 81%) were included in the health check at 24 months of age. The highest number of preterm infants underwent the health check at 36 months (n = 26,338, 93%). The distribution of a number of infants who participated in the infant health check according to birth weight group were shown in Table 1.

Table 1. The population characteristics at the health checkup according to birth-weight group.

Age at Exam	Total Infants	<1000 g	1000–1499 g	1500–1999 g	2000–2499 g	2500–4500 g	Preterm
6 months	311,446 (72.3)	137 (0.0)	693 (0.2)	2332 (0.7)	11,539 (3.7)	295,989 (95.0)	11,398 (3.7)
12 months	313,235 (72.8)	196 (0.1)	819 (0.3)	2487 (0.8)	11,826 (3.8)	297,151 (94.9)	10,919 (3.5)
24 months	347,153 (80.6)	314 (0.1)	1376 (0.4)	3050 (0.9)	13,320 (3.8)	328,176 (94.5)	12,355 (3.6)
36 months	344,468 (80.0)	643 (0.2)	1959 (0.6)	3495 (1.0)	13,240 (3.8)	324,086 (94.1)	26,338 (7.6)
48 months	323,958 (75.2)	606 (0.2)	1425 (0.4)	3747 (1.2)	12,809 (4.0)	304,361 (94.0)	26,028 (8.0)
60 months	286,331 (66.5)	662 (0.2)	1174 (0.4)	4584 (1.6)	12,288 (4.3)	266,669 (93.1)	23,542 (8.2)

Data are presented as Number (%).

The mean percentile of weight, height, and HC according to age at health check was seen in Figure 1. Longitudinal analysis showed a significant difference in height, weight, and HC according to age, birth-weight group, and the combination of age and birth weight, respectively ($p < 0.0001$). The lower birth weight group showed a lower mean percentile of weight, height, and HC. There was a significant difference in height, weight, and HC between the low birth weight infants (<1000 g, 1000–1499 g, 1500–1999 g, 2000–2499 g) and the reference group with birth weight of 2500–4500 g according to age at health checkup.

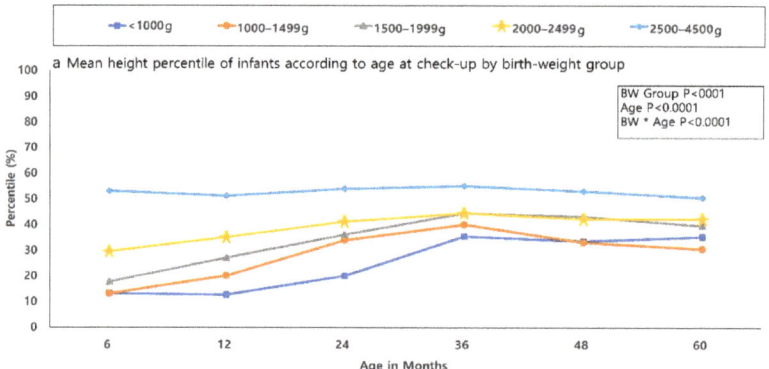

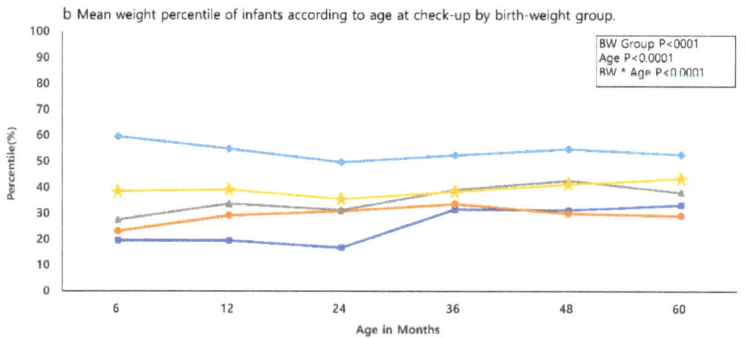

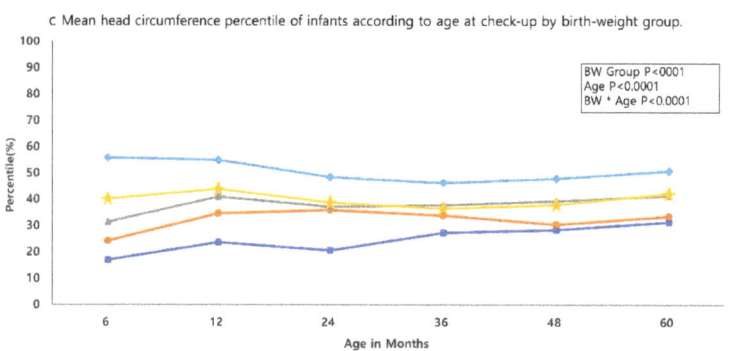

Figure 1. Mean growth percentile of infants according to age at check-up by birth-weight group. (**a**) Height. (**b**) Weight. (**c**) Head circumference (HC). Significant differences in height, weight, and HC between the low birth weight infants groups and the reference group according to age at health checkup were shown. *p*-values were significant in height, weight, and head circumference between each low birth weight group and the reference group compared at age of health check-up.

A total of 10,227 (7.4%) infants had a poor HC growth at 60 months of age, 10,950 (7.92%) infants had poor height growth, and 12,481 (9.03%) infants had a poor weight growth. Using longitudinal analysis, this study found a significant difference in the incidence of poor height, weight, and HC growth according to age at health check, birth-weight group, and combination of age and birth weight, respectively ($p < 0.0001$) (Figure 2). The lower birth-weight groups showed a higher incidence of poor weight, height, and HC growth. There was a significant difference in height, weight, and HC between the low birth weight group (<1000 g, 1000–1499 g, 1500–1999 g, and 2000–2499 g) and the reference group with birth weight of 2500–4500 g according to age at health checkup.

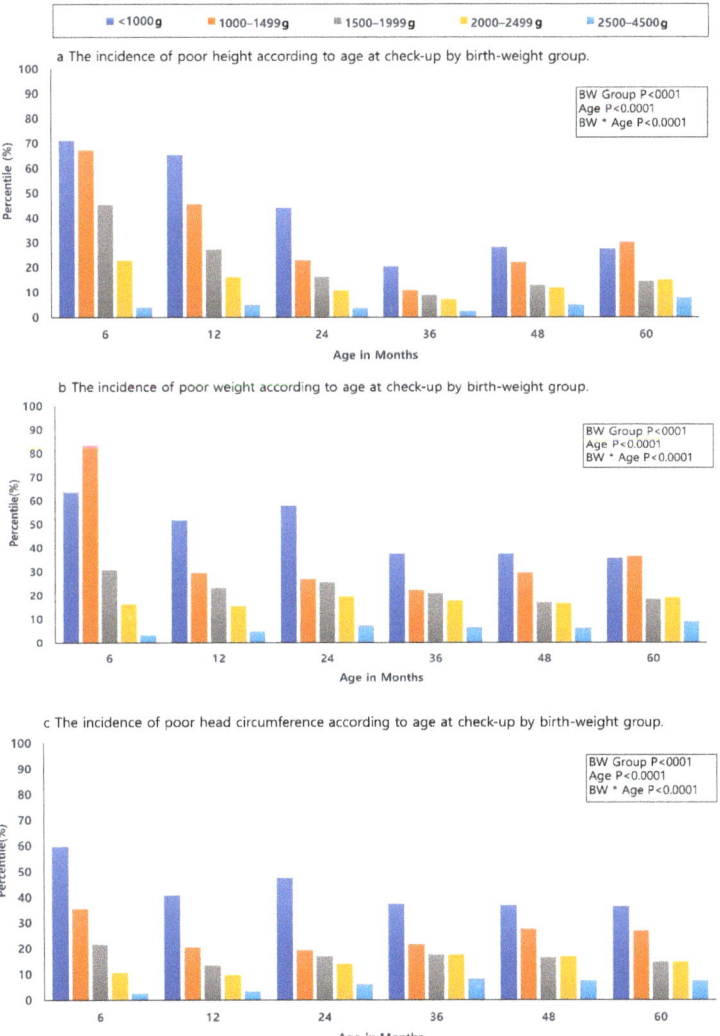

Figure 2. The incidence of poor growth (below 10th percentile) according to age at check-up by birth-weight group. (**a**) Height. (**b**) Weight. (**c**) Head circumference. A higher incidence of poor weight, height, and HC growth in the lower birth-weight groups was noted. A significant difference in height, weight, and HC between the low-birth-weight groups and the reference group according to age at health checkup were shown. *p*-values were significant in height, weight, and head circumference between each low-birth-weight group and the reference group compared at age of health check-up.

The Pearson correlation coefficient of the growth percentiles (the height, weight, and HC percentile) at 6 and 60 months of age obtained using correlation analysis is shown as Figure 3. Figure 3a was the results for the whole study population. Among the infants below 1000 g of birth weight, only weight showed a highly positive correlation (coefficient = 0.72) between 6 and 60 months of age, height (coefficient = 0.65) and HC (coefficient = 0.64) showed a moderate positive correlation. Pearson correlation coefficient analysis between 6 and 60 months of age was performed only among the infants who fell below 10th percentile in terms of height, weight, and HC at 60 months of age, and the results were shown in Figure 3b. Among the infants below 1000 g of birth weight, weight, height, and HC showed a weakly positive correlation; otherwise, there was no association.

a

Birth Weight	WT	HT	HC
<1000 g	0.71	0.65	0.64
1000 – 1499 g	0.45	0.35	0.53
1500 – 1999 g	0.46	0.45	0.57
2000 – 2499 g	0.55	0.56	0.59
2500 – 4500 g	0.52	0.56	0.60

b

Birth Weight	WT	HT	HC
<1000 g	0.41	0.36	0.35
1000 – 1499 g	0.22	0.11	0.19
1500 – 1999 g	0.39	0.26	0.27
2000 – 2499 g	0.29	0.18	0.33
2500 – 4500 g	0.26	0.22	0.24

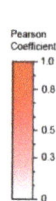

Figure 3. Pearson correlation coefficient between 6 months of age and 60 months of age for birth-weight groups among whole population (**a**) and among infants who were below the 10th percentile of height, weight, and HC at 60 months of age (**b**).

To analyze the relation between the growth at 6 months and 60 months, the risk of poor growth in the infants below 10th percentile of growth at 6 months was compared to the infants within 10–90th percentile of growth. The infant below the 10th percentile of HC and height at 6 months of age, respectively, showed the higher risk of HC and height below the 10th percentile at 60 months of age (HC, OR (95% CI) 1.62 (1.32–1.98); Height, 1.64 (1.38–1.95)). However, weight status at 6 months showed no significant association with the risk of weight below the 10th percentile at 60 months of age.

3.2. Developmental Outcome

The incidence of suspected developmental delay result at 60 months of age was 10% (29,020). In particular, further evaluation was recommended for 4572 (1.5%) infants, and the 'follow-up test' for 24,448 (8.5%) infants. According to the birth-weight group, K-DST results were presented in Table 2. The smaller birth weight group had a greater number of 'further evaluation' results. The infants below 1000 g of birth weight were only 0.2% of the screened population, but among them, 14.8% of this group had 'further evaluation' and 21.0% of this group had 'follow-up test' recommendations. The lower birth-weight groups showed a higher incidence of suspected developmental delay.

There is a significant difference in the incidence of suspected developmental delay results between the infants with poor weight, height, and HC growth and above 10th percentile at 60 months of age by birth weight group (Table 3). The infants with poor weight, height, and HC growth demonstrated higher frequency of suspected developmental delay results at 60 months of age.

Lower birth weight, male sex, poor HC, poor height, and poor weight were confirmed as factors associated with suspected developmental delay results at 60 months of age using multivariate logistic regression analysis (Table 4). Infants with poor HC at 60 months of age had more suspected developmental delay results (OR 1.81, 95% CI 1.66–1.98), and the infants who weighed less than 1000 g at birth had more suspected developmental delay (OR 5.05, 95% CI 3.79–6.73) compared to infants with 2500–4500 g birth weight.

Table 2. The results of developmental screening test at 60 months of age according to birth weight group.

BW Group	Number of Infants	Further Evaluation							Follow-Up Test						
		Total	Gross Motor	Fine Motor	Cognition	Communication	Social Interaction	Self-Control	Total	Gross Motor	Fine Motor	Cognition	Communication	Social Interaction	Self-Control	Peer & High Level
<1000 g	529	56 (11)	48	48	45	47	39	42	91 (17)	59	47	44	40	25	30	382 (72)
1000–1499 g	1067	63 (6)	56	53	46	48	45	46	142 (13)	65	62	54	57	35	53	862 (81)
1500–1999 g	2316	96 (4)	68	64	65	72	59	56	285 (12)	111	123	104	95	75	93	1935 (84)
2000–2499 g	9381	254 (3)	143	168	184	198	156	127	947 (10)	332	383	369	342	269	293	8180 (87)
2500–4500 g	263,579	4094 (2)	2201	2603	2825	3089	2454	2111	22,930 (9)	7394	8234	8848	8820	5938	7013	236,555 (89)

Data are presented as Number or Number (%). BW, birth weight.

Table 3. Poor growth outcomes (below 10th percentile) at 60 months of age according to birth-weight group among the infants with suspected developmental delay results.

BW Group	Number of Infants	WT Poor	HT Poor	HC Poor
<1000 g	147	96 (65)	73 (50)	86 (59)
1000–1499 g	205	71 (35)	88 (43)	83 (40)
1500–1999 g	381	112 (29)	117 (31)	146 (38)
2000–2499 g	1201	319 (27)	342 (28)	393 (33)
2500–4500 g	27,024	2520 (9)	2663 (10)	2958 (11)

Data are presented as No. (%). BW, birth weight; WT, weight; HT, height; HC, head circumference.

Table 4. Multivariate logistic regression analysis for the suspected development delay results at 60 months of age.

Variable	OR (95% CI)	p Value
Poor HC at 60 months of age	1.81 (1.66–1.98)	<0.001
Poor HT at 60 months of age	1.63 (1.48–1.80)	<0.001
Poor WT at 60 months of age	1.18 (1.07–1.30)	<0.001
BW 1000 g vs. 2500–4500 g	5.05 (3.79–6.73)	<0.001
1000–1499 g vs. 2500–4500 g	3.05 (2.35–3.96)	
1500–1999 g vs. 2500–4500 g	2.37 (1.92–2.92)	
2000–2499 g vs. 2500–4500 g	1.64 (1.44–1.87)	
Male vs. Female	2.02 (1.90–2.15)	<0.001

HC, head circumference; HT, height; WT, weight; BW, birth weight.; OR, odds ratio; CI, confidence interval.

4. Discussion

This is the first large study showing the longitudinal growth and developmental patterns of children born with low birth weight in Korea. LBW infants are subject to a significant burden of morbidities, such as postnatal growth failure and neurodevelopmental impairments. However, extreme preterm infants have been the primary focus of the research over the years. In this study, longitudinal growth outcome in LBW infants from birth to 60 months was shown using nationwide population-based health check-up data. We confirmed an association between poor post-natal growth and developmental delay, both of which are persisting on long term follow-up, especially among LBW infants.

Our findings are consistent with those of previous international studies, which reported that a lot of preterm infants born lighter and shorter than full-term infants remain growth-restricted beyond the catch-up period [14]. We found that some degree of catch-up growth did occur with time; however, the difference remained until 60 months of age compared to the infants with 2500–4500 g. As shown in Figure 1, the smaller birth-weight group showed lower catch-up growth even at 60 months. Mean weight, height, and HC percentiles were persistently below 40 percent among LBW infants, as well as VLBW infants. Among children with poor growth, there is a decreasing trend in the incidence of poor growth until the 36 months of age, which then showed a stable or slightly increasing trend in the 48- and 60-months of age. Relatively poor growth can be seen in more preterm infants due to limitation of chronologic age up to 3 years of age; however, the difference in growth has persisted from 3 to 6 years old. Poor growth is still a serious problem in preterm infants, although there is an increase in survival and morbidity free survival in Korea. Therefore, close check-ups and support for catch-up growth until school age should be provided for preterm infants, as well.

Both the severity and duration of the growth retardation are related to the degree of prematurity of an infant [15]. We found the smaller the birth weight, the lower the mean growth percentiles, and the higher the incidence of poor growth. SGA children have a higher risk of growth failure throughout the follow-up period [16]. A 6-year follow-up study of very preterm infants showed the catch-up growth was mostly achieved before 2 months of age; however, it was continued until 6 years of age in SGA infants [17]. There have been reports of risk factors for growth failure that persist even after the catch-up period, and there are reports that SGA infants and more premature infants with morbidities are more vulnerable to growth failure [18–20]. In this study, SGA infants showed a higher risk for growth failure at 60 months of age than non-SGA infants did. In terms of height, most infants born SGA can catch-up by 2 years but around 15 % of them cannot achieve catch-up growth and remain short-heighted in adulthood. [19,21].

Children with poor growth have greater neurodevelopmental functioning problems than those with normal growth [22]. A nationwide Japanese population-based study analyzed the association of SGA infants with poor postnatal growth at 2 years of age with neurobehavioral development both at 5.5 and 8 years of age and reported that the findings warranted early detection and intervention for attention problems among these group [23]. Consistent with the other study, this research found that, children born with smaller birth weight showed poorer developmental results, and children with weight, height, HC less than 10th percentile at 60 months of age also showed higher incidence of the poor development, confirming growth is related to neurodevelopmental functioning.

Early postnatal growth is positively related to neurodevelopmental outcomes, especially Intelligence Quotient [22]; Postnatal growth rate of infants with intrauterine growth restriction has been associated with later cognitive outcomes, specifically Pylipow et al. reported that growth in the first 4 postnatal months is a risk factor for cognitive outcome at age 7 years [24]. Neurodevelopmental score at 8 year was related to weight, height, and HC at 8 years [25]. We confirmed the mean percentile of weight, height, and HC at 60 months of age were correlated with the mean growth percentile of 6 months of age. Therefore, close monitoring from early infant period and proper intervention for growth are important.

Previous studies reported that growth restriction was more common in preterm infants but recent studies have shown positive reports of catch-up growth through nutritional support and quality improvement [26]. Small for gestational age infants with less than 28 week's gestation had appropriate catch-up growth at term, improved with postnatal nutrition and care [27]. Early HC growth failure in very preterm infants can be improved by optimizing parenteral nutrition [28]. Although an aggressive nutritional strategy including using human milk fortifier or preterm formula, and high amino acid composition of parenteral nutrition were adopted in Korea, in this study we confirmed postnatal growth impairment is common in LBW infants, and catch-up growth may be delayed and incomplete in some.

Children who fail to achieve catch up growth within 2 years of life remain short after childhood so an early initiation of growth hormone treatment was recommended by previous research [29,30]. The length Z and changes of scores at 12 months of corrected age may be correlated with catch-up height at 3 years and so it is useful for earlier initiation of growth hormone treatment in VLBW infants [31]. We found that the infants with a height below 10th percentile at 60 months of age were more numerous in VLBW (25%) group than in LBW (14%) or 2500–4500 g (5%) group. At 60 months of age, the mean percentile of height had correlations with the mean height percentile of 6 months of age.

The main strength of this study was that it was a nationwide study with a large population and it was able to report an association between growth and neurodevelopmental outcomes overtime. A total of 99% of eligible infants participated in the national health screening program for infants and children, so these results are an accurate representation of the growth of the infant population in Korea. These nationwide data accounts for all infants, including LBW but not VLBW infants, who participated in health check-ups during the first five years of life in addition to the infants weighing 2500–4500 g infants as a reference.

There are some limitations to this study. Since weight is the most important factor in the growth assessment of newborns and infants, this study design was analyzed based only on birth weight. Because birth weight is usually related with gestation, and SGA status can make some discrepancy, we just display the infants dividing birth weight rather than gestational age. Poor growth was defined as weight, height, and HC individually below the 10th percentile. VLBW infants accounted for 0.7% of total birth infants in this cohort, which is a very small proportion. Preterm infants with intraventricular hemorrhage or post-hemorrhagic hydrocephalus have larger HC but the effect isn't considered due to a small population. There are many factors having affecting on growth including nutrition and co-morbidities, but we lack detailed data that may provide information on important confounders. For the integrity of data on growth in preterm infants, we included the growth parameter at only postnatal age, but not the corrected age.

5. Conclusions

This Korean population-based study showed that a significant number of LBW infants did not achieve catch up growth even at 60 months of age. Close monitoring of appropriate weight gain, nutritional intervention, and early intervention programs will be needed for improving children's growth and developmental outcomes. Our findings provide guidance for developing a nationwide follow-up program for infants with perinatal risk factors.

Author Contributions: Conceptualization, S.M.L. and S.J.Y.; methodology, S.M.L. and S.J.Y.; validation, J.L. and J.H.H.; formal analysis, S.M.L. and S.J.Y.; writing—original draft preparation, S.M.L. and S.J.Y.; writing—review and editing, J.L., J.H.H., J.E.S., H.S.E., M.S.P. and K.I.P.; supervision, S.M.L. and M.S.P. All authors have read and agreed to the published version of the manuscript.

Funding: This research received no external funding.

Institutional Review Board Statement: The study was conducted according to the guidelines of the Declaration of Helsinki, and approved by the Institutional Review Board of Gangnam Severance Hospital (IRB No. 3-2019-0147).

Informed Consent Statement: Not applicable.

Data Availability Statement: Not applicable.

Acknowledgments: The authors thank MID (Medical Illustration & Design) for helping to design Figure 3.

Conflicts of Interest: The authors declare no conflict of interest.

References

1. Deng, Y.; Yang, F.; Mu, D. First-year growth of 834 preterm infants in a Chinese population: A single-center study. *BMC Pediatr.* **2019**, *19*, 403–410. [CrossRef]
2. Kunz, S.N.; Bell, K.; Belfort, M.B. Early Nutrition in Preterm Infants: Effects on Neurodevelopment and Cardiometabolic Health. *NeoReviews* **2016**, *17*, e386–e393. [CrossRef]
3. Euser, A.; De Wit, C.; Finken, M.; Rijken, M.; Wit, J.M. Growth of Preterm Born Children. *Horm. Res. Paediatr.* **2008**, *70*, 319–328. [CrossRef]
4. Guellec, I.; Lapillonne, A.; Marret, S.; Picaud, J.-C.; Mitanchez, D.; Charkaluk, M.-L.; Fresson, J.; Arnaud, C.; Flamand, C.; Cambonie, G.; et al. Effect of Intra- and Extrauterine Growth on Long-Term Neurologic Outcomes of Very Preterm Infants. *J. Pediatr.* **2016**, *175*, 93–99.e1. [CrossRef] [PubMed]
5. Dotinga, B.M.; Eshuis, M.S.; Bocca-Tjeertes, I.F.; Kerstjens, J.M.; Van Braeckel, K.N.; Reijneveld, S.A.; Bos, A.F. Longitudinal Growth and Neuropsychological Functioning at Age 7 in Moderate and Late Preterms. *Pediatrics* **2016**, *138*, 138. [CrossRef] [PubMed]
6. Saigal, S.; Stoskopf, B.; Streiner, D.L.; Paneth, N.S.; Pinelli, J.; Boyle, M. Growth Trajectories of Extremely Low Birth Weight Infants From Birth to Young Adulthood: A Longitudinal, Population-Based Study. *Pediatr. Res.* **2006**, *60*, 751–758. [CrossRef]
7. Ong, K.K. Catch-up growth in small for gestational age babies: Good or bad? *Curr. Opin. Endocrinol. Diabetes Obes.* **2007**, *14*, 30–34. [CrossRef] [PubMed]
8. Icd-10 Version. 2019. Available online: https://icd.who.int/browse10/2019/en (accessed on 25 July 2020).
9. KOrean Statistical Information Service. National Statistics. Available online: http://kosis.kr/statisticsList/statisticsListIndex.do?menuId=M_01_01&vwcd=MT_ZTITLE&parmTabId=M_01_01#SelectStatsBoxDiv (accessed on 25 July 2020).
10. Moon, J.S. Review of National Health Screening Program for Infant and Children in Korea. *J. Korean Med. Assoc.* **2010**, *53*, 377. [CrossRef]
11. Jang, C.H.; Kim, S.W.; Jeon, H.R.; Jung, D.W.; Cho, H.E.; Kim, J.; Lee, J.W. Clinical Usefulness of the Korean Developmental Screening Test (K-DST) for Developmental Delays. *Ann. Rehabil. Med.* **2019**, *43*, 490–496. [CrossRef]
12. Chung, H.J.; Yang, D.; Kim, G.-H.; Kim, S.K.; Kim, S.W.; Kim, Y.K.; Kim, J.S.; Kim, J.K.; Kim, C.; Sung, I.-K.; et al. Development of the Korean Developmental Screening Test for Infants and Children (K-DST). *Clin. Exp. Pediatr.* **2020**, *63*, 438–446. [CrossRef]

13. Kim, C.Y.; Jung, E.; Lee, B.S.; Kim, K.-S.; Kim, E.A.-R. Validity of the Korean Developmental Screening Test for very-low-birth-weight infants. *Korean J. Pediatr.* **2019**, *62*, 187–192. [CrossRef] [PubMed]
14. Van de Pol, C.; Allegaert, K. Growth patterns and body composition in former extremely low birth weight (elbw) neonates until adulthood: A systematic review. *Eur. J. Pediatr.* **2020**, *179*, 757–771. [PubMed]
15. Pilling, E.; Elder, C.; Gibson, A. Growth patterns in the growth-retarded premature infant. *Best Pr. Res. Clin. Endocrinol. Metab.* **2008**, *22*, 447–462. [CrossRef] [PubMed]
16. Saenger, P.; Czernichow, P.; Hughes, I.; Reiter, E.O. Small for Gestational Age: Short Stature and Beyond. *Endocr. Rev.* **2007**, *28*, 219–251. [CrossRef] [PubMed]
17. Toftlund, L.H.; Halken, S.; Agertoft, L.; Zachariassen, G. Catch-Up Growth, Rapid Weight Growth, and Continuous Growth from Birth to 6 Years of Age in Very-Preterm-Born Children. *Neonatology* **2018**, *114*, 285–293. [CrossRef]
18. Liao, W.-L.; Lin, M.-C.; Wang, T.-M.; Chen, C.-H.; Taiwan Premature Infant Follow-up Network. Risk factors for postdischarge growth retardation among very-low-birth-weight infants: A nationwide registry study in Taiwan. *Pediatr. Neonatol.* **2019**, *60*, 641–647. [PubMed]
19. Clayton, P.E.; Cianfarani, S.; Czernichow, P.; Johannsson, G.; Rapaport, R.; Rogol, A. Management of the Child Born Small for Gestational Age through to Adulthood: A Consensus Statement of the International Societies of Pediatric Endocrinology and the Growth Hormone Research Society. *J. Clin. Endocrinol. Metab.* **2007**, *92*, 804–810.
20. Farooqi, A.; Hägglöf, B.; Sedin, G.; Gothefors, L.; Serenius, F. Growth in 10- to 12-Year-Old Children Born at 23 to 25 Weeks' Gestation in the 1990s: A Swedish National Prospective Follow-up Study. *Pediatrics* **2006**, *118*, e1452–e1465. [CrossRef]
21. Labarta, J.I.; Ruiz, J.A.; Molina, I.; De Arriba, A.; Mayayo, E.; Longás, A.F. Growth and growth hormone treatment in short stature children born small for gestational age. *Pediatr. Endocrinol. Rev.* **2009**, *6*, 350–357.
22. Taine, M.; Charles, M.; Beltrand, J.; Rozé, J.-C.; Léger, J.; Botton, J.; Heude, B. Early postnatal growth and neurodevelopment in children born moderately preterm or small for gestational age at term: A systematic review. *Paediatr. Périnat. Epidemiol.* **2018**, *32*, 268–280. [CrossRef]
23. Takeuchi, A.; Yorifuji, T.; Hattori, M.; Tamai, K.; Nakamura, K.; Nakamura, M.; Kageyama, M.; Kubo, T.; Ogino, T.; Kobayashi, K.; et al. Catch-up growth and behavioral development among preterm, small-for-gestational-age children: A nationwide Japanese population-based study. *Brain Dev.* **2019**, *41*, 397–405. [CrossRef] [PubMed]
24. Pylipow, M.; Spector, L.G.; Puumala, S.E.; Boys, C.; Cohen, J.; Georgieff, M.K. Early Postnatal Weight Gain, Intellectual Performance, and Body Mass Index at 7 Years of Age in Term Infants with Intrauterine Growth Restriction. *J. Pediatr.* **2009**, *154*, 201–206. [CrossRef] [PubMed]
25. Casey, P.H.; Whiteside-Mansell, L.; Barrett, K.; Bradley, R.H.; Gargus, R. Impact of Prenatal and/or Postnatal Growth Problems in Low Birth Weight Preterm Infants on School-Age Outcomes: An 8-Year Longitudinal Evaluation. *Pediatrics* **2006**, *118*, 1078–1086. [CrossRef] [PubMed]
26. Andrews, E.T.; Ashton, J.J.; Pearson, F.; Beattie, R.M.; Johnson, M.J. Early postnatal growth failure in preterm infants is not inevitable. *Arch. Dis. Child. Fetal Neonatal Ed.* **2019**, *104*, F235–F241. [CrossRef]
27. Ng, S.M.; Pintus, D.; Turner, M.A. Extreme premature small for gestational age infants have appropriate catch-up growth at term equivalence compared with extreme premature appropriate for gestational age infants. *J. Clin. Res. Pediatr. Endocrinol.* **2019**, *11*, 104–108.
28. Morgan, C.; McGowan, P.; Herwitker, S.; Hart, A.E.; Turner, M.A. Postnatal Head Growth in Preterm Infants: A Randomized Controlled Parenteral Nutrition Study. *Pediatrics* **2013**, *133*, e120–e128. [CrossRef]
29. Olbertz, D.M.; Mumm, R.; Wittwer-Backofen, U.; Fricke-Otto, S.; Pyper, A.; Otte, J.; Wabitsch, M.; Gottmann, P.; Schwab, K.O.; Scholten, M.; et al. Identification of growth patterns of preterm and small-for-gestational age children from birth to 4 years—Do they catch up? *J. Périnat. Med.* **2019**, *47*, 448–454. [CrossRef]
30. Jung, H.; Rosilio, M.; Blum, W.F.; Drop, S.L.S. Growth hormone treatment for short stature in children born small for gestational age. *Adv. Ther.* **2008**, *25*, 951–978. [CrossRef]
31. Arai, S.; Sato, Y.; Muramatsu, H.; Yamamoto, H.; Aoki, F.; Okai, Y.; Kataoka, S.; Hanada, Y.; Hamada, M.; Morimoto, Y.; et al. Risk factors for absence of catch-up growth in small for gestational age very low-birthweight infants. *Pediatr. Int.* **2019**, *61*, 889–894. [CrossRef]

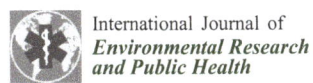

Article

Vision Development Differences between Slow and Fast Motor Development in Typical Developing Toddlers: A Cross-Sectional Study

Elena Pinero-Pinto [1], Verónica Pérez-Cabezas [2,*], Concepción De-Hita-Cantalejo [3], Carmen Ruiz-Molinero [2], Estanislao Gutiérrez-Sánchez [4], José-Jesús Jiménez-Rejano [1], José-María Sánchez-González [3] and María Carmen Sánchez-González [3]

1. Department of Physiotherapy, University of Seville, 41009 Seville, Spain; epinero@us.es (E.P.-P.); jjjimenez@us.es (J.-J.J.-R.)
2. INDESS (Instituto Universitario para el Desarrollo Social Sostenible), Department of Nursing and Physiotherapy, University of Cadiz, 11009 Cadiz, Spain; carmen.ruizmolinero@uca.es
3. Department of Physics of Condensed Matter, Optics Area, University of Seville, 41012 Seville, Spain; mhita@us.es (C.D.-H.-C.); jsanchez80@us.es (J.-M.S.-G.); msanchez77@us.es (M.C.S.-G.)
4. Department of Surgery, Ophthalmology Area, University of Seville, 41009 Seville, Spain; egutierrez1@us.es
* Correspondence: veronica.perezcabezas@uca.es; Tel.: +34-676-719119; Fax: +34-956-252426

Received: 16 April 2020; Accepted: 18 May 2020; Published: 20 May 2020

Abstract: Many studies have established a relationship between visual function and motor development in toddlers. This is the first report to study two-year-olds via an assessment of their visual and motor skills. The purpose of this study is to describe the possible changes that can occur between visual and motor systems in typical developing toddlers. A total of 116 toddlers were included in this observational, descriptive, and cross-sectional study. Their mean age was 29.57 ± 3.45 months. Motor development variables studied were dominant hand/foot; stationary, locomotion, object manipulation, grasping, visual motor integration percentiles; gross motor, fine motor, and total motor percentiles; and gross motor, fine motor, and total motor quotients. Visual development variables were assessed including visual acuity, refractive error, ocular alignment, motor fusion and suppression, ocular motility, and stereopsis. Our findings demonstrated that typical developing toddlers with slow gross motor development had higher exophoria and further near point of convergence values compared to toddlers with fast gross motor development ($p < 0.05$). No statistically significant differences were found in visual acuity and stereopsis between slow and fast gross motor development toddlers.

Keywords: child development; motor skills; vision disorders; evaluation; physical therapy; optometry

1. Introduction

Visual and motor development involves a physical and physiological process that allows perceiving precise details of an image (eyesight) and a perceptual process (vision) that requires multisensory integration: vision, hearing, touch, and proprioception for the interpretation of visual information. Vision delivers a key sensory input required for the proper functioning of neural circuits and is therefore a brain process of sensory integration [1] that offers important information in most daily activities [2]. Binocular vision offers improvements over monocular vision. It allows precise depth perception (stereopsis). It also enables the exploration of the visual scene during movement planning of the hands and feet directed at a target in space, such as the hand to grasp items [3] and the feet to walk [4], climb obstacles [5], or even for sitting postural control [6]. Three- and six-month-old babies can better assess if objects are within reach and move toward them using both eyes instead of one [7], as demonstrated during crawling [8].

Toddlers follow a pattern of skill development that allows them to know when they are progressing adequately. The first years of life are critical to a child's overall development. The central nervous system grows at a very fast rate, similar to the skills that the child develops. During this period, the development of postural reflexes and reactions, basic motor skills, and gross voluntary motor skills lay the foundation for mature motor behavior [9]. Many developmental tests are based on motor activity, such as the Peabody Developmental Motor Scale-II (PDMS) [10]. Gross motor development assesses muscle control, coordination, and locomotion. Fine motor skills include the development of control and coordination of body segments to perform more precise and complex tasks, integrating muscle coordination and perceptual skills [11]. Motor development can be influenced by other areas of development above and beyond sensory systems during childhood [12] For example, babies learns motor skills through observation [13].

Many studies have established a relationship between visual function and motor development [14–19]. They claim that binocular vision disorders such as amblyopia and strabismus can adversely affect skills that depend on eye movements, including reading. Many of these studies assessed only fine motor skills or eye-hand coordination in school-age children and their relationship to amblyopia. They studied groups of participants with different age ranges, between 5–9 years [14], 8–12 years [15–17], and 10–30 years [18]. Other research determined that children with poor stereoacuity have significant visuomotor deficits compared to typical developing children [20], while other reports affirmed that stereoacuity may be limited to specific tasks. In a group of children aged 5 to 13 years without visual impairment, Alramis et al. [21] showed that binocular vision and stereoacuity were associated with higher performance of certain fine motor tasks, and task performance decreased in younger children. They concluded that the role of vision in the performance of fine motor skills depends on both the task and age.

In addition to fine motor skills, few studies measured postural stability and control or gross motor skills in typical developing children. Some reported a delay in motor development and skill acquisition in children with visual disabilities and described a delay in gross motor skills such as control of the head and ability to sit, crawl, and walk during the first year of life [12,22]. Souza et al. [23] observed that a group of 15- to 22-month-old toddlers with visual impairment presented an overall delay in neuropsychomotor development, mainly in coordination. Celano et al. [24] suggested that there may have been a delay in fine motor function and balance in a group of 4.5-year-old children with unilateral visual impairment secondary to congenital cataracts. Chakraborty et al. [25] demonstrated a close relationship between stereopsis and fine and gross motor skills in a group of 4.5-year-old toddlers. Thompson et al. [26] studied a large group of 2-year-olds to fully evaluate the state of vision (visual acuity, stereopsis, alignment of visual axes, eye motility, and self-refraction) and its possible relationship with motor development. Their results demonstrated that global perception of movement and binocular vision are associated with motor function at an early stage of development as measured by the Bayley Scale of Infant and Toddler Development 3rd edition (BSID-III). All of the scientific literature reviewed included babies and toddlers [12,22–24] with some form of visual impairment or born with risk factors for neurological development [25,26]. To the best of our knowledge, this is the first report to study visual and motor development in a sample of between two and three-year-olds both visually and from the perspective of motor development.

The purpose of this study was to describe the vision development differences between slow and fast motor development in typical developing toddlers. Vision study included ocular health screening, visual acuity, refractive errors, ocular alignment, motor fusion and suppression, ocular motility and stereopsis. Among motor development parameters, we studied fine motor development through grasping and hand-eye coordination and gross motor development, analyzing static, locomotion, and object manipulation.

2. Materials and Methods

2.1. Design

This observational, descriptive, and cross-sectional study was conducted from October 2019 to January 2020 in toddlers at the facilities of the University of Seville's (Spain) nursery schools. This study followed the Declaration of Helsinki's tenets. The parents were written and orally informed about the study characteristics, benefits, and risks. Written informed consent was obtained after explaining the nature and possible consequences of the study. The Institutional Review Board of the University Hospital Virgen Macarena of the University of Seville approved this research.

2.2. Subjects

The sample consisted of 116 typical developing participants. Inclusion criteria were toddlers with normal or corrected-to-normal vision, and exclusion criteria were toddlers with previous history of disorder, toddlers with learning disabilities, and preterm toddlers.

2.3. Measurements and Materials

A physiotherapist's measurements were blinded to an optometrist's measurements and vice versa. A first examination was conducted in an individual room. After one hour, second measurements were completed. If the toddlers reported signs of fatigue, they were given a 30-min break before the second set of measurements was obtained.

2.4. Developmental Motor Assessment

The Peabody Developmental Motor Scale-Second Version (PDMS-II), the motor subscale [10] was used to evaluate motor development. This scale evaluates gross and fine motor development in toddlers from birth to five years. The gross motor component included three subtests for toddlers ages two to three: stationary (standing balance, sit-ups, and push-ups), locomotion (walking, running, jumping, and hopping), and object manipulation (throwing and taking different size balls). The fine motor component is composed of two subtests, grasping and visual motor integration. The mean between both scales is considered the total motor development score. The test requires the child to perform specific motor activities that are scored with a 2, 1, or 0 depending on whether the child partially or correctly completes an activity according to the description. Results obtained are standard scores, percentiles, age equivalents, quotient scores in fine and gross motor areas, and total motor development.

The mean value of the development quotients is 100 [10]. Above 100 (quotient > 100), motor development is considered rapid and below 100 (quotient < 100), development is considered slower. We presented two groups, toddlers with fast gross motor development (quotient > 100) and a group of toddlers with slow gross motor development (quotient < 100) based on the variable gross motor quotient (GMQ). The entire PDMS-II can be finished in 45 to 60 min. Separate fine or gross motor subtest administration takes 20 to 30 min.

The PDMS-II is primarily designed to examine and evaluate motor development, but as a secondary objective, it was developed as a research tool. The general test administration procedure is standardized, and formal training is not required. Griffiths et al. [27] reviewed the characteristics and psychometric properties of different tools for evaluating motor development. They determined that the PDMS-II has good psychometric characteristics to evaluate motor development. Hua et al. [28] reported that the scale's internal consistency is excellent. Folio and Fewwell [10] determined that it is good (24–35 months, α = 0.97). Wuang et al. [29] reported that the test has good reliability (test-retest n = 141, ICC = 0.97), and excellent validity. The content and the structural validity are also excellent [10,28]. The minimal detectable change was 7.76 (sensitivity 60.65%, specificity 74.13%) [29] and standard error mean (SEM) for 24–59 months was 3 [10].

2.5. Visual Development Assessment

2.5.1. Visual Acuity and Refraction

External structures of the eye were examined with a pen flashlight and head loupe. Red reflex testing [30] was measured with a direct ophthalmoscope with the lens power set at 0. The red reflex brightness should be identical in both eyes. Any absence of the red reflex, difference between the eyes, or abnormal pupil color may indicate a serious eye condition. The quantification of visual acuity was measured using Cardiff cards [31] and broken wheel tests [32]. Refractive errors were assessed with the non-cycloplegic method and measured with Mohindra retinoscopy [33]. The retinoscope light was the only stimulus for the toddler and did not induce accommodation. The unexplored eye was occluded, and the optometrist was 50 cm from the child. Shadows observed were neutralized with positive or negative spherical or cylindrical lenses. The spherical equivalent (SE) was calculated to homogenize the refraction variables.

2.5.2. Ocular Alignment

Very young toddlers, such as our toddlers, cannot fixate on a target long enough for a valid cover test. In such cases, the optometrist estimated the degree of ocular alignment with the corneal reflex test and diopter prisms (the Krimsky test) or without diopter prisms (the Hirschberg test and kappa angle) [34]. The kappa angle was described as the angle between the visual axis and pupil axis. Each eye has a different Kappa angle, usually less than five degrees. A positive Kappa angle (displacement toward the nose) is physiologic up to five degrees. A negative kappa angle represents a temporal displacement (toward the ear). A large kappa angle may cause ocular alignment disorders [35]. Angles that were zero or no differences between the visual and pupil axis were reported as centered.

2.5.3. Motor Fusion, Suppression, and Stereopsis

For convergence/divergence test, a fixed target was presented at 25 cm. First, a 20Δ base-out (BO) prism was placed in front of one of the child's eyes. Next, a 20Δ base-in (BI) prism was placed in front of one of the child's eyes. The child should direct his/her hand in front of or behind the fixed target [36]. The near point of convergence (NPC) was determined by placing a fixed target 30 cm from the eye in the midplane of the child's head. The child was asked to maintain fixation on the target. The toddlers were asked to describe the picture that they looked at during the measurement. The target was moved slowly toward the eyes until one eye lost fixation and turned out. The distance between the fixed target and the nose bridge was measured with a string and ruler. It was repeated twice for each child [37,38]. To test ocular motility using binocular fixation, the toddler fixed on a small dot for 20 s [17]. Next, smooth movement without restrictions was assessed via smooth pursuit to a moving target located 30 to 40 cm away [36]. Saccades eye movements were also studied. The toddlers were instructed to look at a target point as quickly and accurately as possible using their index finger. Target appeared randomly at four eccentricities ± 5 degrees or ± 10 degrees from central fixation in the horizontal plane [39]. The Lang stereo test II was used to measure stereopsis. The test consisted of three three-dimensional images, a moon, truck, and elephant, and one two-dimensional image, a star that is seen without stereoscopic vision (visible with only one eye) that serves to capture the patient's attention. The test was placed with the observer in front of the child to observe his/her eye movements. The toddlers were told to look at the picture lying perpendicular to approximately 40 cm from the child's face and asked if he/she saw anything, observing the eye movements. If the child was unable to name the images, he/she was asked to locate an area on the card where there appeared to be something different and try to describe their differences [40].

2.6. Statistical Analysis

The data were analyzed with SPSS statistical software (version 26.0 for Windows; SPSS Inc., Chicago, IL, USA). Descriptive analysis was conducted with values expressed as mean ± SD. The data normality distribution was assessed with the Kolmogorov-Smirnov test. Gross, fine, and total motor quotients were divided into two groups (fast motor development when the GMQ, FMQ, and TMQ was ≥ 100 and slow motor development when the GMQ, FMQ, and TMQ was 100). Differences in visual development between the fast and slow motor development groups were assessed with Student's t-test for quantitative variables and the chi-squared test for qualitative variables. For all of the tests, the level of significance was established at 95% (P < 0.05).

3. Results

This study included 116 toddlers, 53 males (45.68%) and 63 females (54.31%). The mean ages of the toddlers were 29.57 ± 3.45 (24.16 to 36.90) months. Population flow chart diagram is shown in Figure 1. In the gender comparison, no statistically significant differences were found in any variable except for the fine motor quotient (FMQ) where the males toddlers obtained 100.56 ± 16.64 and the females toddlers obtained 108.09 ± 12.21 (t = 2.79, $p < 0.01$). Motor development variables included the dominant hand and foot, stationary percentile, locomotion percentile, object manipulation percentile, grasping percentile, visual motor integration percentile, gross motor percentile (GMP), fine motor percentile (FMP), total motor percentile (TMP), gross motor quotient (GMQ), fine motor quotient (FMQ), and total motor quotient (TMQ). They are presented in Table 1. Visual development variables included the Cardiff visual acuity (VA) test for right, left, and both eyes; broken wheels VA test for right eye, left eye, and both eyes; retinoscopy refraction in the mean spherical equivalent; kappa angle for right and left eyes; Hirschberg reflex for right and left eyes; near point of convergence; base-out and base-in test; Lang stereopsis test; Bruckner test; fixation, accuracy, and head tests for tracking movements; and reflection and head tests for saccades movements. These are also presented in Table 1.

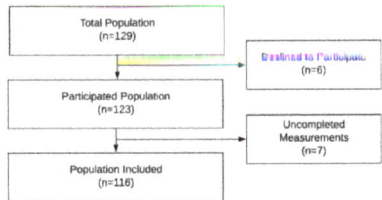

Figure 1. Population flow chart diagram.

Visual development differences between the fast and slow GMQ development groups (GMQ > 100 and GMQ ≤100, respectively) are presented in Table 2. The GMP demonstrated identical results for the GMQ groups. We found no significant differences in visual development between the fast and slow FMP, TMP, FMQ, and TMQ development groups. In the right eye kappa angle, only 17.5% of the toddlers had a centered reflex in the slow gross motor development group (GMQ ≤ 100), while 36.8% of the toddlers had a centered reflex in the fast motor development group (GMQ < 100) ($\chi^2 = 8.28$, P = 0.01). Similar results were found in the right eye Hirschberg test: only 17.95% of the toddlers had a centered corneal reflex in the slow motor development group, whereas 39.5% of the toddlers had the same type of corneal reflex in the fast motor development group ($\chi^2 = 7.64$, P = 0.02). The same situation was found in the kappa angle and Hirschberg test for the left eye, although the results were not statistically significant ($\chi^2 = 4.74$, P = 0.09, $\chi^2 = 4.88$, and P = 0.08, respectively).

The Krimsky and Bruckner tests obtained similar findings. In the slow motor development group, 87.5% and 88.8% of the toddlers had a normal test while 12.5% and 11.3% had a deviated test, respectively. However, in the fast motor development group, all of the toddlers had normal Krimsky (Figure 2) and Bruckner tests and none had any deviations in their eyes ($\chi^2 = 4.92$ and P = 0.02 for the Krimsky test and $\chi^2 = 4.39$ and P = 0.03 for the Bruckner test). The last statistically significant visual development variable was near point of convergence (Figure 3C). The slow motor development group had 2.46 ± 4.07 cm, whereas better results were reported in the fast motor development group, 1.00

± 2.02 (t =2.56, P = 0.01). For visual acuity (Figure 3A), retinoscopy refraction (Figure 3B), base-out and base-in test, stereopsis test, fixation test, accuracy and head position for tracking movements, and reflection and head position for saccades movements, there were non-statistically significant differences between slow and fast motor development including gross, fine, and total percentiles and quotients.

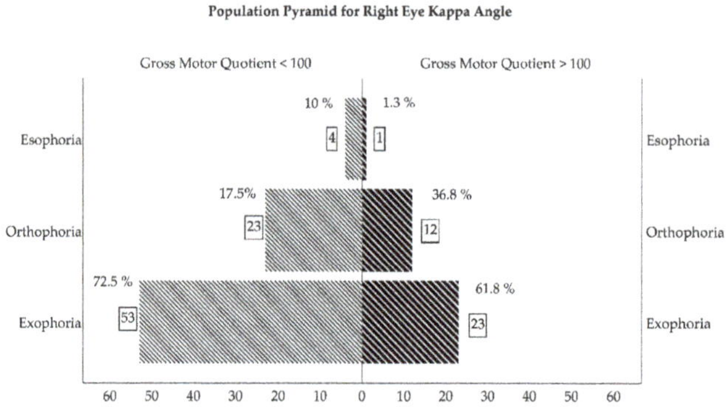

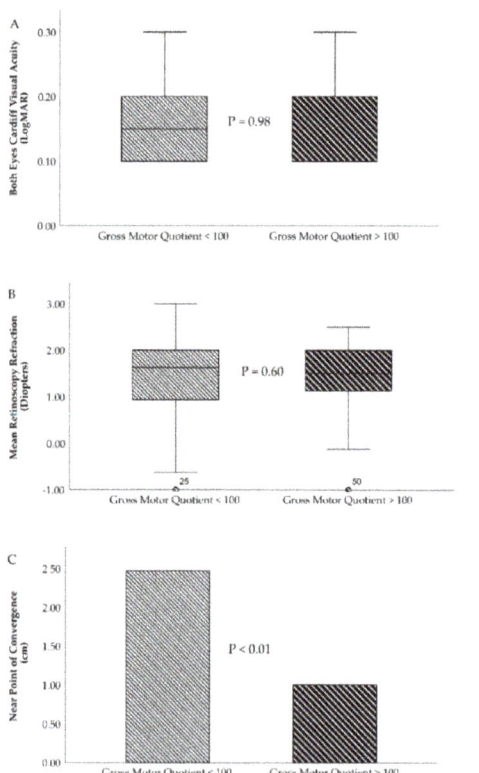

Figure 2. Population pyramid for kappa angle (expressed in percentage and count of toddlers in square).

Figure 3. Slow and fast motor development characteristics for main optometry variables. (**A**)—Box and plot graph for both eyes' visual acuity (Cardiff test, expressed in LogMAR). (**B**)—Box and plot graph for mean retinoscopy refraction (expressed in diopters). (**C**)—Near point of convergence (expressed in cm).

Table 1. Population characteristics for motor and visual development.

Motor Development Parameter (n = 116)	Value	Visual Development Parameter (n = 116)	Value		
			Right Eye	Left Eye	Both Eye
Age (Months)	29.57 ± 3.45 (24.16 to 36.90)	Visual Acuity (Cardiff Test—LogMAR)	0.18 ± 0.10 (0.10 to 0.70)	0.18 ± 0.10 (0.10 to 0.70)	0.17 ± 0.10 (0.10 to 0.70)
Dominant Hand (Right/Left)	113 (97.4%)/3 (2.6)	Visual Acuity (Broken Wheels—LogMAR)	0.36 ± 0.04 (0.20 to 0.40)	0.37 ± 0.49 (0.20 to 0.40)	0.37 ± 0.49 (0.30 to 0.40)
Dominant Foot (Right/Left)	109 (94%)/7 (6%)	Retinoscopy Refraction (Diopters D) Spherical Equivalent Refraction	+1.30 ± 0.85 (−1.00 to +3.00)	+1.39 ± 0.87 (−2.00 to +3.00)	-
Static Percentile	72.04 ± 19.90 (9.00 to 99.00)	Kappa Angle (Negative/0/Positive)	5 (4.3%) 35 (30.2%) 76 (65.5)	5 (5.2%) 34 (29.3) 76 (65.5)	-
Locomotion Percentile	15.87 ± 11.08 (2.00 to 50.00)	Hirshberg Reflex (n = 115 y 114) (Temporal/Centered/Nasal)	4 (3.4%) 37 (31.9%) 74 (63.8%)	5 (4.3%) 38 (32.8%) 71 (61.2%)	-
Handling Percentile	43.43 ± 21.20 (5.00 to 95.00)	Krismky Test (Normal/Deviated)		106 (91.4%)/10 (8.6%)	
Grasp Percentile	73.53 ± 24.16 (5.00 to 99.00)	Near Point of Convergence (centimeter, cm)		2.01 ± 3.62 (0.00 to 20.00)	
Coordination Percentile	37.79 ± 18.76 (2.00 to 84.00)	Base-Out 6Δ Prism Test (prism diopters, Δ) (Negative/Positive)		43 (37.1%)/73 (62.9%)	
Thick Motor Percentile (TMP)	42.40 ± 21.00 (8.00 to 95.00)	Base-In 6Δ Prism Test (prism, diopters, Δ (Negative/Positive)		86 (74.1%)/30 (25.9%)	
Fine Motor Percentile (FMP)	56.68 ± 24.33 (12.00 to 99.00)	Stereopsis Lang Test (Second arc) (200″, 400″ y 600″)		297.29 ± 139.77 (200.00 to 600.00)	
Overall Motor Percentile (OMP)	49.71 ± 22.32 (4.00 to 96.00)	Bruckner Test (Normal/Deviated)		107 (92.2%)/9 (7.8%)	
Thick Motor Quotient (TMQ)	96.81 ± 9.15 (79.00 to 124.00)	Fixation Test (Passed/Not passed)		90 (77.6%)/26 (22.4%)	
Fine Motor Quotient (FMQ)	104.52 ± 14.90 (14.00 to 151.00)	Accuracy and Head (Tracking Movements)		Smooth 34 (29.3%)/Loss 45 (38.8%)/Jumps 27 (23.3%)/Continuous Loss 10 (8.6%) Motionless 17 (14.7%)/Slight 49 (42.2%)/Medium 32 (27.6%)/Strong 18 (15.5%)	
Overall Motor Quotient (OMQ)	98.66 ± 14.55 (0.00 to 126.00)	Reflection and Head (Saccades Movements)		Negative 67 (57.8%)/Positive 49 (42.2%) Motionless 15 (12.9%)/Slight 54 (46.6%)/Medium 30 (25.9%)/Strong 17 (14.7%)	

Values were presented with mean ± SD (standard deviation) and (Range) in quantitative variables or expressed with frequency and percentage in qualitative variable.

Table 2. Visual development differences between over and under mean quotient for gross motor quotient development.

Visual Development Parameter	Gross Motor Quotient < 100 (n = 80)	Gross Motor Quotient > 100 (n = 36)	p Value *
Cardiff VA (RE)/(LE)	0.18 ± 0.10/0.18 ± 0.10	0.18 ± 0.10/0.18 ± 0.09	0.98/0.98
Broken Wheels VA (RE)/(LE)	0.36 ± 0.05/0.36 ± 0.04	0.37 ± 0.04/0.37 ± 0.04	0.26/0.34
Retinoscopy Rx (RE)/(LE)	+1.27 ± 0.91/+1.35 ± 0.92	+1.35 ± 0.73/+1.49 ± 0.74	0.66/0.43
Kappa Angle (RE) (Negative/0/Positive)	4 (10%) 7 (17.5%) 29 (72.5%)	1 (1.3%) 28 (36.8%) 47 (61.8%)	0.01
Kappa Angle (LE) (Negative/0/Positive)	4 (10%) 8 (20%) 28 (70%)	2 (2.26%) 26 (34.3%) 48 (63.2%)	0.09
Hirschberg Reflex (RE) (Temporal/Centered/Nasal)	3 (7.7%) 7 (17.95) 29 (74.4%)	1 (1.3%) 30 (39.5%) 45 (59.2%)	0.02
Hirschberg Reflex (LE) (Temporal/Centered/Nasal)	3 (7.9%) 8 (21.1%) 27 (71.1%)	2 (2.6%) 30 (39.5%) 44 (57.9%)	0.08
Krimsky Test (Normal/Deviated)	70 (87.5%) 10 (12.5%)	36 (100%) 0 (0%)	0.02
NPC (centimeter, cm)	2.46 ± 4.07	1.00 ± 2.02	0.01
Base-Out 6Δ Prism Test (prism diopters, Δ) (Negative/Positive)	27 (33.8%) 53 (66.3%)	16 (44.4%) 20 (55.6%)	0.27
Base-In 6Δ Prism Test (prism, diopters, Δ (Negative/Positive)	60 (75%) 20 (25%)	26 (72.2%) 10 (27.8%)	0.75
Stereopsis Lang Test (Second arc) (Negative, 550″, 600″ and 1200″)	303.89 ± 143.67	282.35 ± 131.35	0.45
Bruckner Test (Normal/Deviated)	71 (88.8%) 9 (11.3%)	36 (100%) 0 (0%)	0.03
Fixation Test (Passed/Not passed)	64 (80%) 16 (20%)	26 (72.2%) 10 (27.8%)	0.35
Accuracy (Tracking Movements) (Smooth/Loss/Jumps/Continuous Loss)	22(27.5%)/33(41.3%) 20(25%)/5(6.3%)	12(33.3%)/12 (33.3%) 7(19.4%)/5(13.9%)	0.44
Head (Tracking Movements) (Motionless/Slight/Medium/Strong)	12(15%)/32(40%) 24(30%)/12 (15%)	5(13.9%)/17(47.2%) 8(22.2%)/6(16.7%)	0.82
Reflection (Saccades Movements) (Negative/Positive)	46 (57.5%) 34 (42.5%)	21 (58.3%) 15 (41.0%)	0.31
Head (Saccades Movements) (Motionless/Slight/Medium/Strong)	12(15%)/33(41.3%) 24(30%)/11(13.85)	3(8.3%)/21(58.3%) 6(16.7%)/6(16.7)	0.23

VA: Visual Acuity; NPC: Near point of convergence; RE: Right eye; LE: Left eye. Quantitative value with mean ± SD and qualitative with frequency (percentage).

4. Discussion

This study evaluated the visual function and motor development in typical developing toddlers. The objective was to determine the possible presence of visual dysfunction and/or motor disorders and analyze possible differences between slow and fast motor development for visual system variables. Visual acuity, alignment of visual axes, stereopsis, and ocular motor skills were included in the present study. The percentiles and quotients of gross, fine, and total motor development in a group of 116 toddlers aged from two to three years were also reported. Two main GMQ groups were established, a slow motor development group (GMQ < 100) and fast motor development group (GMQ > 100). We found statistically significant differences between slow and fast motor development for certain visual system variables. Toddlers with slow gross motor development had a greater tendency of exophoria and a further near point of convergence (NPC) than toddlers with fast gross motor development. These findings agree with previous studies that demonstrated the link among the visual and motor systems in babies, toddlers, and children [4,13–17,19,21,24–26].

Similar to our outcomes, Thompson et al. [26] studied a two-year-old large toddlers group. They fully evaluated vision state (visual acuity, stereopsis, visual axes alignment, ocular motility, and auto-refraction) and its possible relationship with motor development. They measured using the Bayley Scale of Infant and Toddler Development 3rd edition (BSID-III), which has an excellent correlation with the PDMS-II [41,42]. Their outcomes revealed that global movement perception and binocular vision were associated with motor function at an early development stage. This study included toddlers born with risk factors for neurological development. Thus, their early development rates differ from ours since our sample was based on toddlers with neurotypical development. To the best of our knowledge, our study is the first that analyzed typical developing toddlers two- to three-year-old both in motor and visual function.

To date, the prevalence of visual, accommodative, and non-strabismic binocular dysfunction has increased in the pediatric population [43–45]. Early diagnosis and proper management can improve vision-related life in this population, thus guaranteeing its correct evolutionary development in all areas. Different symptoms and signs can be used to diagnose visual function [46,47].

4.1. Visual Acuity Differences between Slow and Fast Gross Motor Development

Amblyopia refers to the unilateral or bilateral reduction of the best corrected visual acuity that is not directly attributed to a structural alteration of the eye or visual pathways [48]. It constitutes one of the main causes of visual impairment in children, with prevalence values ranging from 1% to 4% [49]. Amblyopia is related to the presence of strabismus, refractive errors, astigmatism, and anisometropia. Determination of visual acuity is generally the first clinical step to identify the presence of amblyopia [50]. When we classified the subjects according to their GMQ values, we found no differences in visual acuity values between the two groups. Visual acuity was identical in the RE and LE (0.18 ± 0.10 LogMAR) measured with the Cardiff test, and there were no statistically significant differences between both eyes (OD = 0.36 ± 0.05 LogMAR, OI = 0.37 ± 0.04 LogMAR) when evaluated with broken wheels. Similar findings were obtained in binocular visual acuity values and did not differ between the two groups. Many studies link visual acuity deficits with motor delays [14–17,21,51,52]. The presence of refractive errors, mainly hyperopia, is common in children with amblyopia, which is normally associated with mild delays in many aspects of development [53]. In our study, the sample consisted of toddlers without visual impairment whose objective refraction did not exceed +1.50 diopters in either of the two eyes, which could be why we did not find differences between the slow and fast motor development groups.

4.2. Ocular Alignment Differences between Slow and Fast Gross Motor Development

Heterophoria is ocular misalignment in the absence of fusional vergence. Exophoria is a divergent misalignment, while esophoria is a convergent misalignment [54]. The measurement of heterophoria is an important clinical test since it indicates the demand of the fusional vergence system [55]. It has been fully evaluated in adults and older children, but is difficult to measure in toddlers younger than five years because of their limited cooperation [38,54,56,57]. We found authors who established that many toddlers under five years old were orthophoric [38,56]. However, our results are in line with more recent studies showing that the phoria of children without visual impairment between two and seven years old was mainly exophoric, with small differences in that age range [54,55,57].

Our study found that all of toddlers had clear exophoria, which significantly increased their slow motor development. Overall, 72.5% in the slow gross motor development group had a right eye kappa angle that was more positive (exophoric) than 61.8% in the fast development group (P = 0.01). The left eye kappa angle had significant differences (P = 0.09). Correspondingly, the right eye Hirschberg reflex was significantly more nasal (exophoric) (P = 0.02) and considerable (P = 0.08) in the slow motor development toddlers. Furthermore, the slower gross motor development toddlers had an NPC of 2.46 ± 4.07 cm, significantly higher than in the fast-gross motor development group, where the NPC was 1.00 ± 2.02 cm (P = 0.01).

The findings of Jeon et al. [58] were very revealing. They reported that the prevalence of exotropia was higher in toddlers with several motor impairments. Motor function was studied using gross motor function. In this case, our patients were typical developing, and we did not have cases of strabismus but had cases of exophoria. In this sense, the slow motor development group had greater exophoria than the fast motor development group. In addition, we found a decrease in the ability to merge with an NPC increase in the slow gross motor development group. These results agree with Jeon et al. [58]; however, they found the same prevalence in exotropia and esotropia.

On the one hand, exophoria is characterized by a divergent deviation in the line of sight when the visual axes are at rest. Exotropia is defined as a more serious, manifest, and fixed situation of ocular exodeviation [59]. On the other hand, Barbosa et al. [60,61] categorized infants by the degree of motor performance in three motor levels: cerebral palsy, motor delay, and typical development. Therefore, our results could be very useful for anticipating below average cases of motor development in which a higher prevalence of exophoria is demonstrated.

4.3. Stereopsis Differences between Slow and Fast Gross Motor Development

Stereopsis allocates depth calculations based on the binocular disparity between the images of an object in the left and right eyes [62]. Toddler stereopsis determination allows rapid detection of visual disturbances, mainly cases of amblyopia with a history of strabismus [63]. Previous studies concluded that toddlers with deficient stereopsis have developmental disorders [20]. Other studies showed that stereopsis is associated with higher performance of certain fine motor tasks at very young ages [21]. We also found studies that showed that many toddlers perform well on manual skill assessments even with poor stereopsis [64]. Previous research demonstrated that toddlers who underwent strabismus surgery showed postoperative improvements in motor performance that were not correlated with stereopsis improvements [65]. Our stereopsis findings were similar in the toddlers' fine and gross motor development. This was probably because the toddlers in the sample did not present any type of visual alterations. Stereopsis was positive in both groups, with a slight non-statistically significant difference in the fast-gross motor development group (282.35 ± 131.35) second arc, compared to the slow gross motor development group (303.89 ± 143.67) second arc with P = 0.45.

4.4. Future Research and Limitations

Future research could be assessed by visual and therapy programs. Visual therapy has been shown to be a useful treatment option in subjects with visual disturbances [66,67] and assesses how it affects motor development quotients. We also proposed the reverse option, conducting an intervention to promote and enhance motor development in toddlers with slow gross motor development to ascertain how it affects binocular vision development. Within the limitations, sample follow-up was missing because this was a cross-sectional study. Future research should include longitudinal gross and fine motor development changes in this sample. The toddlers enrolled were in their last year of nursery school. This issue could limit sample follow-up.

5. Conclusions

Neurotypical developing toddlers and without visual impairment with slow gross motor development had higher exophoria and further near point of convergence values compared with fast gross motor development toddlers. No statistically significant differences were found in visual acuity and stereopsis between both slow and fast gross motor development toddlers.

Author Contributions: Conceptualization, E.P.-P., V.P.-C., C.D.-H.-C., C.R.-M., E.G.-S., J.-J.J.-R., J.-M.S.-G., and M.C.S.-G.; methodology, E.P.-P., V.P.-C., C.D.-H.C., C.R.-M., E.G.-S., J.-J.J.-R., J.-M.S.-G., and M.C.S.-G.; validation, E.P.-P., V.P.-C., C.D.-H.-C., C.R.-M., E.G.-S., J.-J.J.-R., J.-M.S.-G., and M.C.S.-G.; formal analysis, E.P.-P., V.P.-C., C.D.-H.-C., C.R.-M., E.G.-S., J.-J.J.-R., J.-M.S.-G., and M.C.S.-G.; investigation, E.P.-P., V.P.-C., C.D.-H.-C., C.R.-M., E.G.-S., J.-J.J.-R., J.-M.S.-G., and M.C.S.-G.; resources, E.P.-P., V.P.-C., C.D.-H.-C., C.R.-M., E.G.-S., J.-J.J.-R., J.-M.S.-G., and M.C.S.-G.; data curation, E.P.-P., V.P.-C., C.D.-H.-C., C.R.-M., E.G.-S., J.-J.J.-R., J.-M.S.-G., and M.C.S.-G.; writing—original draft preparation, E.P.-P., V.P.-C., C.D.-H.-C., C.R.-M., E.G.-S., J.-J.J.-R., J.-M.S.-G., and M.C.S.-G.; writing—review and editing, E.P.-P., V.P.-C., C.D.-H.-C., C.R.-M., E.G.-S., J.-J.J.-R., J.-M.S.-G., and M.C.S.-G.; visualization, E.P.-P., V.P.-C., C.D.-H.-C., C.R.-M., E.G.-S., J.-J.J.-R., J.-M.S.-G., and M.C.S.-G.; supervision, E.P.-P., V.P.-C., C.D.-H.-C., C.R.-M., E.G.-S., J.-J.J.-R., J.-M.S.-G. and M.C.S.-G.; project administration, E.P.-P., V.P.-C., C.D.-H.-C., C.R.-M., E.G.-S., J.-J.J.-R., J.-M.S.-G., and M.C.S.-G.; funding acquisition, E.P.-P., V.P.-C., C.D.-H.-C., C.R.-M., E.G.-S., J.-J.J.-R., J.-M.S.-G., and M.C.S.-G. All authors have read and agreed to the published version of the manuscript.

Funding: This research received no external funding.

Conflicts of Interest: The authors declare no conflict of interest.

References

1. Niechwiej-Szwedo, E.; Colpa, L.; Wong, A.M.F. Visuomotor Behaviour in Amblyopia: Deficits and Compensatory Adaptations. *Neural Plast.* **2019**, *2019*, 6817839. [CrossRef] [PubMed]
2. Hayhoe, M.M. Vision and Action. *Annu. Rev. Vis. Sci.* **2017**, *3*, 389–413. [CrossRef] [PubMed]
3. Goodale, M.A. Transforming vision into action. *Vis. Res.* **2011**, *51*, 1567–1587. [CrossRef] [PubMed]
4. Logan, D.; Kiemel, T.; Dominici, N.; Cappellini, G.; Ivanenko, Y.; Lacquaniti, F.; Jeka, J.J. The many roles of vision during walking. *Exp. Brain Res.* **2010**, *206*, 337–350. [CrossRef]
5. Chapman, G.J.; Scally, A.; Buckley, J.G. Importance of binocular vision in foot placement accuracy when stepping onto a floor-based target during gait initiation. *Exp. Brain Res.* **2012**, *216*, 71–80. [CrossRef]
6. Kyvelidou, A.; Stergiou, N. Visual and somatosensory contributions to infant sitting postural control. *Somatosens. Mot. Res.* **2018**, *35*, 240–246. [CrossRef]
7. von Hofsten, C.; Fazel-Zandy, S. Development of visually guided hand orientation in reaching. *J. Exp. Child Psychol.* **1984**, *38*, 208–219. [CrossRef]
8. Anderson, D.I.; He, M.; Gutierrez, P.; Uchiyama, I.; Campos, J.J. Do balance demands induce shifts in visual proprioception in crawling infants? *Front. Psychol.* **2019**, *10*. [CrossRef]
9. Veldman, S.L.C.; Santos, R.; Jones, R.A.; Sousa-Sá, E.; Okely, A.D. Associations between gross motor skills and cognitive development in toddlers. *Early Hum. Dev.* **2019**, *132*, 39–44. [CrossRef]
10. Folio, M.; Fewell, R. *Peabody Developmental Motor Scales–Second Edition (PDMS-2): Examiner's Mmanual*; Pro-Ed: Austin, TX, USA, 2000.
11. Hadders-Algra, M. Variation and Variability: Key Words in Human Motor Development. *Phys. Ther.* **2010**, *90*, 1823–1837. [CrossRef]
12. Prechtl, H.F.R.; Cioni, G.; Einspieler, C.; Bos, A.F.; Ferrari, F. Role of vision on early motor development: Lessons from the blind. *Dev. Med. Child Neurol.* **2001**, *43*, 198–201. [CrossRef] [PubMed]
13. Fagard, J.; Rat-Fischer, L.; Esseily, R.; Somogyi, E.; O'Regan, J.K. What does it take for an infant to learn how to use a tool by observation? *Front. Psychol.* **2016**, *7*. [CrossRef] [PubMed]
14. Grant, S.; Suttle, C.; Melmoth, D.R.; Conway, M.L.; Sloper, J.J. Age- and stereovision-dependent eye-hand coordination deficits in children with amblyopia and abnormal binocularity. *Investig. Opthalmology Vis. Sci.* **2014**, *55*, 5687–57015. [CrossRef] [PubMed]

15. Webber, A.L.; Wood, J.M.; Gole, G.A.; Brown, B. The effect of amblyopia on fine motor skills in children. *Investig. Opthalmol. Vis. Sci.* **2008**, *49*, 594–603. [CrossRef]
16. Kelly, K.R.; Jost, R.M.; De La Cruz, A.; Birch, E.E. Amblyopic children read more slowly than controls under natural, binocular reading conditions. *J. AAPOS* **2015**, *19*, 515–520. [CrossRef]
17. Kelly, K.R.; Jost, R.M.; De La Cruz, A.; Dao, L.; Beauchamp, C.L.; Stager, D.; Birch, E.E. Slow reading in children with anisometropic amblyopia is associated with fixation instability and increased saccades. *J. AAPOS* **2017**, *21*, 447–451.e1. [CrossRef]
18. O'Connor, A.R.; Birch, E.E.; Anderson, S.; Draper, H. FSOS Research Group The functional significance of stereopsis. *Investig. Opthalmology Vis. Sci.* **2010**, *51*, 2019–2023. [CrossRef]
19. Hemptinne, C.; Aerts, F.; Pellissier, T.; Ruiz, C.R.; Cardoso, V.A.; Vanderveken, C.; Yüksel, D. Motor skills in children with strabismus. *J. Am. Assoc. Pediatr. Ophthalmol. Strabismus* **2020**. [CrossRef]
20. Kulp, M.T.; Schmidt, P.P. A pilot study. Depth perception and near stereoacuity: Is it related to academic performance in young children? *Binocul. Vis. Strabismus Q.* **2002**, *17*, 129–134.
21. Alramis, F.; Roy, E.; Christian, L.; Niechwiej-Szwedo, E. Contribution of binocular vision to the performance of complex manipulation tasks in 5-13 years old visually-normal children. *Hum. Mov. Sci.* **2016**, *46*, 52–62. [CrossRef]
22. Elisa, F.; Josée, L.; Oreste, F.-G.; Claudia, A.; Antonella, L.; Sabrina, S.; Giovanni, L. Gross motor development and reach on sound as critical tools for the development of the blind child. *Brain Dev.* **2002**, *24*, 269–275. [CrossRef]
23. Souza, T.A.; Souza, V.E.; Lopes, M.C.B.; Kitadai, S.P.S. Description of the neuropsychomotor and visual development of visually impaired children. *Arq. Bras. Oftalmol.* **2010**, *73*, 526–530. [CrossRef] [PubMed]
24. Celano, M.; Hartmann, E.E.; Dubois, L.G.; Drews-Botsch, C. Motor skills of children with unilateral visual impairment in the Infant Aphakia Treatment Study. *Dev. Med. Child Neurol.* **2016**, *58*, 154–159. [CrossRef] [PubMed]
25. Chakraborty, A.; Anstice, N.S.; Jacobs, R.J.; Paudel, N.; LaGasse, L.L.; Lester, B.M.; McKinlay, C.J.D.; Harding, J.E.; Wouldes, T.A.; Thompson, B. Global motion perception is related to motor function in 4.5-year-old children born at risk of abnormal development. *Vis. Res.* **2017**, *135*, 16–25. [CrossRef] [PubMed]
26. Thompson, B.; McKinlay, C.J.D.; Chakraborty, A.; Anstice, N.S.; Jacobs, R.J.; Paudel, N.; Yu, T.Y.; Ansell, J.M.; Wouldes, T.A.; Harding, J.E. Global motion perception is associated with motor function in 2-year-old children. *Neurosci. Lett.* **2017**, *658*, 177–181. [CrossRef]
27. Griffiths, A.; Toovey, R.; Morgan, P.E.; Spittle, A.J. Psychometric properties of gross motor assessment tools for children: A systematic review. *BMJ Open* **2018**, *8*, 21734. [CrossRef]
28. Hua, J.; Gu, G.; Meng, W.; Wu, Z. Age band 1 of the Movement Assessment Battery for Children-Second Edition: Exploring its usefulness in mainland China. *Res. Dev. Disabil.* **2013**, *34*, 801–808. [CrossRef]
29. Wuang, Y.-P.; Su, C.-Y.; Huang, M.-H. Psychometric comparisons of three measures for assessing motor functions in preschoolers with intellectual disabilities. *J. Intellect. Disabil. Res.* **2012**, *56*, 567–578. [CrossRef]
30. Bowman, R.; Foster, A. Testing the red reflex. *Community Eye Health* **2018**, *31*, 23.
31. Sathar, A.; Abbas, S.; Nujum, Z.T.; Benson, J.L.; Sreedevi, G.P.; Saraswathyamma, S.K. Visual outcome of preterm infants screened in a tertiary care hospital. *Middle East Afr. J. Ophthalmol.* **2019**, *26*, 158–162. [CrossRef]
32. Schmidt, P.P. Allen figure and broken wheel visual acuity measurement in preschool children. *J. Am. Optom. Assoc.* **1992**, *63*, 124–130. [PubMed]
33. Mohindra, I. A non cycloplegic refraction technique for infants and young children. *J. Am. Optom. Assoc.* **1977**, *48*, 518–523. [PubMed]
34. Rutstein, R.P.; Author Martin Cogen, P.S.; Cotter, S.A.; Kent Daum, O.M.; Mozlin, R.L.; Julie Ryan, O.M.; Heath, D.A.; Diane Adamczyk, C.T.; John Amos, O.F.; Brian Mathie, M.E.; et al. *Optometric clinical practice guideline care of the patient with strabismus: Esotropia and Exotropia*; American Optometric Association: St. Louis, MO, USA, 2010.
35. Basmak, H.; Sahin, A.; Yildirim, N.; Papakostas, T.D.; Kanellopoulos, A.J. Measurement of angle kappa with synoptophore and Orbscan II in a normal population. *J. Refract. Surg.* **2007**, *23*, 456–460. [CrossRef] [PubMed]

36. Yu, T.Y.; Jacobs, R.J.; Anstice, N.S.; Paudel, N.; Harding, J.E.; Thompson, B. Global motion perception in 2-year-old children: A method for psychophysical assessment and relationships with clinical measures of visual function. *Investig. Opthalmology Vis. Sci.* **2013**, *54*, 8408–8419. [CrossRef] [PubMed]
37. Ostadimoghaddam, H.; Hashemi, H.; Nabovati, P.; Yekta, A.; Khabazkhoob, M. The distribution of near point of convergence and its association with age, gender and refractive error: A population-based study. *Clin. Exp. Optom.* **2017**, *100*, 255–259. [CrossRef] [PubMed]
38. Chen, A.H.; O'Leary, D.J.; Howell, E.R. Near visual function in young children. Part I: Near point of convergence. Part II: Amplitude of accommodation. Part III: Near heterophoria. *Ophthalmic Physiol. Opt.* **2000**, *20*, 185–198. [CrossRef] [PubMed]
39. Niechwiej-Szwedo, E.; Goltz, H.C.; Chandrakumar, M.; Hirji, Z.A.; Wong, A.M.F. Effects of anisometropic amblyopia on visuomotor behavior, I: Saccadic eye movements. *Investig. Opthalmology Vis. Sci.* **2010**, *51*, 6348–6354. [CrossRef]
40. Budai, A.; Czigler, A.; Mikó-Baráth, E.; Nemes, V.A.; Horváth, G.; Pusztai, Á.; Piñero, D.P.; Jandó, G. Validation of dynamic random dot stereotests in pediatric vision screening. *Graefe's Arch. Clin. Exp. Ophthalmol.* **2019**, *257*, 413–423. [CrossRef]
41. Connolly, B.H.; McClune, N.O.; Gatlin, R. Concurrent validity of the bayley-III and the peabody developmental motor scale-2. *Pediatr. Phys. Ther.* **2012**, *24*, 345–352. [CrossRef]
42. Gill, K.; Osiovich, A.; Synnes, A.; Agnew, J.; Grunau, R.E.; Miller, S.P.; Zwicker, J.G. Concurrent Validity of the Bayley-III and the Peabody Developmental Motor Scales-2 at 18 Months. *Phys. Occup. Ther. Pediatr.* **2019**, *39*, 514–524. [CrossRef]
43. Hussaindeen, J.R.; Rakshit, A.; Singh, N.K.; George, R.; Swaminathan, M.; Kapur, S.; Scheiman, M.; Ramani, K.K. Prevalence of non-strabismic anomalies of binocular vision in Tamil Nadu: Report 2 of BAND study. *Clin. Exp. Optom.* **2017**, *100*, 642–648. [CrossRef] [PubMed]
44. Jang, J.U.; Park, I.J. Prevalence of general binocular dysfunctions among rural schoolchildren in South Korea. *Taiwan J. Ophthalmol.* **2015**, *5*, 177–181. [CrossRef] [PubMed]
45. Cacho-Martínez, P.; García-Muñoz, Á.; Ruiz-Cantero, M.T. Do we really know the prevalence of accomodative and nonstrabismic binocular dysfunctions? *J. Optom.* **2010**, *3*, 185–197. [CrossRef]
46. Cacho-Martínez, P.; Cantó-Cerdán, M.; Carbonell-Bonete, S.; García-Muñoz, Á. Characterization of Visual Symptomatology Associated with Refractive, Accommodative, and Binocular Anomalies. *J. Ophthalmol.* **2015**, *2015*, 895803. [CrossRef] [PubMed]
47. Cacho-Martínez, P.; García-Muñoz, Á.; Ruiz-Cantero, M.T. Is there any evidence for the validity of diagnostic criteria used for accommodative and nonstrabismic binocular dysfunctions? *J. Optom.* **2014**, *7*, 2–21. [CrossRef]
48. DeSantis, D. Amblyopia. *Pediatric Clin. N. Am.* **2014**, *61*, 505–518. [CrossRef]
49. Kiorpes, L. Understanding the development of amblyopia using macaque monkey models. *Proc. Natl. Acad. Sci. USA* **2019**, *116*, 26217–26223. [CrossRef]
50. Guo, X.; Fu, M.; Lü, J.; Chen, Q.; Zeng, Y.; Ding, X.; Morgan, I.G.; He, M. Normative distribution of visual acuity in 3- to 6-year-old Chinese preschoolers: The Shenzhen kindergarten eye study. *Investig. Opthalmology Vis. Sci.* **2015**, *56*, 1985–1992. [CrossRef]
51. Birch, E.E.; Castañeda, Y.S.; Cheng-Patel, C.S.; Morale, S.E.; Kelly, K.R.; Beauchamp, C.L.; Webber, A. Self-perception of School-aged Children with Amblyopia and Its Association with Reading Speed and Motor Skills. *JAMA Ophthalmol.* **2019**, *137*, 167. [CrossRef]
52. Birch, E.E.; Castañeda, Y.S.; Cheng-Patel, C.S.; Morale, S.E.; Kelly, K.R.; Beauchamp, C.L.; Webber, A. Self-perception in Children Aged 3 to 7 Years with Amblyopia and Its Association with Deficits in Vision and Fine Motor Skills. *JAMA Ophthalmol.* **2019**, *137*, 499–506. [CrossRef]
53. Atkinson, J.; Nardini, M.; Anker, S.; Braddick, O.; Hughes, C.; Rae, S. Refractive errors in infancy predict reduced performance on the movement assessment battery for children at 3 1/2 and 5 1/2 years. *Dev. Med. Child Neurol.* **2005**, *47*, 243–251. [CrossRef] [PubMed]
54. Babinsky, E.; Sreenivasan, V.; Rowan Candy, T. Near heterophoria in early childhood. *Investig. Opthalmology Vis. Sci.* **2015**, *56*, 1406–1415. [CrossRef] [PubMed]
55. Troyer, M.E.; Sreenivasan, V.; Peper, T.J.; Candy, T.R. The heterophoria of 3–5 year old children as a function of viewing distance and target type. *Ophthalmic Physiol. Opt.* **2017**, *37*, 7–15. [CrossRef] [PubMed]

56. Lam, S.R.; LaRoche, G.R.; De Becker, I.; Macpherson, H. The range and variability of ophthalmological parameters in normal children aged 4 1/2 to 5 1/2 years. *J. Pediatric Ophthalmol. Strabismus* **1996**, *33*, 251–256.
57. Sreenivasan, V.; Babinsky, E.E.; Wu, Y.; Candy, T.R. Objective measurement of fusional vergence ranges and heterophoria in infants and preschool children. *Investig. Opthalmol. Vis. Sci.* **2016**, *57*, 2678–2688. [CrossRef]
58. Jeon, H.; Jung, J.H.; Yoon, J.A.; Choi, H. Strabismus Is Correlated with Gross Motor Function in Children with Spastic Cerebral Palsy. *Curr. Eye Res.* **2019**. [CrossRef]
59. Jampolsky, A. Differential Diagnostic Characteristics of Intermittent Exotropia and True Exophoria. *Am. Orthopt. J.* **1954**, *4*, 48–55. [CrossRef]
60. Barbosa, V.M.; Campbell, S.K.; Smith, E.; Berbaum, M. Comparison of Test of Infant Motor Performance (TIMP) item responses among children with cerebral palsy, developmental delay, and typical development. *Am. J. Occup. Ther.* **2005**. [CrossRef]
61. Barbosa, V.M.; Campbell, S.K.; Berbaum, M. Discriminating infants from different developmental outcome groups using the Test of Infant Motor Performance (TIMP) item responses. *Pediatr. Phys. Ther.* **2007**. [CrossRef]
62. Read, J.C.A. Stereo vision and strabismus. *Eye* **2014**, *29*, 214–224. [CrossRef]
63. Levi, D.M.; Knill, D.C.; Bavelier, D. Stereopsis and amblyopia: A mini-review. *Vis. Res.* **2015**, *114*, 17–30. [CrossRef] [PubMed]
64. Murdoch, J.R.; McGhee, C.N.G.; Glover, V. The relationship between stereopsis and fine manual dexterity: Pilot study of a new instrument. *Eye* **1991**, *5*, 642–643. [CrossRef] [PubMed]
65. Caputo, R.; Tinelli, F.; Bancale, A.; Campa, L.; Frosini, R.; Guzzetta, A.; Mercuri, E.; Cioni, G. Motor coordination in children with congenital strabismus: Effects of late surgery. *Eur. J. Paediatr. Neurol.* **2007**, *11*, 285–291. [CrossRef] [PubMed]
66. Iwasaki, T.; Nagata, T.; Tawara, A. Potential preventive effects of a new visual intervention for accommodative insufficiency and asthenopia due to sustained near task. *Ophthalmologica* **2012**, *228*, 181–187. [CrossRef]
67. Ma, M.M.-L.; Scheiman, M.; Su, C.; Chen, X. Effect of Vision Therapy on Accommodation in Myopic Chinese Children. *J. Ophthalmol.* **2016**, *2016*, 1202469. [CrossRef]

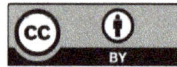

© 2020 by the authors. Licensee MDPI, Basel, Switzerland. This article is an open access article distributed under the terms and conditions of the Creative Commons Attribution (CC BY) license (http://creativecommons.org/licenses/by/4.0/).

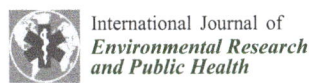

Article

Does Maternal Depression Undermine Childhood Cognitive Development? Evidence from the Young Lives Survey in Peru

Magdalena Bendini and Lelys Dinarte *

The World Bank, Washington, DC 20433, USA; mbendini@worldbank.org
* Correspondence: ldinartediaz@worldbank.org

Received: 14 August 2020; Accepted: 1 October 2020; Published: 3 October 2020

Abstract: This paper studies the effect of maternal depression on early childhood cognition in Peru, where rates of depression are around 50%. By using an instrumental variables approach, this study exploits variation in the exogeneity of the exposure to shocks during early life to instrument for maternal depression. The empirical strategy exploits a novel longitudinal data—the Young Lives survey—that includes information on cognitive outcomes of children and variation in their mothers' mental health status between rounds of data collection. Results suggest that maternal depression is detrimental to a child's vocabulary at age 5, but effects fade out by age 8. Effects do not vary by maternal education but are significant only for children living in disadvantaged households. Estimations indicate that the presence of a partner worsens the effect of maternal depression on vocabulary development, results that are driven mainly by households with heavy-drinking partners. Our findings make a strong case for recognizing maternal mental health problems as disorders of public health significance and guide maternal and infant health policies in Peru.

Keywords: child development; child vocabulary; maternal mental health; Peru

1. Introduction

Maternal depression is a major global public health challenge due to its high prevalence and direct and indirect consequences. Globally, depression is experienced by about 10 percent of pregnant women, and by 13 percent of women who have just given birth [1]. In developing countries, the prevalence of depression is almost 50 percent higher than in developed contexts: Around 15.6 percent of women experience it during pregnancy and 19.8 percent after childbirth [1]. Given the limited availability of data on maternal depression in developing countries [2] and that it remains under-diagnosed and undertreated, these figures likely represent a lower bound of the scale of the problem.

Existing studies on maternal mental health warrant concern about the economic and human costs of maternal depression, not only to the women suffering from it but also to the children in their care, given the crucial role mothers traditionally play in childrearing, particularly when children are younger [3,4]. Maternal depression is characterized by sadness, negative affect, loss of interest in daily activities, fatigue, difficulty thinking clearly, and bouts of withdrawal and intrusiveness, and may interfere with the consistent, attentive, and responsive caregiving associated with effective parenting [5]. Because mother-child interactions during early life shape foundational neural circuits [6,7], neglect or maltreatment associated with maternal depression can undermine children's brain development and lead to worse health (physical and mental), cognitive, and behavioral outcomes [8–10]. Given that it often "goes hand in hand with poverty" [6], a major concern about maternal depression is that it may increase poverty and contribute to its intergenerational transmission. In particular, maternal depression can intensify the negative effects of material deprivation and exposure to exogenous shocks associated with poverty, and confine children to substandard developmental trajectories and hence worse outcomes later in life. However, despite the potentially far-reaching harmful effects of maternal depression on mothers and child welfare, there is still a limited amount of rigorous evidence that quantifies its consequences on child development, the channels through which it acts, and how to mitigate its impact on children, particularly in developing countries.

The present paper aims to provide causal evidence of the effects of maternal mental health on children's human capital accumulation in a developing country. We study the under-explored relationship between maternal depression and child cognition, a dimension of child development that has been extensively documented as a crucial determinant of life outcomes [11–13]. We focus our analysis on the context of Peru, a developing country with a high prevalence of maternal depression.

To shed light on the issue, we conducted our analysis using information from the Young Lives (YL) survey in Peru, a rich longitudinal household survey that follows households with at least one child born between 2001 and 2002 (index child). For our analysis, we used YL's first three rounds: A baseline round in 2002, when the index child was 6–20 months old, the first follow-up when the child was 4–6 years old, and the last round in 2009–2010, when the child index was 7–8 years of age. The YL also has the novelty that includes questions related to maternal mental health and a child's vocabulary, along with a wealth of information on child, family, and community characteristics.

Inspired by the literature that links the exposure to shocks during pregnancy, maternal mental health, and children's outcomes, we employed an instrumental variable (IV) approach as an estimation strategy. This approach helps us to address the reverse causality bias in the estimation of the effect of maternal depression on a child's vocabulary. We exploit the richness and longitudinal nature of the data to better capture the dynamic nature of maternal mental health on child cognitive development at the age of 5 and 8 years old. In particular, we instrument maternal depression with having experienced a shock (loss of crop or livestock) at baseline (when the child was in utero or recently born). We also strengthen the robustness of the analysis by considering variations of the indicator used for maternal depression, exploring heterogeneous effects of household characteristics, such as mother's education, household wealth, and the presence of a male partner and some of his characteristics. Given the large set of potential controls, and to avoid overfitting the model or omitted variables bias, we used a machine learning procedure to select the instruments and controls to include in our model.

The remainder of the paper is organized as follows. In the next section, we describe our research design, including details on the data we are using for our analysis and some descriptive statistics. In Results, we present the main results, including some robustness checks. Finally, in Discussion and Conclusions, we discuss the policy implications, this paper's contribution to the literature, and conclude.

2. Materials and Methods

In this section, we briefly described the data we used to assess the impact of maternal depression on early child vocabulary in Peru. Then, we presented some descriptive statistics of the different rounds of data used in our analysis. Since we restricted our study to the sample that had information across all rounds, we also briefly described the results from the sample attrition analysis.

2.1. Data

2.1.1. Description

To measure the effects of MMH on child development, we used the first 3 rounds of the Young Lives Peru Survey (YL), conducted by the University of Oxford and core-funded by the UK Department for International Development. The YL survey was also being conducted in Vietnam, Ethiopia, and India (Andra Pradesh region). As of now, 5 rounds of data have been collected, which can be publicly accessible through the Young Lives website (https://www.younglives.org.uk/content/data-research). This was a rich longitudinal survey that included a complete set of individual, parental, household, and community characteristics, including early developmental, economic and demographic indicators, as well as information about social assistance programs in every community. The baseline sample of YL was cluster stratified, with 20 districts randomly selected across the country. Because the YL project was particularly interested in children living in poorer households, the sampling frame excluded the top 5 percent of districts as measured by a district poverty ranking. Despite excluding the least poor, it has been documented that the data reflects the Peruvian population in a broad range of indicators. Within each of the selected districts, 100 households with at least one child born between 2001 and 2002 (index child) were chosen randomly to participate in the project. Within each household, YL surveyed an index child who was born in 2000–2001 and was followed from infancy until they reached their mid-teens. The baseline round was conducted in 2002 when the index children were aged 6–20 months, the first follow-up conducted in 2006/2007, when they were between 4 and 6 years old, and the last round in 2009/2010, when they were between 7 and 8 years of age. The attrition rate between the 3 rounds of data collection was approximately 4 percent, which was low by international standards [14].

Of the 2000 index children in the baseline round, we focused our analysis on the sample of 1095 of them that were present in the first 3 waves for whom data on maternal mental health and Peabody Picture Vocabulary Test (PPVT) scores were available. We presented below tests for differences in some characteristics between the included and excluded samples.

2.1.2. Measures of a Dimension of Child Development

We use PPVT scores [15] as the measure of early vocabulary skills, a strong predictor of later cognitive ability, including writing and reading skills, schooling, and labor market outcomes later in life [13,16–18]. In the YL survey, this outcome was measured using the Spanish version of the PPVT instrument. The PPVT measures receptive vocabulary; children are shown slides, each of which has 4 pictures, and were asked to identify the picture that corresponded to objects or actions named by the test administrator. Children did not need to name the objects or actions or be able to read or write them. It was just an object identification or association process. The test continued until the child had made 6 mistakes in the last 8 slides. The number and the level of difficulty of questions differed according to children's age (see [19]). We, therefore, constructed age-specific z-scores by subtracting the month-of-age-specific mean of the raw score and dividing by the month-of-age-specific standard deviation. PPVT scores were available in the 2nd and 3rd rounds of the YL survey, i.e., when children were 4–6 and 7–8 years.

2.1.3. Measures of Maternal Mental Health

The explanatory variable was constructed using the information on maternal common mental disorders from the Self Reporting Questionnaire 20 items (SRQ20), a screening (case-finding) tool included in the YL survey. The SRQ20 consisted of 20 yes/no questions with a reference period of the previous 30 days. The tool had a number of limitations, including the small number of items, the fact that it was not diagnostic, and could not separate out anxiety from depression. Still, the tool had been recommended by the World Health Organization and has acceptable levels of reliability and validity in developing countries. To the extent that depression and anxiety are closely related, and both of them can undermine the quality of care mothers provide to their children, the information gathered from the questionnaire was very valuable. Henceforth, we will use the term mental health to refer to both cases of depression and/or anxiety.

Using the responses to the questionnaire, we estimated 3 mental health indexes: The simple average of all items and 2 standardized items using factor analysis and principal components analysis. As we explain below, we used the information on maternal mental health from the first round of the YL survey.

2.1.4. External Shocks

We exploited the availability of data on exposure to external shocks in the first round of the Peruvian YL. Caregivers were asked about events or changes that negatively affected the household welfare, and that occurred since the mother of the index child was pregnant until the day of the interview. The survey respondents described the event, and the enumerator classified it among the 14 categories. We grouped these categories into 6 groups of shocks, including natural disaster, crop or livestock loss, decrease in food availability, job or income loss, death or severe illness, and birth/new household member.

2.1.5. Other Relevant Variables

In addition to the outcomes of interest and data on shocks, we used additional variables available in the survey that we used to address potential concerns to our identification strategy, as we explained in the following section. These additional variables consist of indexes that captured information on wealth, housing quality, and consumption of durable goods. These indexes were created using information reported by the caregivers. In each round, they were asked about the assets they own, characteristics of the household (materials of the floor, walls, etc.), among others. To collect consumption data, caregivers were asked how much they spent on non-food items during the last 30 days or on durable goods over the last 12 months.

2.2. Descriptive Statistics

Table 1 reports the summary statistics of the variables used in this paper for the sample under analysis. We separated the variables into 4 panels by mother, child, household, and community characteristics. Columns 1–3 presented mean, standard deviation, and the number of observations for the sample in the 2006/2007 round. Similarly, columns 4–6 showed the same statistics for the 3rd YL round (2009/2010).

Table 1. Descriptive Statistics by Survey Round.

Variables	(1)	(2)	(3)	(4)	(5)	(6)
	Year 2006/2007			Year 2009/2010		
	Mean	S.D.	N	Mean	S.D.	N
Panel A. Maternal characteristics						
Age of the mother (years)	31.43	6.64	1095	33.71	6.64	1095
Indigenous ethnic group	0.16	0.37	1095	–	–	–
Less than primary school	0.57	0.50	1095	–	–	–
Literate	0.79	0.41	1095	–	–	–
Attended antenatal care in 2002	0.94	0.23	1095	–	–	–
Mother has Mental Health Problems in 2002	0.30	0.46	1095			
Panel B. Child characteristics						
Child is a boy	0.50	0.50	1095	–	–	–
Weight at birth (kg)	3.21	0.51	1095	–	–	–
Long-term health problems	0.09	0.09	1095	–	–	–
Age (in months)	63.5	4.71	1095	94.9	3.58	1095
Child is the eldest	0.16	0.37	1095	0.23	0.42	1095
Height for age Z-score	−1.42	1.08	1095	−1.05	1.02	1095
PPVT score (raw)	29.9	17.4	1095	47.6	12.9	1095
PPVT Z-score	0.06	0.98	1095	0.07	0.95	1095
Panel C. Household characteristics						
Wealth index	0.49	0.22	1095	0.56	0.20	1095
Housing quality index	0.41	0.24	1095	0.44	0.24	1095
Consumption of durable goods index	0.37	0.23	1095	0.45	0.23	1095
Live in urban area	0.58	0.49	1095	0.76	0.43	1095
Household size	5.52	2.13	1095	5.44	1.94	1095
School aged children in the household (n)	1.33	1.25	1095	1.09	1.05	1095
Panel D. Community characteristics						
Violent crime in community	0.33	0.47	1095	0.36	0.48	1095
Social assistance (education) available	0.95	0.22	1095	0.98	0.13	1095

Table 1 present summary statistics (mean and standard deviation) of the variables used in the analysis. These variables are available in the first three rounds of the Peruvian Young Lives Survey. The sample is restricted to children with available information on maternal mental health in 2002 and PPVT scores in 2006 and 2009.

As presented in Panel A, mothers were 31–35 years old on average between the 2 rounds. On average, 16% of these mothers reported being of indigenous origin, and although 79% of them reported they were literate, 57% had not completed primary school. Finally, statistics showed that 30% of mothers had mental health issues in 2002, and 94% of them reported that they attended antenatal care while they were pregnant from the index child. In terms of children's characteristics (Panel B), half of index children were boys and 16% of them were the eldest. Cognitive outcomes, as measured by PPVT Z-scores, were practically unchanged between the 2 rounds, even if, as expected, the mean score increased as the children age, reflecting a larger vocabulary. The average child in the sample scored 0.06 standard deviations above the mean PPVT score of a reference child in both 2006/2007 and 2009/2010. Children's height-for-age Z-scores, on the other hand, showed an improving trend.

To summarize information at the household level, we created some indexes that captured information on wealth, housing quality, and consumption of durable goods (see Panel C). Each of these indexes took values between 0 to 1. A household with an index level close to 0 (1) indicated that the family was worse (better) in the particular dimension that the index was measuring. In 2007, the average household in the sample under analysis was below the median of the distribution in all indexes. The wealth and housing quality indexes of the average household from our sample remained similar between the 2 rounds. Only the consumption of durable goods index increased between 2006–2009, which can be related to an increase in the number of older household members that consumed more expensive durable goods. Moreover, 58% of households under analysis lived in urban areas and had 5.5 members on average, 1.3 of them were school-aged children in 2006/2007. Three years after, 18% of households were more likely to live in urban areas.

Appendix A compared the sample under analysis with the observations excluded from the study. There are only 2 differences in maternal characteristics between these 2 sub-samples, and the difference remained statistically significant at 10%: Mothers in the sample were less likely to have completed primary school and were less likely to live in urban areas.

2.3. Empirical Strategy

What were the ways in which maternal depression can undermine children's cognitive outcomes? We framed our analysis following Frank and Meara's Model (FMM) [20] of maternal depression effects on the formation of children's skill, which was inspired by Cunha and Heckman's inter-generational model of human capability formation [13,21]. FMM assumed that a skill S was constituted in period t, through a production function f and several determinants that occurred in the previous period ($t-1$). In sum, the model can be represented as follows:

$$S_t = f(S_{t-1}, I_{t-1}, PS; M_{t-1},) \qquad (1)$$

where S is the level of skill formation, PS represents parental skill attributes (education, cognitive abilities, etc.), I_{t-1} indicates monetary and non-monetary investments in child capabilities, and M_{t-1} is maternal mental health status at time $t-1$. Mental health problems that interfered with mother-child interactions or undermined maternal behavior during $t-1$ could potentially undercut the effectiveness of parental skills and/or reduce the productivity of investments and result in deficient children's cognitive ability later in life.

To empirically estimate this theoretical model, we exploited information on maternal mental health during the 1st round and data on cognitive outcomes for our sample of 1095 children for which we have information of PPVT Z-scores from the 2nd and 3rd rounds of data collection. A naïve estimation of the effects of exposure to lagged maternal stress on cognitive development will regress a measure of maternal stress in 2002 on the PPVT Z-scores in 2006/2007 and 2009/2010, using the following specification:

$$PPVT_{i,t} = \alpha_0 + \alpha_1 MH_{i,t-1} + \alpha_2 C_{i,t} + \alpha_3 M_{i,t} + \alpha_4 H_{i,t} + \epsilon_{it} \qquad (2)$$

where $PPVT_{i,t}$ represents the PPVT Z-scores for child i in period t (i.e., 2006/2007 or 2009/2010). $MH_{i,t-1}$ captures the value of any of the three maternal mental health indexes we estimated using data from 2002. $C_{i,t}$, $M_{i,t}$, and $H_{i,t}$ are vectors of child, mother, and household/community observable and time-varying characteristics that can lead to differences in cognitive ability across children and influence their parents' investments in them. These vectors include all the variables presented in Table 1, all of which have been documented to affect children cognition (for a review, see [6]). ϵ_{it} represents a random, idiosyncratic error term.

Under the assumption of complete exogeneity of $MH_{i,t-1}$, the parameter of interest, $\hat{\alpha}_1$, measures performance in the PPVT at each period t for children whose mothers were depressed in 2002. The fact that the specification used measures of maternal depression and child's vocabulary taken at different points in time addressed, to a large extent, the possibility of reverse causality. However, the probability that there were unobserved factors, such as pollution, access to services, or changes that had affected the household between rounds—that influenced maternal mental health and children's outcomes cannot be entirely ruled out. Consequently, we used an instrumental variable (IV) approach to address the possibility of omitted variable bias.

In addition, the IV estimation helped to remedy the problem of measurement error in the main explanatory variable, which could be a relevant factor in the context of this paper. In particular, our main explanatory variable captured symptoms of mental health issues that affected mothers 30 days prior to the survey in 2002. We used those symptoms and estimated indexes of mental health, which constituted proxies of the unobserved, latent variable $MH^*_{i,t-1}$. Thus, estimations of Equation (2) that incorporated the proxy for maternal depression can produce inconsistent estimators of α_1 and lead to attenuation bias of these coefficients if $MH_{i,t-1}$ and the error term $\epsilon_{i,t}$ are negatively correlated [22,23].

The IV approach hinges on finding observable covariates that are correlated with maternal mental health, but which do not affect child cognitive status or other possible omitted variables. Considering this, we define our instrument by relying on the existing evidence that identifies the negative effect of exposure to exogenous shocks during pregnancy or during the first months after birth on children cognitive outcomes [3,24–29]. Some of these papers find that the main mechanism driving this relationship is maternal stress induced by the shock. Therefore, by exploiting the fact that the first round of YL asked caregivers about exposure to shocks, we use them to instrument maternal mental health. We excluded natural disasters and decreases in food availability due to lack of variation (less than 0.18% of households reported any of these shocks) and job or income loss because it can be highly correlated with the fact that the woman just gave birth. Hence, we restricted our analysis to the remaining three shocks–loss of crop or livestock, death or severe illness, or changes in their household composition—as potential instruments of maternal mental health. In this sense, Equation (2) corresponds to our second stage estimation, and our first stage will be given by the following:

$$MH_{i,t-1} = \beta_0 + \beta_1 S^j_{i,t-1} + X_i + \epsilon_i \qquad (3)$$

where $S^j_{i,t-1}$ indicates if the mother of child i was affected by shock j and X_i represent the vectors of child, mother, and household characteristics described in Equation (2).

The validity of the instrument had to meet 2 conditions. First, it had to be relevant. In other words, the correlation between the shock and maternal mental health had to be high and statistically different from zero. To test this condition, we presented statistics of the shocks and measures of maternal mental health in Table 2, panels A and B. Panel C summarizes the correlations between each measure of maternal mental health and the three shocks under analysis. All correlations were statistically significant. In particular, the correlation between the loss of crop or livestock and the different indexes of maternal mental health ranges between 0.34 to 0.70.

The second condition for the instrument to be valid was exogeneity. In other words, suffering a shock during pregnancy or during the 1st months after birth should not have an impact on children's vocabulary at the age of 5 other than through the impact on maternal mental health in the period when the shock occurred. There were 3 potential concerns that might affect this assumption, but we aimed to address those concerns with our specification. First, there was the concern of the nutritional effect of an income shock. A past shock can affect children's nutritional status in $t-1$, which can then translate into worse cognitive development later in life. To address this concern, we controlled for several children anthropometric measures. A 2nd concern was the learning resources: The shock could limit the exposure of the child to enriching opportunities or materials that might help her to improve her vocabulary development during childhood. To control for this potential channel, we included in our specification some measures of household wealth and consumption in $t-1$. Finally, the 3rd concern was that the shock limited additional stimulation that might have been provided to her by other members in the household, in addition to the mother and her partner. For example, in extended households, non-working relatives tended to contribute to childcare duties. The shock may forced these other household members to find a job, which could, in turn, limit opportunities for child stimulation and consequent development. Since extended households were larger than the non-extended ones, we controlled for that characteristic by including the variable household size in our model. Alternatively, we tested the exogeneity assumption in our model by estimating the correlation between the measure of vocabulary and the shock, conditional on the variables that captured differences in availability of learning resources, child's nutritional status, and the rest of the control variables. These results are presented in Appendix B.

Table 2. Correlations between Shocks and Maternal Mental Health Indexes (MHI) in 2002.

	(1)	(2)	(3)
Panel A. Descriptive statistics of Maternal MHI	Mean	S.D.	N
MHI-1	−0.02	0.50	1095
MHI-2	−0.04	0.98	1095
MHI-3	−0.04	0.92	1095
Panel B. Shocks experienced by mothers during pregnancy or within the first year after the child was born (in 2002)	Mean	S.D.	N
Crop or livestock loss	0.03	0.16	1095
Death, severe illness, divorce	0.13	0.34	1095
Birth/new household member	0.06	0.24	1095
Panel C. Correlations between shocks and Maternal MHI in 2002	MHI-1	MHI-2	MHI-3
Crop or livestock loss	0.34 ***	0.70 ***	0.65 ***
Death, severe illness, divorce	0.15 ***	0.32 ***	0.29 ***
Birth/new household member	0.13 **	0.27 **	0.24 **

Table 2 presents summary statistics (mean and standard deviation) of maternal mental health indexes and shocks experienced by mothers of our sample of analysis. These variables are available in the first round of the Peruvian Young Lives Survey (2002). The sample is restricted to children with available information on maternal mental health in 2002 and PPVT scores in 2006 and 2009. Mental health index 1 is the standardized average of the SRQ-20 items. Panel A presents statistics of mental health indexes. Mental health index 2 and 3 are standardized indexes estimated using principal components and factor analysis, respectively. Panel B presents the % of mothers reporting being exposed to any of the four shocks. Panel C shows correlations between the mental health indexes and shocks. *** and ** indicate statistical significance at 1% and 5%, respectively.

Finally, having at least three instruments and a large set of potential control variables posited the challenge of selecting the "right" set of them. On the one hand, using too few controls or the wrong ones may lead to omitted variable bias. However, by using too many, our model may be affected by overfitting. To address this issue, we estimate the parameters of interest using the Instrumental Variables Least Absolute Shrinkage and Selection Operator (IV-LASSO), a routine for estimating structural parameters in linear models with many controls and/or instruments. In particular, we used the post-double selection (PDS) methodology [30,31] that was applied in Stata's built-in commands by Ahrens et al. [32].

3. Results

We found three main results. First, maternal depression was detrimental to a child's vocabulary at the age of 5, but the effect faded out by age 8. Our estimations indicated that 1 standard deviation of maternal depression during pregnancy and postpartum reduced the vocabulary of 5-year-old children—measured through PPTV scores—in 0.54 standard deviations. This impact is no longer statistically significant at the age of 8, even considering different measures of maternal depression. The magnitude of these effects is large and consistent with the upper bound found in the existing literature.

Second, heterogeneity analysis by household wealth shows that these effects were driven by children living in disadvantaged households. When the impact of maternal depression was analyzed separately by household wealth, there was evidence of worse effects for less wealthy households, providing suggestive evidence that maternal mental illness may contribute to the intergenerational transmission of poverty given the high rates of depression among low-income mothers cited in the literature.

Finally, we explored if the presence of household members that supported mothers can dampen the effect of experiencing a shock that affects maternal mental health. We focused on the presence of a partner in the household when the woman was pregnant or during the first year after childbirth. Our estimations indicated that mental health issues of women living with a partner when they experienced a shock effect more their child's vocabulary than those without a partner. Upon further exploration, we found that women living with heavy-drinking partners were the ones driving the negative impacts on the child's cognitive development. In this sense, this set of results indicates that it is not the presence of a partner in itself that matters, but the quality of such partners.

3.1. Main Results

Table 3 reports the main results of the paper. Columns 1–3 present results for Ordinary Least Squares (OLS) with PDS-selected variables and full regressor set. Each column shows the results for a measure of mental health, as defined above. Columns 4–6 show results for the IV with PDS-selected variables and full regressor set as depicted in Equation (2).

First-stage estimates for the exposure to an external shock on maternal mental health are presented in Panel B. Selected instrument by the LASSO regression was suffering crop or livestock loss during pregnancy or within the first year of the index child. The outcome variable was a measure of maternal mental health in 2002. The coefficient indicated changes in maternal mental health after experiencing a shock of crop or livestock loss during pregnancy or after giving birth. Across columns, the precision of the estimate does not change, but the size of the coefficients is sensible to the measure of mental health used.

As presented in Panel A, our IV estimations indicate that poor maternal mental health has a negative impact on child cognition. An increase by one standard deviation in maternal mental health problems when children were 1-year-old or younger was associated with a reduction of 0.5–0.54 standard deviations in vocabulary Z-scores when children were 5 years old. This effect corresponds to a reduction of 31 percent of the mean PPVT raw score. These large estimated effects were consistent with existing evidence. For example, Aizer et al. [3] found that exposure to stress hormones in utero negatively affects cognition (verbal IQ at age 7), behavior, and motor development. Specifically, the authors found that exposure to cortisol in the top quintile of the distribution was associated with a 43 percent of a standard deviation reduction in verbal IQ.

The LASSO regression selected the following controls: Mother's age, wealth index, living in an urban area, child's age, consumption of durable goods index, household size, number of children younger than 5 years in the household, and height for age Z-score. The effects on child cognition of demographic controls (not shown in the table) are in the expected direction. Z-scores of children living in urban areas were higher than those of children living in an urban area. In addition, children's nutritional status also affected performance in the PPVT. The coefficients for wealth were positive, statistically significant, and among the highest, which was in line with research that points to socioeconomic status gradients of cognition as measured by vocabulary [16,33–35].

Table 3. Effect of maternal mental health on children's vocabulary at age 5.

	Dependent Variable: Standardized PPVT					
	(1)	(2)	(3)	(4)	(5)	(6)
Panel A. Estimated coefficients from OLS and IV estimation approaches	OLS with PDS-selected variables and full regressor set			IV with PDS-selected variables and full regressor set		
	MHI-1	MHI-2	MHI-3	MHI-1	MHI-2	MHI-3
Maternal Mental Health	−0.0314	−0.0157	−0.0173	−1.025 *	−0.499 *	−0.536 **
	(0.0513)	(0.0254)	(0.0275)	(0.527)	(0.255)	(0.274)
Observations	1095	1095	1095	1095	1095	1095
Mother controls	Yes	Yes	Yes	Yes	Yes	Yes
Child controls	Yes	Yes	Yes	Yes	Yes	Yes
Household controls	Yes	Yes	Yes	Yes	Yes	Yes
Panel B. First-stage estimation				MHI-1	MHI-2	MHI-3
Shock: Crop or livestock loss				0.573 ***	0.616 ***	0.300 ***
				(0.165)	(0.179)	(0.088)
Observations				1095	1095	1095
Mother controls				Yes	Yes	Yes
Child controls				Yes	Yes	Yes
Household controls				Yes	Yes	Yes
Weak identification F-Stats (Full IV set)				11.53	11.69	11.75

Panel A in Table 3 presents the estimated impacts of maternal mental health on children vocabulary at the age of 5 years obtained from Equation (2), using Ordinary Least Squares (OLS) and Instrumental Variables (IV) as estimation approaches. The dependent variable was measured using the standardized value of the PPVT test. Mental health indexes are standardized values of the SRQ-20 items using three different estimation approaches. Columns (1–3) present estimated coefficients using OLS and columns (4–6) show coefficients using IV. Both approaches were implemented using the option PDS-selected variables and full regressor available in the LASSO command. The selected instrument was suffering crop or livestock loss during pregnancy or within the first year of the index child. Selected controls are mother's age, wealth index, living in an urban area, child's age, consumption of durable goods index, household size, number of children younger than 5 years in the household, and height for age Z-score. The sample is restricted to children with available information on maternal mental health in 2002 and PPVT scores in 2006 and 2009. *, ** and *** indicate statistical significance at 10%, 5% and 1%, respectively. Confidence intervals at the 95% confidence are presented in Appendix C. Robust standard errors in parentheses.

We then explored if these negative impacts were held three years after the first measure of vocabulary. Using data of child vocabulary at the age of 8, we estimated the model presented in Equations (2) and (3). The main results are presented in Table 4. Our estimations showed that maternal depression had no effect on the child's vocabulary at the age of 8. Not only were the estimated coefficients not statistically significant, but also their sizes were very small—that is, the vocabulary of children whose mothers' experienced mental health problems when they were 1-year-old caught up with the vocabulary of children whose mothers did not suffer mental health problems. As we present in the table in Appendix D, the effects of a shock on maternal mental health are not statistically significant a year after the woman experienced the shock. These results suggest that the effect of exposure to maternal depression during early childhood need not undermine language development permanently, and exposure to rich vocabulary environments later on during childhood can compensate for earlier developmental gaps. For our sample, it is possible that the convergence in vocabulary development is explained by the fact that by the time they reached age 8, all children had had exposure to formal education opportunities (99.9% of children in our sample), which may have a compensatory effect on children's vocabulary development. Still, given that early vocabulary constitutes a foundational skill that facilitates the development of other cognitive skills, based on our results, we cannot rule out the possibility that exposure to maternal depression during early life does not undermine cognitive development and academic achievement.

3.2. Heterogeneity by Household Characteristics

We explore heterogeneous effects by a number of maternal characteristics that have been identified in the literature as moderators of the effect of mental health, using our main model and all measures of mental health.

Table 4. Effect of maternal mental health on children's vocabulary at age 8.

	Dependent Variable: Standardized PPVT					
	(1)	(2)	(3)	(4)	(5)	(6)
Panel A. OLS and IV second-stage estimations	OLS with PDS-selected variables and full regressor set			IV with PDS-selected variables and full regressor set		
	MHI-1	MHI-2	MHI-3	MHI-1	MHI-2	MHI-3
Maternal Mental Health	0.006	0.006	0.008	−0.065	−0.032	−0.034
	(0.0471)	−0.0233	(0.0253)	(0.501)	(0.245)	(0.265)
Observations	1095	1095	1095	1095	1095	1095
Mother controls	Yes	Yes	Yes	Yes	Yes	Yes
Child controls	Yes	Yes	Yes	Yes	Yes	Yes
Household controls	Yes	Yes	Yes	Yes	Yes	Yes
Panel B. First-stage estimation				MHI-1	MHI-2	MHI-3
Shock: Crop or livestock loss				0.338 ***	0.689 ***	0.639 ***
				(0.091)	(0.184)	(0.172)
Observations				1095	1095	1095
Mother controls				Yes	Yes	Yes
Child controls				Yes	Yes	Yes
Household controls				Yes	Yes	Yes
Weak identification F-Stats (Full IV set)				13.61	13.65	11.75

Table 4 presents the effects of maternal mental health on children's vocabulary at the age of 8 years. The dependent variable was measured using the standardized value of the PPVT test. Mental health indexes are standardized values of the SRQ-20 items using three different estimation approaches. Columns (1–3) present estimated coefficients using OLS and columns (4–6) show coefficients using IV. Both approaches were implemented using the option PDS-selected variables and full regressor available in the LASSO command. The selected instrument was suffering crop or livestock loss during pregnancy or within the first year of the index child. Selected controls are mother's age, the mother is indigenous, mother literacy, wealth index, living in an urban area, consumption of durable goods index, and height for age Z-score. *, ** and *** indicate statistical significance at 10%, 5% and 1%, respectively.

First, we run separated regressions by different levels of household wealth, which, it is generally agreed, influences the extent to which maternal mental health affects children [3,6,36]. For our analysis, we compared the vocabulary of children living with mothers with different mental health levels within the upper or lower half of the wealth distribution. Using data from the 2002 round, we estimated three indexes: Housing quality, consumer durables, and services indexes. Then, we created a wealth index for each household of our sample that consisted of the average of the three first ones mentioned above. Using the wealth index distribution, we separated our sample by the median of the wealth index distribution. The results are presented in Table 5. Our estimations indicate that 1 standard deviation of maternal mental health issues reduces vocabulary by 0.58 to 0.63 standard deviations of children living in less wealthy households (columns 4–6). This is around 0.08 standard deviations more than the impacts in the total sample. The effects of maternal mental health on the vocabulary of children living in wealthier households are not statistically significant.

These results are an important contribution to the evidence of intergenerational transmission of poverty. Poor households are less able to protect themselves from external shocks, such as crop or livestock losses, which then increases stress levels for household heads. In low-income families where there is a pregnant woman or with a child younger than 1-year-old, our results indicate that the negative shock translates into a reduction in the child's cognitive skills in the short term. Giving that the development of these skills during early childhood is the foundation of future ones [13,16–18], this negative effect can have long-lasting impacts in terms of human capital accumulation, which is in line with existing literature indicating that events before five years old can have large long-term impacts on adult outcomes [3,37].

The existing literature has also found that maternal schooling levels may modulate the impact of depression [6,38]. A recent paper by Aizer et al. [3] finds that mothers with low levels of human capital are characterized by higher stress levels and that the negative impact of their elevated stress levels on their children is greater. We explore this heterogeneity using the YL data by separating the sample into two groups: Mothers with less than primary education and mothers with at least primary education completed. Our estimations are presented in Table 6. Unlike the existing literature, there are no apparent differences in the effect of maternal mental health for mothers who have completed or not primary education.

Table 5. Heterogeneous effects of Maternal Mental Health on Children Vocabulary at Age 5 by HH Wealth Level.

	Dependent Variable: Standardized PPVT					
	(1)	(2)	(3)	(4)	(5)	(6)
	IV with PDS-selected variables and full regressor set					
	Effects on children from wealthier HH			Effects on children from less wealthy HH		
	MHI-1	MHI-2	MHI-3	MHI-1	MHI-2	MHI-3
Maternal Mental Health	−2.971	−1.427	−1.509	−1.194 *	−0.581 *	−0.625 *
	(4.212)	(2.009)	(2.111)	(0.661)	(0.319)	(0.342)
Constant	1.098	1.101	1.098	1.147 **	1.157 **	1.158 **
	(0.869)	(0.854)	(0.839)	(0.583)	(0.576)	(0.574)
Observations	514	514	514	581	581	581
Mother controls	Yes	Yes	Yes	Yes	Yes	Yes
Child controls	Yes	Yes	Yes	Yes	Yes	Yes
Household controls	Yes	Yes	Yes	Yes	Yes	Yes

Table 5 presents estimated effects of maternal mental health on child vocabulary at age 5, separated by whether the HH is in the upper or lower wealth half of the distribution. We estimate the model selected from LASSO procedure. The selected control regressor set includes the mother's age, wealth index, living in an urban area, child's age, consumption of durable goods index, household size, number of children younger than 5 years in the household, and height for age Z-score. The sample is restricted to children with available information on maternal mental health in 2002 and PPVT scores in 2006 and 2009. Robust standard errors in parentheses. * and ** indicate statistical significance at 10%, and 5%, respectively.

Table 6. Heterogeneous effects of maternal mental health on children's vocabulary at age 5 by the educational level of the mother.

	Dependent Variable: Standardized PPVT					
	(1)	(2)	(3)	(4)	(5)	(6)
	IV with PDS-selected variables and full regressor set					
	Effects on children from mothers with primary incomplete			Effects on children from mothers with at least primary education complete		
	MHI-1	MHI-2	MHI-3	MHI-1	MHI-2	MHI-3
Maternal Mental Health	−0.799	−0.389	−0.419	−1.829	−0.889	−0.949
	(0.513)	(0.249)	(0.268)	(1.848)	(0.885)	(0.937)
Constant	1.292 ***	1.299 ***	1.300 ***	0.739	0.736	0.739
	(0.401)	(0.398)	(0.397)	(0.778)	(0.771)	(0.763)
Observations	719	719	719	376	376	376
Mother controls	Yes	Yes	Yes	Yes	Yes	Yes
Child controls	Yes	Yes	Ye	Yes	Yes	Yes
Household controls	Yes	Yes	Yes	Yes	Yes	Yes

Table 6 presents the estimated effects of maternal mental health on child vocabulary at age 5, separated by whether the mother has completed at least primary education or not. We estimate the model selected from LASSO procedure. The selected control regressor set includes the mother's age, wealth index, living in an urban area, child's age, consumption of durable goods index, household size, number of children younger than 5 years in the household, and height for age Z-score. The sample is restricted to children with available information on maternal mental health in 2002 and PPVT scores in 2006 and 2009. Robust standard errors in parentheses. *** indicates statistical significance at 1%.

However, when we combine the heterogeneity by household wealth and maternal education, we find out that our results are still in line with the existing literature for two reasons. First, the papers finding that lower maternal education exacerbates the negative effect of maternal mental health on early vocabulary argue that this low maternal education can be associated with sub-optimal childcare practices or to restricted access to quality material inputs and opportunities. Access to quality inputs that help to improve children's vocabulary is restricted to less wealthy households as well. Second, there is extensive evidence of a strong correlation between a mother's education and socioeconomic status. In this sense, the expected differences in terms of lack of resources that allow overcoming the negative effects of maternal mental health on child language are captured not by maternal education but by household wealth in this particular context.

In addition, we explore whether the effects of exposure to maternal mental health issues during a child's young age varies depending on whether the mother has a partner, given that this factor may modulate the impact of depression. The literature suggests that the presence of other members in the household that provide support to the mother can buffer the effect of depression on children. Our results are presented in Table 7. Our estimates suggest that having a partner can actually worsen the negative effects of maternal mental health issues on a child's vocabulary (Columns 1–3).

Table 7. Heterogeneous effects of maternal mental health on children vocabulary at age 5 by the mother's marital status and partner's drinking behavior.

	Dependent Variable: Standardized PPVT								
	(1)	(2)	(3)	(4)	(5)	(6)	(7)	(8)	(9)
	IV with PDS-selected variables and full regressor set								
	Effects on children from mothers with a partner			Effects on children from mothers with a drinking partner			Effects on children from mothers with a heavily-drinking partner		
	MHI-1	MHI-2	MHI-3	MHI-1	MHI-2	MHI-3	MHI-1	MHI-2	MHI-3
Maternal Mental Health	−0.889 *	−0.433 *	−0.465 *	−1.070 **	−0.518 **	−0.556 **	−1.150 **	−0.549 **	−0.587 **
	(0.459)	(0.222)	(0.239)	(0.511)	(0.246)	(0.264)	(0.573)	(0.270)	(0.287)
Constant	1.144 ***	1.147 ***	1.148 ***	1.195 ***	1.201 ***	1.200 ***	1.653 ***	1.642 ***	1.633 ***
	(0.339)	(0.337)	(0.336)	(0.379)	(0.376)	(0.375)	(0.439)	(0.434)	(0.432)
Observations	963	963	963	770	770	770	486	486	486
Mother controls	Yes	Yes	Yes	Yes	Yes	Yes	Yes	Yes	Yes
Child controls	Yes	Yes	Yes	Yes	Yes	Yes	Yes	Yes	Yes
Household controls	Yes	Yes	Yes	Yes	Yes	Yes	Yes	Yes	Yes

Table 7 presents the estimated effects of maternal mental health on child vocabulary at age 5, separated by whether the mother lives with a partner and his drinking likelihood. We estimate the model selected from LASSO procedure. The selected control regressor set includes the mother's age, wealth index, living in an urban area, child's age, consumption of durable goods index, household size, number of children younger than 5 years in the household, and height for age Z-score. The sample is restricted to children with available information on maternal mental health in 2002 and PPVT scores in 2006 and 2009. Robust standard errors in parentheses. *, ** and *** indicate statistical significance at 10%, 5% and 1%, respectively.

To understand these unexpected results, we further explore the characteristics of the partner. First, we separate the sample of women living with a drinking (columns 4–6) and a heavily-drinking partner (columns 7–9). Our estimations indicate that Z-scores of children with mothers whose mental health was 1sd worse at $t-1$ and lived with a drinking partner was, on average, 0.52 to 0.56 standard deviations lower than Z-scores of children of mothers who were also living with a drinking partner. These coefficients were statistically significant at the five percent level. Moreover, the estimated coefficients for the effects of mentally ill mothers living with heavily-drinking partners indicated that this group was driving the effects described before.

A potential explanation of these results was the alcohol-induced physical intimate partner violence (AIPIPV). Existing evidence from psychology shows that Intimate Partner Violence (IPV) is a major predictor of post-traumatic stress disorder in abused women [39] and can drive to negative interactions between mother and children [40], directly affecting child development [41]. Using YL data, Bedoya et al. [41] found that IPV was one of the main forms of violence against women in Peru. The authors also found that early-life exposure to AIPIPV was indeed associated with lower test scores in vocabulary.

A second explanation was budget constraints. Allocating household income to consume alcohol reduces the availability of resources in the household for other needs, including inputs that help to support child development. This creates a vicious cycle for mothers with mental health issues since it can impose additional stressors.

4. Discussion

Results in this paper underscore children's incredible resilience, while at the same time provide further evidence that maternal depression can undermine children's development. Moreover, the heterogeneous findings by household wealth and quality of partner, combined with extensive evidence in the literature of the disproportionally high prevalence rates of anxiety and depression among households with low socio-economic status around the world cited in this paper's introduction, suggests that maternal mental illness may contribute to the intergenerational transmission of poverty. In addition, stress, in general, and associated maternal mental illness in particular, constitute yet another pathway from poverty to substandard developmental trajectories and potentially worse outcomes later in life.

What are the implications of these findings for policymakers? To the extent that the maternal depression-child cognitive development relationship is causal, findings suggest that a two-pronged approach may be necessary for protecting children's cognitive development from maternal depression. First, given its disease burden and the associated deleterious effects, a strong case can be made for recognizing maternal mental health problems as disorders of public health significance and integrated as such into maternal and infant health policies [38]. For this to occur, the public health commitment to mental health problems should increase, particularly in developing countries, where the current commitment is minimal [42].

Cost-effective interventions to effectively treat mental health issues that affect women in poorer households have been successfully implemented in developed and developing countries. Most relevant to this paper, evaluations of interventions that, in addition, to addressing maternal depression, also included children reported improved mother-infant interaction and better cognitive development [43]. Considering cultural differences and local sensitivities, similar initiatives could prove effective and efficient in improving maternal mental health in developing countries such as Peru and improving the livelihoods of children whose early development is hindered by maternal depression.

The heterogeneous results in this paper suggest that the child cognition nexus is a complex one, determined not only by maternal illness but also maternal and household characteristics that interact in ways that are not yet fully understood. Consequently, the most effective way to protect children's welfare may be to target children themselves and build support systems at the household, community, or institutional level that protect vulnerable children's outcomes. Programs and policies that promote poor children's cognitive development directly, such as by improving access to quality pre-school programs or indirectly, by promoting cognitive stimulation at home and improving the quality of their home environments, may help prevent and compensate for early deficits related to maternal depression. In addition, given the hierarchical and interdependent nature of development, the earlier in life the intervention, the better. In recent years, there have been a number of interventions in Latin America that have successfully boosted the cognitive development of poor young children, including cash transfers to very poor households in Nicaragua [44], programs that increase preschool availability in Argentina and Uruguay [45,46], and a program of home visits in Colombia [47].

Contributions to the Global Literature on Early Child Development

This paper makes several contributions to the literature that studies how parents influence children's developmental outcomes. First, it uniquely identifies the impact of maternal depression on child cognition in a developing country, which, to our knowledge, has not been done before, as previous studies have focused on the effects of maternal depression on child health outcomes [48]. Findings from previous research of the effect of maternal depression on cognitive development are mixed and mostly use data from developed countries. In a study in England [14], the authors found that children of mothers who were depressed in the first year had reliably lower cognitive skills as measured by a test score at age 4 than children whose mothers had not been ill. Petterson and Albers [15] also reported lower cognitive outcomes for children exposed to depression in the U.S. In addition, Kurstjens and Wolke [16] concluded that maternal depression is linked with a higher probability of long-term effects for boys and neonatal risk born, chronic cases of depression, or if the family is exposed to other social risks. Our study, which focuses on Peru, provides much needed empirical evidence of the deleterious impact of maternal depression on child cognition in a region where the causal nexus between maternal depression and child cognition has not been studied before despite maternal depression prevalence rates that range between 35% and 50% [17].

Second, the paper focuses on an important marker of early cognition, the accumulation of vocabulary, which has been extensively shown to predict reading comprehension throughout school and into early adulthood [18]. To capture vocabulary competence, we use performance in the Peabody Picture Vocabulary Test (PPVT), a test of receptive vocabulary, which has been widely used and translated to Spanish and Quechua, the two most widely spoken languages in Peru.

Finally, this paper contributes to the literature on the protective effect that other household members can have on the development of children exposed to maternal depression. Our results suggest that, in and of itself, the presence of other household members does not attenuate the effect of maternal depression on child vocabulary development. In fact, the presence of heavy-drinking partners appears to worsen the effect of maternal depression. This latter result may be explained by the increased risk of Intimate Partner Violence (IPV) associated with high alcohol consumption. Evidence from psychology suggests that IPV constitutes a major predictor of post-traumatic stress disorder in abused women [39] and can lead to negative interactions between mother and children [40], directly affecting child development [41]. Using YL data, Bedoya et al. [41] found that IPV was one of the main forms of violence against women in Peru. The authors also found that early-life exposure to alcohol-induced IPV was indeed associated with lower test scores in vocabulary. Our results suggest that maternal depression is a mechanism through which alcohol-induced IPV leads to worse child vocabulary outcomes.

5. Conclusions

In this paper, we explore the extent to which maternal depression affects child cognition in Peru. The identification strategy exploits variation in the exogeneity of the exposure to a particular shock between pregnancy and when the child was 1 year old. Exposure to shock can affect maternal mental health and children's vocabulary development. The paper's main results indicate that exposure to a crop or livestock loss in 2002 increases maternal depression in that period. Moreover, a standard deviation of maternal mental health in 2002 negatively affects a child's vocabulary up to 0.54 standard deviations when children are 5 years old, a result that fades out by the children are 8 years old. That is, our results suggest the negative effects of maternal depression on child receptive vocabulary do not persist beyond children's early school years. However, given that vocabulary size in kindergarten and earlier predicts reading comprehension throughout school and into early adulthood, facilitating the development of other cognitive skills [18], we cannot rule out the possibility that exposure to maternal depression during early life does not undermine other markers of cognitive development in the medium to long term.

In addition to the main results discussed above, this paper also estimates heterogeneous effects by household wealth, maternal education level, and the presence of a partner in the household. When the impact of maternal depression is analyzed separately by household wealth, we find that the effects of maternal mental health issues are worse for children living in less wealthy households during the period when the shock occurred. These results shed light on the negative complementarities between poverty and maternal mental health. Somewhat surprisingly, we found no heterogenous effects by maternal education. Given that our estimations control for a host of important household characteristics that tend to be associated with maternal education (household wealth, consumption, size, number of young children), our results suggest that maternal education may not be the main conduit through which maternal depression undermines children's vocabulary development.

The heterogeneity analysis, in terms of whether the mother has a partner, is enlightening. We find that having a partner does not attenuate the effect of maternal depression on child vocabulary, a result that is driven mostly by partners that are heavy alcohol drinkers. This result is consistent with the literature on domestic violence, which defines low-quality partners as those reported to consume high quantities of alcohol. This literature argues that having a drinking partner is positively correlated with IPV, maternal stress, and worse child vocabulary outcomes. Our results suggest that maternal depression is a mechanism through which alcohol-induced IPV leads to worse child vocabulary outcomes.

Author Contributions: L.D. and M.B. contributed to the conceptualization, methodology, software, validation, formal analysis, investigation, data curation, and writing—original draft preparation, review and editing. L.D. and M.B. have read and agreed to the published version of the manuscript.

Funding: This research received no external funding.

Acknowledgments: We are very grateful to Omar Arias, Monserrat Bustello, Rafael de Hoyos, Carol Graham, Asif Islam, Kabir Malik, Amparo Palacios, Pamela Surkan, Deon Filmer, John Giles, Marianne Fay, the team of the World Bank in Peru, Veronica Schiariti (academic editor), and three anonymous referees, whose comments and suggestions improved different drafts of the paper. We also gratefully acknowledge the Young Lives Project for permission to use the data. The findings, interpretations, and conclusions expressed in this paper are entirely ours and not those of the Young Lives Project, the University of Oxford, DFID, or any other funders. They also do not represent the views of the World Bank.

Conflicts of Interest: The authors declare no conflict of interest.

Appendix A

Table A1. Tests for differences between included and excluded subsamples.

Variables	(1)	(2)	(3)
	Mean and Tests for Differences in Means between Included and Excluded Samples		
	Included	Excluded	p-Value
Panel A. Maternal characteristics			
Age of the mother (years)	31.43	33.73	0.235
Indigenous ethnic group	0.16	0.16	0.995
Less than primary school	0.57	0.42	0.085
Literate	0.79	0.77	0.567
Attended antenatal care in 2002	0.94	0.92	0.734
Panel B Child characteristics			
Child is a boy	0.50	0.51	0.847
Weight at birth	3.21	3.20	0.835
Long-term health problems	0.09	0.08	0.123
Age (in months)	63.5	63.42	0.568
Child is the eldest	0.16	0.17	0.723
Height for age Z-score	−1.42	−1.62	0.167
Panel C Household characteristics			
Wealth index	0.49	0.49	0.934
Housing quality index	0.41	0.42	0.76
Consumption of durable goods index	0.37	0.35	0.582
Live in urban area	0.58	0.62	0.073
Household size	5.52	5.60	0.382
School-aged children in the household (n)	1.33	1.32	0.923
Panel D. Community characteristics			
Violent crime in community	0.33	0.35	0.634
Social assistance (education) available	0.95	0.97	0.913

Table A1 presents the mean of the variables used in the analysis from the included sample (children with available information on maternal mental health in 2002 and PPVT scores in 2006 and 2009) and excluded one (the rest of the sample).

Appendix B

Table A2. Test for exogeneity assumption of the IV.

Dependent Variable: Standardized PPVT	
Shock: Crop or livelihoods loss	
Coefficient	−0.194
Standard error	(0.117)
CI: Upper limit	0.036
CI: Lower limit	−0.424
Observations	1095
R-squared	0.362

Table A2 presents an alternative test for exogeneity of the instrument. We estimate a model that tests the independence between the shock under analysis (instrument) and the vocabulary measure, conditional on all variables that account for the availability of learning resources and child's nutritional status. The estimated coefficient is not statistically significant. CI stands for "confidence interval." R-squared indicates that 36% of the variance for the vocabulary measure is explained by the shock and the rest of independent variables.

Appendix C

Table A3. Confidence intervals of Table 3.

	Dependent Variable: Standardized PPVT					
	(1)	(2)	(3)	(4)	(5)	(6)
Panel A. Estimated coefficients from OLS and IV estimation approaches	OLS with PDS-selected variables and full regressor set			IV with PDS-selected variables and full regressor set		
	MHI-1	MHI-2	MHI-3	MHI-1	MHI-2	MHI-3
Upper bound	0.069	0.034	0.036	0.008	0.000	0.000
Lower bound	−0.132	−0.065	−0.071	−2.057	−0.999	−1.073
Panel B. First-stage estimation				MHI-1	MHI-2	MHI-3
Upper bound				0.472	0.968	0.899
Lower bound				0.128	0.264	0.247

Table A3 Panel A presents the confidence intervals of the estimated impacts of maternal mental health on children's vocabulary at the age of 5 years obtained from Equation (2), using Ordinary Least Squares (OLS) and Instrumental Variables (IV) as estimation approaches. Panel B also presents confidence intervals obtained from the first stage of the IV estimation.

Appendix D

Table A4. Correlations between Shock in 2002 and Maternal Mental Health Index in 2006/2007.

	(1)	(2)	(3)
	MHI-1	MHI-2	MHI-3
Experienced shock of crop or livestock	0.176	0.354	0.335
Loss in 2002	(0.126)	(0.256)	(0.239)
Observations	1095	1095	1095
Mother controls	Yes	Yes	Yes
Child controls	Yes	Yes	Yes
Household controls	Yes	Yes	Yes
R-squared	0.074	0.075	0.076

Table A4 presents correlations between maternal mental health indexes and the main shock under analysis experienced by mothers of our sample. The sample is restricted to our group of interest. Mental health indexes are the standardized measures described in the data section using the SRQ-20 items.

References

1. World Health Organization. *Maternal and Child Mental Health Topic*; WHO: Geneva, Switzerland, 2020.
2. Parsons, C.E.; Young, K.S.; Rochat, T.J.; Kringelbach, M.L.; Stein, A. Postnatal depression and its effects on child development: A review of evidence from low-and middle-income countries. *Br. Med. Bull.* **2012**, *101*, 57–79. [CrossRef] [PubMed]

3. Aizer, A.; Stroud, L.; Buka, S. Maternal stress and child outcomes: Evidence from siblings. *J. Hum. Resour.* **2016**, *51*, 523–555. [CrossRef] [PubMed]
4. Wachs, T.D.; Black, M.M.; Engle, P.L. Maternal depression: A global threat to children's health, development, and behavior and to human rights. *Child. Dev. Persp.* **2009**, *3*, 51–59. [CrossRef]
5. Paulson, J.F.; Dauber, S.; Leiferman, J.A. Individual and combined effects of postpartum depression in mothers and fathers on parenting behavior. *Pediatrics* **2006**, *118*, 659–668. [CrossRef]
6. Phillips, D.A.; Shonkoff, J.P. *From Neurons to Neighborhoods: The Science of Early Childhood Development*; National Academies Press: Washington, DC, USA, 2000.
7. OECD. *Babies and Bosses: Reconciling Work and Family Life: A Synthesis of Findings for OECD Countries*; Organization for Economic Co-operation and Development: Paris, France, 2007.
8. Stratakis, C.A. Cortisol and growth hormone: Clinical implications of a complex, dynamic relationship. *Pediatr. Endocrinol. Rev.* **2006**, *3*, 333–338.
9. Gunnar, M.; Quevedo, K. The neurobiology of stress and development. *Annu. Rev. Psychol.* **2007**, *58*, 145–173. [CrossRef]
10. Center on the Developing Child, Harvard University. Maternal Depression Can Undermine the Development of Young Children. Working Paper No. 8. 2009. Available online: https://developingchild.harvard.edu/resources/maternal-depression-can-undermine-the-development-of-young-children/ (accessed on 10 August 2020).
11. Currie, J.; Thomas, D. *Early Test Scores, Socioeconomic Status and Future Outcomes*; National Bureau of Economic Research, Inc.: Cambridge, MA, USA, 1999.
12. Feinstein, L. Inequality in the Early Cognitive Development of British Children in the 1970 Cohort. *Economica* **2003**, *70*, 73–97. [CrossRef]
13. Cunha, F.; Heckman, J. The Technology of Skill Formation. *Am. Econ. Rev.* **2007**, *97*, 31–47. [CrossRef]
14. Outes-Leon, I.; Dercon, S. Survey Attrition and Attrition Bias in Young Lives. 2008. Available online: https://www.younglives.org.uk/sites/www.younglives.org.uk/files/YL-TN5-OutesLeon-Survey-Attrition.pdf (accessed on 1 July 2020).
15. Dunn, L.M.; Padilla, E.R.; Lugo, D.E.; Dunn, L.M. *Test de Vocabulario en Imágenes Peabody*; American Guidance Service (AGS), Inc.: Circle Pines, MN, USA, 1986.
16. Schady, N. Parental Education, Vocabulary, and Cognitive Development in Early Childhood: Longitudinal Evidence from Ecuador. *Am. J. Public. Health* **2011**, *101*, 2299–2307. [CrossRef]
17. Case, A.; Paxson, C. Stature and Status: Height, Ability, and Labor Market Outcomes. *J. Political Econ.* **2007**, *116*, 499–532. [CrossRef]
18. Powell, D.R.; Diamond, K.E. Promoting early literacy and language development. *Early Child. Edu.* **2012**, *2*, 194–216.
19. Cueto, S.; Leon, J. *Psychometric Characteristics of Cognitive Development and Achievement Instruments in Round 2 of Young Lives*; Young Lives, University of Oxford: Oxford, UK, 2009.
20. Frank, R.G.; Meara, E. *The Effect of Maternal Depression and Substance Abuse on Child Human Capital Development*; National Bureau of Economic Research, Inc.: Cambridge, MA, USA, 2009.
21. Cunha, F.; Heckman, J.; Lochner, L. Interpreting the Evidence on Life Cycle Skill Formation. In *Handbook of the Economics of Education*; Hanushek, E., Welch, F., Eds.; North Holland: Amsterdam, The Netherlands, 2006; pp. 697–812.
22. Greene, W.H. *Econometric Analysis*, 6th ed.; Prentice Hall: Upper Saddle River, NJ, USA, 2005.
23. Berger, E.; Spiess, C. Maternal Life Satisfaction and Child Outcomes: Are They Related? *J. Econ. Psychol.* **2011**, *32*, 142–158. [CrossRef]
24. Almond, D.; Edlund, L.; Palme, M. Chernobyl's subclinical legacy: Prenatal exposure to radioactive fallout and school outcomes in Sweden. *Q. J. Econ.* **2009**, *124*, 1729–1772. [CrossRef]
25. Brown, R. The Intergenerational Impact of Terror: Did the 9/11 Tragedy Impact the Initial Human Capital of the Next Generation? *Demography* **2020**, *57*, 1–23. [CrossRef] [PubMed]
26. Carrillo, B. Early Rainfall Shocks and Later-Life Outcomes: Evidence from Colombia. *World Bank Econ. Rev.* **2020**, *34*, 179–209. [CrossRef]
27. Koppensteiner, M.F.; Manacorda, M. Violence and birth outcomes: Evidence from homicides in Brazil. *J. Dev. Econ.* **2016**, *119*, 16–33. [CrossRef]

28. Guantai, F.; Kijima, Y. Ethnic violence and birth outcomes: Evidence from exposure to the 1992 conflict in Kenya. *Demography* **2020**, *57*, 1–22. [CrossRef]
29. Persson, P.; Rossin-Slater, M. Family ruptures, stress, and the mental health of the next generation. *Am. Econ. Rev.* **2018**, *108*, 1214–1252. [CrossRef]
30. Belloni, A.; Chernozhukov, V.; Hansen, C. Inference on treatment effects after selection among high-dimensional controls. *Rev. Econ. Stud.* **2014**, *81*, 608–650. [CrossRef]
31. Chernozhukov, V.; Hansen, C.; Spindler, M. Post-selection and post-regularization inference in linear models with many controls and instruments. *Am. Econ. Rev.* **2015**, *105*, 486–490. [CrossRef]
32. Ahrens, A.; Hansen, C.B.; Schaffer, M. *PDSLASSO: Stata Module for Post-Selection and Post-Regularization OLS or IV Estimation and Inference*; Boston College Department of Economics: Chestnut Hill, MA, USA, 2019.
33. Paxson, C.; Norbert, S. Does Money Matter? The Effects of Cash Transfers on Child Development in Rural Ecuador. *Econ. Dev. Cult. Change* **2010**, *59*, 187–229. [CrossRef] [PubMed]
34. Engle, P.L.; Fernald, L.C.; Alderman, H.; Behrman, J.; O'Gara, C.; Yousafzai, A.; de Mello, M.C.; Hidrobo, M.; Ulkuer, N.; Ertem, I.; et al. Strategies for reducing inequalities and improving developmental outcomes for young children in low-income and middle-income countries. *Lancet* **2011**, *378*, 339–1353. [CrossRef]
35. Naudeau, S.; Martinez, S.; Premand, P.; Filmer, D. Cognitive development among young children in low-income countries. In *No Small Matter: The Impact of Poverty, Shocks, and Human Capital Investments in Early Childhood Development*; Suter, L.E., Smith, E., Denman, D.B., Eds.; SAGE: Thousand Oaks, CA, USA, 2011; pp. 9–50.
36. Lovejoy, M.; Graczyk, P.; O'Hare, E.; Neuman, G. Maternal depression and parenting behavior: A meta-analysic review. *Clin. Psychol. Rev.* **2000**, *20*, 561–592. [CrossRef]
37. Almond, D.; Currie, J. Human Capital Development before Age Five. *Labor Econ.* **2011**, *4*, 1315–1486.
38. Currie, J.; Patel, V.; Rodrigues, M.; de Souza, N. Gender, poverty and post-natal depression: A cohort study from Goa, India. *Am. J. Psychiatry* **2002**, *159*, 43–47. [CrossRef]
39. Pico-Alfonso, M.A. Psychological intimate partner violence: The major predictor of posttraumatic stress disorder in abused women. *Neurosci. Biobehav. Rev.* **2005**, *29*, 181–193. [CrossRef]
40. Taylor, C.A.; Guterman, N.B.; Lee, S.J.; Rathouz, P.J. Intimate partner violence, maternal stress, nativity, and risk for maternal maltreatment of young children. *Am. J. Public Health* **2009**, *99*, 175–183. [CrossRef]
41. Bedoya, M.; Espinoza, K.; Sanchez, A. Alcohol-induced physical intimate partner violence and child development in Peru. *Oxf. Dev. Stud.* **2020**, *4*, 1–16. [CrossRef]
42. Prince, M.; Patel, V.; Saxena, S.; Maj, M.; Maselko, J.; Phillips, M.R.; Rahman, A. No health without mental health. *Lancet* **2007**, *370*, 859–877. [CrossRef]
43. Rahman, A.; Love, H.; Bunn, J. Mothers' mental health and infant growth: A case control study from Rawalpindi, Pakistan. *Br. Med. J.* **2004**, *30*, 21.
44. Barham, T.; Macours, K.; Maluccio, J.A. *More Schooling and More Learning? Effects of a Three-Year Conditional Cash Transfer Program in Nicaragua after 10 Years*; Inter-American Development Bank: Washington, DC, USA, 2013.
45. Berlinski, S.; Galiani, S.; Gertler, P. The effect of pre-primary education on primary school performance. *J. Public Econ.* **2009**, *93*, 219–234. [CrossRef]
46. Berlinski, S.; Galiani, S.; Manacorda, M. Giving children a better start: Preschool attendance and school-age profiles. *J. Public Econ.* **2008**, *92*, 1416–1440. [CrossRef]
47. Attanasio, O.; Baker-Henningham, H.; Bernal, R.; Meghir, C.; Pineda, D.; Rubio-Codina, M. *Early Stimulation and Nutrition: The Impacts of a Scalable Intervention (No. w25059)*; National Bureau of Economic Research: Cambridge, MA, USA, 2018.
48. Surkan, P.J.; Kennedy, C.E.; Hurley, K.M.; Black, M.M. Maternal depression and early childhood growth in developing countries: Systematic review and meta-analysis. *Bull. World Health Organ.* **2011**, *89*, 607–615. [CrossRef] [PubMed]

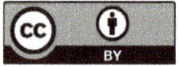

© 2020 by the authors. Licensee MDPI, Basel, Switzerland. This article is an open access article distributed under the terms and conditions of the Creative Commons Attribution (CC BY) license (http://creativecommons.org/licenses/by/4.0/).

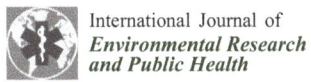

International Journal of
Environmental Research and Public Health

Article

Exploring Factors That Could Potentially Have Affected the First 1000 Days of Absent Learners in South Africa: A Qualitative Study

Carien van Zyl and Carlien van Wyk *

Centre for Child, Youth and Family Studies, COMPRES, Faculty of Health Sciences, North-West University, Potchefstroom 2531, South Africa; carienshalom@gmail.com
* Correspondence: Carlien.VanWyk@nwu.ac.za; Tel.: +27-21-8643593

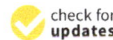

Citation: van Zyl, C.; van Wyk, C. Exploring Factors That Could Potentially Have Affected the First 1000 Days of Absent Learners in South Africa: A Qualitative Study. *Int. J. Environ. Res. Public Health* **2021**, *18*, 2768. https://doi.org/10.3390/ijerph18052768

Academic Editor: Verónica Schiariti

Received: 9 February 2021
Accepted: 26 February 2021
Published: 9 March 2021

Publisher's Note: MDPI stays neutral with regard to jurisdictional claims in published maps and institutional affiliations.

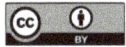

Copyright: © 2021 by the authors. Licensee MDPI, Basel, Switzerland. This article is an open access article distributed under the terms and conditions of the Creative Commons Attribution (CC BY) license (https://creativecommons.org/licenses/by/4.0/).

Abstract: Background: The first 1000 days of life—from conception to the second birthday of children—is widely recognized as the most crucial development phase, which could have long lasting effects on the health and well-being of children throughout their lives. Purpose: The purpose of this study was to qualitatively explore and describe factors that could potentially have affected the first 1000 days of absent learners in the Foundation Phase within the Paarl-East community in the Western Cape of South Africa. Methods: The data for this qualitative descriptive study were collected through semi-structured interviews with 18 biological mothers of absent learners in the Foundation Phase, who resided in Paarl East. The transcribed texts were analyzed by making use of a thematic data analysis. Results: The findings revealed six predominant themes that played a role during the first 1000 days of the lives of these absent learners. Conclusion: It was concluded from the findings in this study that factors, such as health and nutrition of both the mothers and their children, substance use/abuse during pregnancy, toxic stress, support received by the mothers and their children, attachment, attentive care, and stimulation and play, could have affected the first 1000 days of the absent learners in this study. Since this study did not aim to confirm a correlation between the first 1000 days and absenteeism, but solely to explore factors affecting the first 1000 days, conclusions regarding cause and effect was not possible.

Keywords: absent learners; biological mothers; first 1000 days; Foundation phase

1. Introduction

The significance of the first 1000 days as a time-period, is broadly asserted: "The first 1000 days of life—the time spanning roughly between conception and one's second birthday—is a unique period of opportunity when the foundations of optimum health, growth, and neurodevelopment across the lifespan are established" [1].

The first 1000 days is believed to be the greatest development phase where children's physical, cognitive, and socio-emotional development will have a lifelong impact, later in their lives [2]. The infancy period, from birth to two years, is characterized by rapid development of the physical and nervous systems, influencing other domains of children's development. The characteristics infants acquire during this phase are, therefore, fundamental for their lives [3]. The developing brain is particularly vulnerable to prenatal influences during the prenatal period [4]. The brain architecture formed during this critical time-period lays either a strong or weak foundation for the health, learning, and behavior of children later in life [5]. Furthermore, brain development during infancy endures explosive growth, and forms the building blocks of the lives and future of children.

All children must not merely survive but thrive and reach their full potential. It is, therefore, critical to detect risk factors that impact the physical, mental, moral, spiritual, and social development of children [6]. In order for children to reach their full potential, they need nurturing care from birth up until they are two years old, which includes good healthcare, nutrition, security, safety, responsive caregiving, and early learning [7]. The absence of these nurturing care factors during the first 1000 days could result in physical, emotional, and social challenges in the future [8]. A disfavored first 1000 days could, therefore, affect children's neurological and biological adaptations throughout their lives [9].

In South Africa, the Western Cape Government acknowledged the importance of the first 1000 days of life by launching the First 1000 Days campaign, entitled 'Right Start Bright Future' in 2016. The aim of this campaign was to raise awareness regarding the importance of the first 1000 days among health workers, other professionals, as well as the general public, by means of workshops and social media. The intention was to further shift the perceptions of healthcare workers and other professionals, to consequently improve health and social services to children during this crucial time-period [10]. This campaign focused on three key areas, namely—(1) health and nutrition; (2) love and attention; and (3) play and stimulation. These three key areas play a fundamental role in the development of children's physical, social, emotional, and cognitive domains [11]. These distinct key areas respectively involve assorted factors. The first key area, health and nutrition, includes various factors like nutritional deficiency, malnourishment, the physical and mental health of both mothers and their children, and substance use/abuse during pregnancy. The second key area, love and attention, incorporates factors like support to both mothers and their children, nurturing care, and attachment. The last key area, play and stimulation, refers to the stimulation and protection of children [12].

The rational for concentrating on 'absent learners' was motivated by the author's work context at the Khula Development Group, a registered non-governmental organization (NGO), rendering services to absent learners and their families. In South Africa, school absenteeism is a huge concern with alarming statistics of 616,327 learners who were absent in the Cape Winelands District, Western Cape, in 2017 [13]. South African policies include various definitions in terms of absenteeism, including, 'absent' for any learner not in class or participating in school activities when the class register is marked, as well as 'continuous absenteeism' for learners absent from school for ten consecutive days without a valid reason [13]. In this study, the term 'absent learner' refers to any form of absenteeism, whether continuous or irregular. There are numerous reasons for school absenteeism, such as poverty, lack of transport, unsuitable housing, children taking care of their siblings, lack of health care, chronic diseases, disabilities, poor nutrition, children's lack of interest in the curriculum, bullying, lack of family support, working conditions of parents, negative role modeling of parents, parents' lack of understanding regarding the value of school attendance, parents' lack of education, as well as problems within the family structure like divorce or domestic violence [14–16]. In terms of South Africa, the following reasons for school absenteeism is highlighted, namely poverty, parents' inability to afford a school uniform or school fees, lack of transport, poor nutrition, child labor, dysfunctional families, gang violence, chronic illnesses of parents or children, learning disabilities, and psychological challenges [13,17]. The multi-level consequences of school absenteeism include poor academic performance, and an increased school drop-out rate with long-term outcomes, such as inadequate education, unemployment, financial instability, and health-related problems [18].

The authors were particularly interested in the Foundation Phase, as this is the first phase of formal schooling in South Africa. The Foundation Phase in South Africa refers to Grade R to 3, where learners might enroll for Grade R in the year that they turn six and be admitted to Grade 1 when they turn seven years old. [19]. During this first phase of formal schooling, which establishes the starting point for the academic growth of learners [20], children are expected to master the formal curriculum content, including reading, writing, counting, and calculating [21]. The ability of children to succeed in school is determined by their behavior, social engagement with others, and their capacity to obtain literacy and numeracy skills that are interrelated with their physical, motor, social, emotional, moral, and spiritual development [22]. Children struggle with the curriculum in higher phases if they do not acquire basic reading skills during the Foundation Phase [23]. It is, therefore, of the utmost importance that the early development of children is promoted before they enter the formal school system [24].

From the literature, it is evident that there are many factors transpiring during the first 1000 days that can potentially affect the schooling of children later in life. These factors are—(1) nutritional deficiencies; (2) substance abuse during pregnancy; (3) toxic stress; (4) attachment; and (5) stimulation. Malnourishment, including iron deficiency during the first 1000 days, could lead to reduced cognitive abilities, insufficient school achievement, grade repetition, school absenteeism, and school dropout, later in life [25]. Although substance abuse during pregnancy might involve various substances, such as tobacco, alcohol, Marijuana, or other illicit drugs [26], the effects of alcohol are highlighted. Excessive alcohol abuse during pregnancy could lead to Fetal Alcohol Spectrum Disorder (FASD), a collection of physical, cognitive, and neurobehavioral abnormalities [27,28]. Children with FASD might struggle with learning and behavior challenges at school, such as hyperactivity, memory difficulties, problem solving, social problems, reading, lack of attention, disruptive behavior in class, disobeying school rules, absenteeism, suspension, and school dropout [29,30]. Toxic stress weakens the architecture of the developing brain that could result in long-term learning problems [31]. It is further confirmed that extreme exposure to stress during pregnancy could cause long-lasting emotional and cognitive problems, whereas stressful experiences after birth could alter the neurobiology of children that decreases their ability to succeed in school [32]. Secure attachment in infancy is associated with a positive relationship between children and their school teachers, higher self-esteem, and greater resilience, whilst disorganized attachment during infancy correlates with a series of developmental problems in school, including aggressive behavior, poor relations with peers, and cognitive immaturity [33,34]. Adequate stimulation during infancy results in better cognitive and educational performance later in life [35]. However, learning at school is influenced by the lack of learning, and stimulation in the early years [36].

The purpose of this study was to qualitatively explore and describe factors that could potentially have affected the first 1000 days of absent learners in the Foundation Phase in the Paarl-East community in the Western Cape of South Africa. The authors acknowledge the existence of many variables, besides the first 1000 days, that could influence schooling and absenteeism. For this reason, this paper does not aim to confirm a correlation between the first 1000 days and absenteeism, but solely to explore factors that could potentially have affected the first 1000 days of absent learners in the Foundation Phase.

2. Materials and Methods

2.1. Research Approach and Design

A qualitative approach was applied to provide insight into the social world of these biological mothers and their children, by producing descriptive data in the participants own words [37,38]. A qualitative descriptive design was utilized for the purpose of this study to obtain a collection of rich and descriptive information, by conducting individual interviews [39–42].

2.2. Research Setting and Sampling

The study was conducted amidst the NGO sector, specifically within the Khula Development Group's context that renders services to absent learners and their families in the Paarl-East community. The process for service delivery commences when schools in disadvantaged communities refer absent learners to this organization, where they are contacted by the means of home visits. Hereafter, continuous services are rendered, which include home and school visits to provide academic and psychosocial support to absent learners, as well as parental guidance and support to their primary caregivers [43]. The context of the Paarl-East community is characterized by a low-income population, high levels of crime and violence, together with substance abuse [44,45].

A random purposive sampling method was utilized for recruiting 18 biological mothers of the Foundation Phase learners from Grades R to 3, on the database of the Khula Development Group. These learners were referred to the Khula Development Group for a variety of reasons for school absenteeism, such as poverty, social ills like substance abuse, and domestic violence at home, transport challenges, chronic illnesses, poor academic progress, etc. Although the possibility exists that these 18 biological mothers could possibly have older children that was also absent and were recorded on the database of the Khula Development Group, the focus of this study was learners from Grade R to 3. The inclusion criteria were as follows—(1) biological mothers of absent learners in the Foundation Phase; (2) residing in Paarl-East; (3) lived with their child during their child's first 1000 days; (4) currently lives with their child; and (5) were factually capable of giving consent to participate in this research study.

2.3. Procedure

Ethical approval was obtained from the registered Health Research Ethics Committee at the North-West University (NWU-000008-19-A1), South Africa, which conforms to the principles outlined in the Declaration of Helsinki. Written permission to conduct the study at the Khula Development Group was obtained from the chief operational officer of this organization, who acted as a gatekeeper. The branch manager and two other employees at the Khula Development Group fulfilled the role as mediator and independent persons during the recruitment process. The independent persons conducted home visits to recruit participants, and they were also responsible for obtaining written consent forms from all participants. Arrangements were made to conduct the interviews with the participants at the offices of the Khula Development Group.

2.4. Data Collection

Semi-structured individual interviews were conducted with all of the participants, which lasted approximately one hour each. An interview schedule consisted of 12 questions, along with a timeline tool. The interview schedule covered the three key areas of the Western Cape's First 1000 Days campaign—(1) health and nutrition; (2) love and attention; and (3) play and stimulation. During the interview, the participants were asked a variety of questions about the time-period of their child's first 1000 days—from pregnancy until their child's second birthday. The interview schedule contained two sections, the first section covered questions regarding the pregnancy phase, whereas the second section focused on questions relating to the phase from birth to two years. These open-ended questions were formulated in a simple style, and the following were asked—(1) describe your living conditions while you were pregnant with your child; (2) tell me more about your own health during your pregnancy; (3) explain what you ate and drank during your pregnancy; (4) tell me more about the people who helped and supported you during your pregnancy; (5) describe your feelings towards your unborn baby while you were pregnant with your child; (6) how did you experience the pregnancy?; (7) describe your living conditions from the time your child was born until two years of age; (8) tell me more about your child's health from birth until two years; (9) tell me more about your child's nutrition from birth until two years; (10) describe your relationship with your child from birth until two years; (11) how did you play with your child from birth until two years?; and (12) describe any challenges regarding your child since the time he/she was born until two years of age. All interviews were audio-recorded and transcribed verbatim, as preparation for the data analysis.

2.5. Data Analysis

Thematic analysis was utilized to analyze the qualitative data, in order to identify various themes [46]. This involved six phases [47,48], as seen in Figure 1. Additionally, QDA Miner Lite, a free version of the Computer-Aided Qualitative Data Analysis Software

(CAQDAS), version 1.4, Provalis Research, Montreal, QC, Canada, was used to assist with the data analysis process [49].

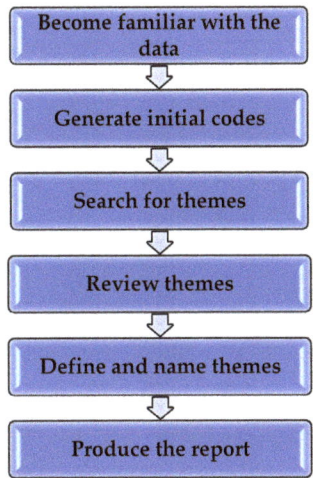

Figure 1. Phases of thematic analysis.

3. Results

The results were based on interviews with 18 biological mothers of absent learners in the Foundation Phase. The biographical data of the participants are presented in Table 1.

Table 1. Biographical data of participants.

Participant	Current Age during the Study	Current Relational Status during the Study	Total Number of Children	Position of Absent Learner in Relation to Other Siblings
Participant 1	31 years	Single	3	Eldest
Participant 2	28 years	Married	3	Eldest
Participant 3	40 years	Married	6	Fourth child
Participant 4	31 years	Single	2	Youngest
Participant 5	26 years	Single	3	Eldest
Participant 6	37 years	Long-term relationship	7	Fifth child
Participant 7	42 years	Married	5	Youngest
Participant 8	39 years	Married	7	Fourth child
Participant 9	31 years	Married	3	Eldest
Participant 10	44 years	Long-term relationship	5	Youngest
Participant 11	37 years	Divorced	4	Third child
Participant 12	29 years	Single	2	Youngest
Participant 13	48 years	Single	4	Youngest
Participant 14	33 years	Married	2	Youngest
Participant 15	28 years	Long-term relationship	2	Eldest
Participant 16	29 years	Long-term relationship	2	Eldest
Participant 17	32 years	Long-term relationship	2	Youngest
Participant 18	34 years	Long-term relationship	3	Middle child

The data analysis revealed six themes, which were further divided into sub-themes. The sub-themes indicated the various factors that could potentially have affected the first 1000 days of the absent learners in the Foundation Phase. See Figure 2.

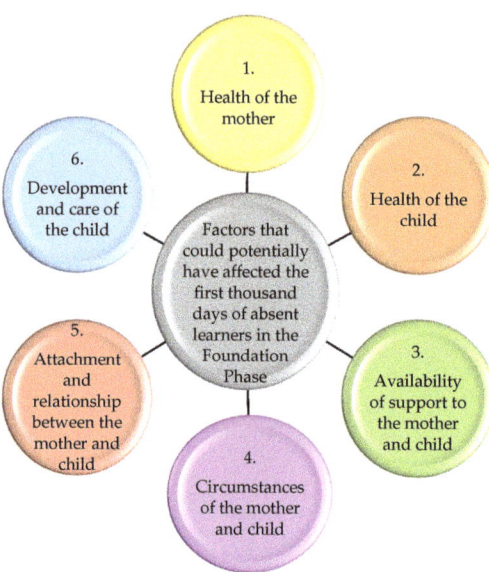

Figure 2. A graphical representation of the six main themes (condensed version) that could potentially have affected the Figure 1000. days of absent learners in the Foundation Phase.

3.1. Theme 1: Health of the Mothers during the First 1000 Days of Their Children's Lives

This theme described the physical and mental well-being of the mothers, and other factors that played a role in their overall health, such as nutrition and substance use/abuse.

3.1.1. Sub-Theme 1.1: Physical Health of the Mothers

Approximately half of the participants indicated having good physical health during their pregnancies, while the rest of the participants recalled some health issues, such as heartburn, morning sickness, high blood pressure, and tuberculosis (TB). Many of participants experienced complications, especially during the birth process, for example, participant 18 shared: " ... but when I went into labor with her, then with the push, then the umbilical cord was stuck around her neck".

3.1.2. Sub-Theme 1.2: Mental Health and Emotional Well-Being of Mothers

Although many participants described their pregnancy experience in a positive light, some defined their pregnancy as a negative experience. The participants expressed a variety of stressors (external, internal, or both). Some participants were still teenagers when they got pregnant, which contributed to excessive stress: "I was still in school ... and I did not know what do to with the child" (Participant 16). Many participants indicated their current circumstances as stressful and overwhelming, such as the relationship with their child's father or intimate partner: "Oh, he hit me that evening. He took the belt. He pulled my hair ... My stomach was blue from how he hit me" (Participant 17).

Some participants also experienced internal stressors, as expressed: "I felt like a disappointment, felt like I've disappointed them [family] with the pregnancy" (Participant 2). Various participants experienced the birth process itself as a strain: " ... it is a fear in you, because if you make a mistake here, then it is your fault. Then I panicked ... " (Participant 18). The poor mental health of Participant 17 was further portrayed by serious indicators of attempts to harm her child: "I cannot anymore. I left the child at the hospital ... I walked out without the child. I do not want the child ... I am tired of being a mother ... ". On another occasion, the same participant tried to kill the baby: "I told myself, throw the child in the dam of water ... we are hungry. We don't have food".

3.1.3. Sub-Theme 1.3: Nutrition of Mothers

Numerous participants felt they ate healthy during their pregnancy, whereas some participants admitted maintaining poor nutrition: "I ate a lot of junk food ... I did not worry about what I was eating" (Participant 4). Many participants experienced various challenges regarding their own nutrition, such as morning sickness: "And all that I could force down was water and potato chips. It was only that which I could get in, up to seven months" (Participant 2). Several participants implied a lack of food or limited food as a major challenge: "Food was scarce. There were places [soup kitchens] that handed out food and then I would go and fetch some" (Participant 8).

3.1.4. Sub-Theme 1.4: Substance Use/Abuse of Mothers during Pregnancy

Many participants consumed alcohol, cigarettes, or illicit drugs during their pregnancies, for example, Participant 14 stated: " ... about five liters ... I just drank a lot". Only a small number of participants declared a total lack of any substance use during pregnancy. More than half of the participants revealed that they smoked cigarettes during their pregnancies, as stated by Participant 11: "I smoked a lot of cigarettes. Smoked cigarettes the whole day". A few participants acknowledged using drugs during their pregnancy, which included dagga (Marijuana), Mandrax, or Methamphetamine, referred to as Tik in South Africa. Although very few participants verbalized an understanding of the harmful effects of their own substance abuse on their child, Participant 17 acknowledged: "Tik and Mandrax, that is why the child was so sickly. And at school too. It is almost as if the drugs left something behind. This is why she takes so long, struggle to think".

3.2. Theme 2: The Health of Children during the First 1000 Days of Life

The participants shared information regarding their child's health, and the challenges experienced due to illnesses or hospitalization. This theme further elaborated on the children's nutrition from birth to two years.

3.2.1. Sub-Theme 2.1: Physical Health of the Children

Many participants mentioned a diversity of illnesses that their child suffered from, including an eye infection, jaundice, gastroenteritis (gastro), respiratory difficulties, kidney disease, colon problems, and TB, some resulting in hospitalization. Four participants who smoked cigarettes while pregnant, revealed that their child endured various types of respiratory difficulties after birth, as described: " ... then there is a wheezing in her chest" (Participant 8). Two participants' children contracted TB before the age of two years. Information about medical check-ups and immunizations also emerged during the interviews. Certain participants confirmed taking their children for their scheduled medical check-ups and immunizations. In addition, numerous participants experienced challenges as a result of their children's illnesses, such as transport problems, lack of communication by medical staff, or stress due to the hospitalization of their children.

3.2.2. Sub-Theme 2.2: Nutrition of Children

Approximately half of the participants breastfed their child from birth, whereas others fed their baby formula milk. Almost half of the participants experienced challenges with regard to breastfeeding, such as not providing an adequate supply of milk, the baby refusing to take the breast, going back to work, and receiving additional TB treatment to prevent the baby from contracting TB through breastfeeding.

The participants indicated various ages when their child started to eat solid foods, including from as young as one month to approximately a year. Several participants reported that their child ate healthy food, whereas some participants listed unhealthy food items, such as "Sweets, very much so" (Participant 4). When some of the children in this study were introduced to solid foods, they encountered various challenges, as described by Participant 14: "There was little food. I had to walk with her [child], looking where we could eat". Several participants referred to their child's weight as healthy and normal, although three of the participants commented on their children being underweight or overweight, as quoted by Participant 11: "She was a little bit overweight".

3.3. Theme 3: Availability of Support to the Mothers and Their Children during the First 1000 Days of the Children's Lives

The participants discussed their experience pertaining to the support they received. They mentioned receiving good to poor support from different groups of people. Furthermore, the participants also mentioned challenges in their relationship with these groups of people, and their child's relationship with them.

3.3.1. Sub-Theme 3.1: The Mothers' Experience Regarding Support

Several participants were unmarried and living with their families when they found out that they were pregnant, which impacted the response from others and the support they received. Participant 16 experienced antagonism from her strict father and shared: "He wanted to put me out [out of the home]". A few participants faced negative responses from their child's father: "He told me it was not his child. ... he degraded me" (Participant 2), whereas two participants revealed positive responses from their children's father. Furthermore, some participants had a positive experience regarding support that contributed to optimistic feelings, as stated by Participant 16: "He [friend] made me feel that there was hope". Some participants had negative experiences regarding support, as indicated: "It is difficult if you are pregnant and you don't have good support" (Participant 12).

3.3.2. Sub-Theme 3.2: Support from the Children's Biological Fathers

During pregnancy, several participants felt supported by the biological father: "Oh, if my feet were swollen, he massaged it. He was there ... if I had my date at the hospital, he came along ... he was always there" (Participant 8). However, some participants did not feel supported by their child's father: "He did not help me. He was only there because he had to, but he never helped me like other dads helped their wives or girlfriends" (Participant 13). A few participants highlighted the practical assistance of the father: "Then he cleans up, and he puts on the rice and peels the potatoes. He helped me with everything" (Participant 7). For one participant, the support was mainly financial, whereas Participant 9 also received personal involvement.

Several participants conveyed challenges pertaining to their relationship with their child's biological father, which included unstable relationships, break-ups, conflict, substance abuse, a psychiatric disorder, physical abuse, criminal activities, distrust, and financial challenges.

Five of the participants revealed that their children had a good relationship with their biological father. However, several participants described a poor or absent relationship between their child and the biological father, as specified by Participant 5: "But he was still with her at three months and then he did not come again ... when she was two years old, he came again, but then she did not want anything to do with him ... ".

3.3.3. Sub-Theme 3.3: Support from Family Members and Others

Most participants identified family members, especially their own biological mothers who supported them during their pregnancy. The support of one participant's mother influenced her thoughts on considering an abortion: "Then my mom said, 'No, abortion is not an option'. She would help me" (Participant 2). Beside their mothers, the participants also mentioned the support received from other family members or other people supporting them, such as neighbors, friends, and colleagues. For one participant, her brother's support made a big difference in her life: "My brother came down [to the hospital] and brought me stuff ... and I knew that he would help me" (Participant 16). However, a few participants reported a total lack of support from others: "Although my mom was there, her cousins, aunts ... they did not help me. I went through everything on my own" (Participant 13).

Referring to the child's relationships with other people, numerous participants elaborated on the integral role family members like grandparents and siblings played in the lives of their child: "He was really spoiled by his sisters. They dressed him up ... they were crazy about him" (Participant 7).

3.4. Theme 4: Circumstances of the Mothers and Their Children during the First 1000 Days of Their Children's Lives

The participants shared information pertaining to their circumstances during their child's first 1000 days that included living and financial circumstances.

3.4.1. Sub-Theme 4.1: Living Circumstances

The type of housing varied and included houses, flats, and even informal structures made from wood or corrugated iron. More than half of the participants reported positive aspects regarding their living circumstances during their pregnancy. On the contrary, many participants lived in informal structures without water or electricity. They experienced various challenges with regard to their living circumstances. Participant 8 lived with the family of her child's father, but the house was overcrowded with 20 occupants in a small house with no electricity. Other challenges mentioned were substance abuse within the home, as stated by Participant 16: "My mom drank. My dad was on Mandrax".

It appears that some participants' living circumstances improved in the time-period after their child's birth. Participant 18 relocated to another home after her child's birth: "It was nice. The structure was small, but is was warm, comfortable and not leaking or so. It was quite okay". Furthermore, several participants expressed increased conflict after the arrival of the baby: "And in the home, my sisters and I had a lot of fighting. The child cried, they couldn't sleep ... and then the other grandchildren felt now they were being neglected ... " (Participant 16).

3.4.2. Sub-Theme 4.2: Financial Circumstances

Most participants indicated the nature of their employment, along with the number of people working in the household. Several participants gave an account of favorable financial circumstances: "He [child's father] also had a full-time job. Financially, it went well during my pregnancy. His income was enough" (Participant 7). However, numerous participants experienced financial strain, as they themselves or their family members only worked part-time: "It was very difficult. My father-in-law did char [part time] jobs ... and my mother-in-law also did char [part time] jobs, but only two times a week or once a week ... " (Participant 8). Some participants were teenagers, and left school when they got pregnant: "Like me, I do not have experience of work and so. Grade 10 out of the school" (Participant 12).

Some participants found employment after the birth of their child that relieved the financial strain: " ... I went working. And then it started to go better" (Participant 16). In contrast, numerous participants experienced severe financial difficulty, and were consequently not able to sufficiently provide for their own needs and the needs of their baby, as expressed by Participant 10: "Then there were those Fridays when we did not even have money for a box of milk for the child. We were not in a financial position to give the child what was due to her".

3.5. Theme 5: Attachment and Relationship between the Mothers and Their Children during the First 1000 Days of Their Children's Lives

The participants discussed their attachment to and relationship between themselves and their child, as seen in the following sub-themes.

3.5.1. Sub-Theme 5.1: Attachment and Relationship between the Mothers and Their Children during Pregnancy

The participants shared their initial responses when they found out they were pregnant: "I was happy" (Participant 5), and "I was thrilled. I was very glad" (Participant 10). More than half of the participants experienced various negative emotions: "First, I panicked. Thought ... 'I already have a child and circumstances are not favorable" (Participant 18).

This study revealed the strong gender preference of many of the participants, and their emotions regarding gender: "Excited, and the day I found out it was a girl, then I was even more happy" (Participant 6), whereas Participant 12 stated: "When I found out it was a girl it was too late already ... I was actually very angry".

Several participants considered abortion or adoption: "In the first place, I wanted an abortion ... " (Participant 4), and Participant 17 shared: "I told myself, 'I am going to let the child be adopted by other people'".

Most participants expressed positive thoughts and emotions towards their unborn baby when they felt the movement of the baby: "I was very happy about the kicks. And to see on the sonar how he was moving and carrying on. It was beautiful. It was nice" (Participant 4), and "I've bonded with him while I was pregnant" (Participant 2). Additionally, many participants described how they interacted with their unborn child: "If I was alone with him and he kicked me, then I talked to him. And I listened to music, always with the phone, then I put the phone next to me ... " (Participant 2).

3.5.2. Sub-Theme 5.2: Attachment and Relationship between the Mothers and Their Children from Birth to Two Years

The participants described their initial response towards their baby after birth: "I was in love with him from day one. That moment when they put him in my arms, I was in love with the child, until now" (Participant 7). Some participants recalled their immediate interactions, as voiced: "When she was lying there after her birth, I played with her or sang for her" (Participant 1). For two participants, the birth of their children created a sense of responsibility and motivation: "Then after that [the child's birth], then I thought to myself, 'I must stand out a bit' and I did stand out for her" (Participant 14).

During the time-period from birth up to two years, many participants expressed their positive responses: "You have that bond with your child" (Participant 8) and "I was very attached to her" (Participant 9). However, some participants experienced negative emotions or thoughts at times: "I don't feel up to baby today" (Participant 11), and " ... can't the child die or something, throw the child away" (Participant 17).

Numerous participants mentioned that their child constantly wanted to be with them with regard to attachment and the relationship from their child's side: "If I am not with her, then she cries. She was very close to me. I could not walk away ... she looked for me" (Participant 1). Two participants distinctively described their children's positive responses and attachment towards them: "And she always clung, grabbed and said, 'Mommy', then grabbed me and held onto me" (Participant 8).

3.6. Theme 6: Development and Care of the Children during the First 1000 Days of Their Lives

This theme described aspects relating to the children's development, the care, and protection the participants provided to their child, as well as the way the participants stimulated and played with their child.

3.6.1. Sub-Theme 6.1: The Children's Development

The participants mentioned various aspects pertaining to their child's physical development, such as hearing, movement, rolling, and crawling: "We wanted to see if she could hear correctly, if she could listen" (Participant 9). Some participants referred to their child's emotional needs, whilst some participants showed insight into their child's linguistic and cognitive development: "She wanted to know about everything. She was at that age where she walked, she experimented with things" (Participant 11).

Relating to their children's milestones, some participants indicated that their child reached some milestones early: "She did not crawl for long, then she started to stand up against things and began to walk. She developed quickly" (Participant 12). A few participants felt their child failed to meet some age-appropriate milestones or had developmental delays: "She does not catch or understand so well what I say. And the one eye is here while the other eye turns that side" (Participant 17).

3.6.2. Sub-Theme 6.2: The Mothers' Care and Protection of the Children

Participants referred to different aspects of caregiving, and many shared examples of how they ensured good caregiving: "So, I must make sure that he has everything, because the nanny must be paid, she must be looked after, her food must be ready—what she eats, her milk, clothing, everything" (Participant 3). Three participants explicitly noted that their children had all they needed, referring specifically to their physical needs: "Provision was always made for him ... he never lacked anything. He was never hungry or so" (Participant 2).

Some participants also indicated that emotional caregiving was important, as stated by Participant 14: "I gave her love". Three participants showed an awareness of risks, and the need to protect their children: "She can maybe just be in the yard at the back, then I would look for her. Don't let her play in the street. Scared the cars will drive over her" (Participant 1).

Furthermore, the participants revealed a range of challenges regarding the caregiving of their children: "Sometimes yes, he was tired, but he always battled to sleep ... when he became older, it was always a struggle to get him to sleep" (Participants 2). Two participants experienced feelings of inadequacy: " ... didn't know what to do ... " (Participant 15). For some participants, their physical or emotional well-being influenced their caregiving: "I think it was the cut [cesarean] that caught me off guard ... I had a lot of pain, so I did not have time for her. So, I neglected her a little bit ... " (Participant 9). An additional challenge for many participants was the lack of baby goods, due to financial strain: "Sometimes, when there was no cereal and I didn't have money, then the child cried the whole day and so. When there were no [nappies]" (Participant 17).

3.6.3. Sub-Theme 6.3: Stimulation and Play

This study revealed different ways in which the participants incorporated stimulation and play into the various stages of their children's lives. During infancy and the first few months, the participants reported the following: " ... tickled him on his chest" (Participant 3), " ... sing for them, then swing them a little bit" (Participant 5), and " ... played hide and seek" (Participant 13). Two participants hanged items in the air for their children to play with: "Then I maybe make the balloons ... with a string to just where his hands could touch, then he plays with it" (Participant 7).

Some participants played with their children when they became older: "I played with him with cars" (Participant 2), or other activities, such as "sang for her, danced" (Participant 5). Some mothers used specific activities to intentionally stimulate and educate their children, such as walking in the garden, or using items in their home to teach them about shapes and colors. However, two participants did not regard it as necessary to play directly with their children, as they felt that their children could play with their siblings, as captured: "No, because most of the time she played with her sisters. So, I did not really play like that, like in play with her ... " (Participant 6). Two participants mentioned their child's father playing with the child, as explained by Participant 18: " ... and then I would go and call the father ... and then we [participant, child and father] played together".

4. Discussion

4.1. Discussion of Findings

The data provided insight into the various factors that could potentially influence the first 1000 days of the lives of children. In the context of this study, these factors relate to the three key areas outlined in the First 1000 Days campaign that was launched in the Western Cape, South Africa, namely (1) health and nutrition; (2) love and attention; and (3) play and stimulation [10].

The health of mothers (Theme 1) involved their physical and mental health, nutrition, and substance abuse of the participants, which played a vital role during their pregnancy and after the birth of their children. Many participants in this study suffered from severe illnesses and medical conditions, such as extreme high blood pressure, a stroke, and TB during their pregnancy. These conditions increased the risk of complications for both the mothers and their children [50–52]. Numerous complications occurred during pregnancy, especially during the birth process, including the following—preterm birth, low birth weight, umbilical cord prolapse, ectopic pregnancy, hypertension, and breech births [53]. In addition, various children in this study suffered from oxygen deprivation after birth, which could have caused disabilities and developmental delays [54,55]. The participants revealed various aspects that influenced their emotional and mental well-being during this time-period. Although some participants encountered positive experiences and emotions during their pregnancy, others endured severe stress, especially since it seemed that all these pregnancies were unplanned. Several participants described their pregnancy experience in a negative light, as a result of morning sickness, swelling, uncertainty, sleeping challenges, and high blood pressure caused by their pregnancy. A mother's well-being during pregnancy influences the baby's well-being [56], which could have long-lasting physical, cognitive, and emotional outcomes for the child [57]. During pregnancy, the participants experienced stressors related to their circumstances. Some participants were teenagers during their pregnancy, and they had to attend school, and the relationship with the biological father also added strain. Numerous participants experienced internal stressors, especially relating to the announcement of the pregnancy to their family, which caused intense emotions. The findings also indicated that a few participants experienced sadness, anxiety, guilt, and feelings of worthlessness, which could possibly be associated with symptoms of depression [58]. Prenatal exposure to maternal depression could affect the brain development of the fetus [59].

During the time from the child's birth to two years, the stressors mentioned were mostly related to motherhood and losing a loved one. One of the mother's mental health after the birth of her child showed signs of postpartum depression [60,61], or even postpartum psychosis [62], as she attempted to kill her baby. Although most participants ate healthy during their pregnancy, poor nutrition occurred amongst some participants. Nutritional deficiencies during pregnancy could affect children's cognition, behavior, and productivity later in life [63,64]. The occurrence of substance use/abuse during pregnancy was considerably high, with cigarette smoking the highest, followed by alcohol use, and lastly, drug abuse. Illicit drugs that were consumed during pregnancy included Methamphetamine (Tik), dagga (Marijuana), and Mandrax. Substance use/abuse during pregnancy poses severe risks to both mothers and their unborn babies, especially physical and neurological damage [65]. Prenatal use of alcohol, as consumed by many participants, could have long-term consequences on their children's cognitive, behavioral, social, and emotional development [66]. The prenatal use of alcohol by the participants in this study corresponds to the high prevalence rates of FASD in South Africa [67].

The health of the children (Theme 2) during the first 1000 days establishes the foundation for optimal health and development later in life [68]. Although a few participants highlighted their children's good health, many of these children in this study experienced poor health. Several children suffered from oxygen deprivation directly after birth, which can cause disabilities, developmental delays, and other long-term effects [55,56]. The children of four participants who smoked during their pregnancy experienced respiratory problems after birth, which could possibly be caused by prenatal cigarette smoking [69]. A number of children of participants suffered more severe illnesses and conditions, such as TB, kidney disease, colon problems, and physical disabilities. A few children were hospitalized, causing sleep deprivation and severe psychological stress. A number of participants confirmed taking their children for their medical check-ups and immunization at the scheduled times, which played a vital role in the health of their children [70]. The study also focused on the children's feeding and nutrition, from birth to two years, and many participants breastfed their babies during the first few months, as recommended by the World Health Organization [71]. Some participants complied with the guidelines set by the Department of Health in South Africa, by introducing solid foods to their infant's diet at six months [72]. Many participants provided good food choices like fruit, vegetables, meat, and dairy products, as suggested by the Australian Government [73]. In terms of the children's weight, several participants regarded their children's weight as healthy, while a few stated that their children were underweight or overweight. Many participants experienced challenges regarding their children's feeding and nutrition, with a lack of or limited food. Nutritional deficiencies occurred, due to poor nutrition and other challenges, which possibly caused stunting in some of these children, which affected their brain development and resulted in learning difficulties at school [74].

Support (Theme 3) from others could influence the health and well-being of individuals [75]. The participants' experience of support during pregnancy was affected by their emotions and thoughts, as well as the announcement of their pregnancy and other people's responses. Many participants were unmarried at the time when they became pregnant, and the announcement of the pregnancy caused anxiety and fear. Several mothers experienced family members not talking to them, threatening to put them out of the house, or the biological father denying fatherhood. Many participants felt supported during their pregnancy and after the birth of their child, while numerous participants experienced a lack of support that resulted in a sense of loneliness. A lack of support caused the participants to be more vulnerable to depression and anxiety. Support from the biological father is paramount [76], as experienced by some participants. A number of participants received support from the child's father, however, several participants experienced no support from the biological father during that time-period. Many participants expressed challenges pertaining to their relationship with the biological father, including an unstable relationship, conflict, drug abuse of the father, and lack of financial support. A few biological fathers engaged with their children, and played an active role in their lives, which could have had a positive influence on these children's social, emotional, and cognitive development [77]. It was clear that other significant people, especially the grandparents, siblings, and the participants' male friends, played a positive role in the lives of their children.

The circumstances of the mothers and their children (Theme 4) referred to their living and financial circumstances during pregnancy and birth to two years. More than half of the mothers described their living circumstances as suitable and pleasant, while others experienced adverse living conditions, such as unsuitable housing, lack of water or electricity, a significant amount of family conflict, and substance abuse in the home, which led to an increased vulnerability experienced by the mothers and their children [78]. The living circumstances remained the same in most cases after the birth of the child, however, there were changes and even improvements for some participants during that time-period. Financial circumstances had a huge impact on the participants, as most of them experienced some form of financial strain, often lacking the resources to supply their child's basic needs.

The attachment and relationship between the participants and their children (Theme 5) during pregnancy, and during the two-year period after birth were influenced by various aspects. Some participants were happy and excited when they found out they were pregnant, whereas many of them initially experienced negative emotions, such as shock, confusion, disappointment, anger, sadness, and panic, due to an unplanned pregnancy [79]. These negative emotions made the mothers more susceptible to the risk of maternal depression [80]. The child's gender influenced the emotional responses of participants. Many participants felt relief, happiness, and excitement when the gender coincided with their preferences. Several participants considered abortion or adoption. The movement of the unborn baby activated various positive emotions, such as happiness, excitement, enjoyment, love, acceptance, and protection. These positive emotions indicated signs of bonding [81,82]. Some participants interacted with their unborn babies in various ways, by talking and singing to them. These interactions promoted the children's development [81], and enhanced bonding between them and their unborn babies [83]. Many participants expressed positive initial responses, interaction, and emotions, directly after the birth of their child, while some experienced an internal motivation for self-improvement. These positive responses immediately after birth influenced them to be more inclined towards their children's needs [84]. It was noticeable that attachment between the participants and their children formed during the two-year period after they were born. However, a few participants expressed certain negative emotions and thoughts towards their child, which included irritation, lack of attachment, and serious harmful emotions and thoughts by one of the participants specifically.

The development and care of the children (Theme 6) involved a variety of aspects. Although most participants showed an understanding of some of their children's developmental needs—especially their physical needs—many participants had a limited understanding about their children's emotional, linguistic, and cognitive developmental needs. Some participants felt that their children met their developmental milestones, while others highlighted their children's rapid development. One of the mothers who abused drugs during her pregnancy, emphasized her child's cognitive and physical developmental challenges. Many participants used 'serve and return' to stimulate and play with their babies, which is beneficial for building a strong foundation in the child's brain architecture [85]. Many participants used educational toys or activities to incorporate stimulation and play into their children's lives. Only some participants played with their children when they were older, since they felt that the children could play with their siblings.

Reflecting on the findings of this study and various theories relating to child development, it appears that these theories play a significant role in the following way. The first two stages of Erikson's Psychosocial theory [86,87] refer to children's development of trust and autonomy. The sensorimotor stage of Piaget's theory of cognitive development was noticeable in the way the participants described their children's understanding of their environment through different activities involving their senses. Attachment between the participants and their children, as indicated by the attachment theory [28], was highlighted as one of the themes and occurred various times in this study. The four phases of the attachment theory [28,86] were also evident during the time from birth to two years, as the participants described the bond between them and their child, and the reaction of their child when separation occurred. However, specific types of attachment [28,86] were not definite. Bronfenbrenner's bioecological theory [88] was clearly evident throughout the study, where both the mothers' and children's interaction with various systems played a vital role. Lastly, Maslow's hierarchy of needs [87,89], mainly the first three needs, namely (1) physiological needs; (2) the need for safety; and (3) the need for love; were strongly visible in the findings. A lack in basic physiological needs, such as food and baby goods due to poverty, had an enormous effect on some of the participants, and were highlighted by many of them.

Finally, it should be noted that although the aim of this study was not to determine a correlation between the first 1000 days and absenteeism, the findings of this study indicated that many factors played a vital role during the first 1000 days of the absent learners in this study. Literature further confirmed that specific aspects revealed in the findings of this study, such as nutritional deficiency [25], substance abuse during pregnancy [29,30], toxic stress [32], attachment, [34] and stimulation [36] could have negative effects on the schooling of children. Some of these aspects include academic, social, emotional problems at school, and school absenteeism.

4.2. Limitations

This study involved participants from a rural community in South Africa, characterized by high rates of poverty. The findings might, therefore, not be representative of all children in other communities, pertaining to their first 1000 days of life. Conducting the study on a small scale with a total of 18 female participants from one area limits the generalizability of the findings in terms of being representative of all children's first 1000 days. The interview schedule that was utilized during the interviews was limited to 12 questions, resulting in some areas not being explored. For example, the age of the mothers during pregnancy, or whether the pregnancy was planned were not specifically asked. Another aspect that was not explored, was the mothers' substance use/abuse after birth while they were breastfeeding, since this was not a definite question, and not mentioned by the mothers.

4.3. Implications for Future Research

Future research should include a larger sample size, or be conducted in other communities besides rural communities. Future qualitative studies should explore other aspects that could have affected the first 1000 days of the lives of children, for example, whether mothers consumed alcohol or used other substances while breastfeeding. Since the first 1000 days are affected by various factors, a quantitative study could provide information with a numerical value relating to these different factors. Future research should evaluate the impact of numerous first 1000 days initiatives worldwide, to provide insight and recommendations regarding the best interventions and strategies.

4.4. Contributions to Communities and Professionals Working in the Field of Early Child Development

This study makes a contribution by increasing our understanding of the various factors that could potentially have affected the first 1000 days of absent learners in the Foundation Phase. These insights could provide Government, NGOs, communities, and professionals working in the field of Early Childhood Development (ECD) with recommendations that could be considered during their planning of future programs and interventions. These recommendations include—(1) educate the broader communities on the importance of the first 1000 days through continual social media campaigns, by making use of platforms like the radio, television, newspapers, and Facebook; (2) incorporate the guidelines set out by the World Health Organization on the identification and management of substance abuse during every antenatal visit, to screen the past and present substance use/abuse of mothers; (3) provide support groups for pregnant mothers and mothers with children up to two years, in order to offer emotional support, education, and practical guidance regarding nurturing care, attachment, and stimulation of children in this time-period; (4) offer workshops and interactive events to biological fathers and extended family members to establish meaningful support to mothers during pregnancy and after their child's birth; (5) add a module that focuses on the first 1000 days to the tertiary training curriculum of social workers, healthcare workers, ECD practitioners and educators; and (6) include first 1000 days initiatives in national and international policies, to compel and guide countries regarding the implementation of these interventions during this critical time-period.

5. Conclusions

Research on a South African and international level highlights the many factors that could influence the first 1000 days of life—between pregnancy and the second birthday of children. Whilst research emphasizes that adequate nutrition and care during this unique time-period determine whether children will thrive and reach their full potential, it is evident that this is not always true for all children. Based on the findings of this study, it was concluded that a substantial number of factors, such as the health and nutrition of both the mothers and their children, substance use/abuse during pregnancy, toxic stress, support to the mothers and their children, attachment, attentive care, stimulation and play could have played a role during the first 1000 days of the absent learners in this study. Most of these factors relate to the Western Cape Government's First 1000 Days campaign launched in South Africa, entitled 'Right Start Bright Future'. It was confirmed by literature that the factors relating to the First 1000 Days campaign could potentially have affected the development of children during their first 1000 days, with a lifelong impact on, amongst others, their schooling.

In addition, it is imperative that support is offered to both mothers and their children during this critical time. It is, therefore, essential that NGOs, practitioners, and even the private sector are educated on the importance of the first 1000 days of life, in order to motivate them to collaborate with government departments to strengthen the support of mothers and children. Greater collaboration and multi-sector partnerships are, therefore, needed to improve services focusing on the first 1000 days of life, enabling all children to thrive and transform.

Author Contributions: Conceptualization, C.v.Z. and C.v.W.; Formal analysis, C.v.Z. and C.v.W.; Investigation, C.v.Z.; Methodology, C.v.Z. and C.v.W.; Project administration, C.v.W.; Supervision, C.v.W.; Visualization, C.v.Z.; Writing—original draft, C.v.Z.; Writing—review & editing, C.v.Z. and C.v.W. All authors have read and agreed to the published version of the manuscript.

Funding: This research received no external funding.

Institutional Review Board Statement: The study was conducted according to the guidelines of the Declaration of Helsinki, and approved by the registered Health Research Ethics Committee of North-West University (NWU-000008-19-A1 approved on 17 April 2019).

Informed Consent Statement: Informed consent was obtained from all subjects involved in the study.

Data Availability Statement: The data presented in this study are available on request from the corresponding author. The data are not publicly available due to privacy.

Acknowledgments: The authors acknowledge the professional services delivered by Mari Grobler (language editor) who has her own academic language practice, and Neville Robertson, who is a research assistant at the North-West University (Potchefstroom Campus), for his assistance with regards to reference and technical aspects. Finally, we would like to thank the biological mothers who participated in this research who helped us to understand the various factors that played a role during the first 1000 days of their children.

Conflicts of Interest: Although one author had a personal interest in absent learners, as a result of her work context, various aspects were incorporated into the study to combat any form of bias that could have inappropriately influenced the interpretation of the research results.

References

1. UNICEF: Office of Research-Innocenti. The First 1000 Days of Life: The Brain's Window of Opportunity. Available online: https://www.unicef-irc.org/article/958-the-first-1000-days-of-life-the-brains-window-of-opportunity.html (accessed on 8 April 2018).
2. Pem, D. Factors affecting early childhood growth and development: Golden 1000 days. *Adv. Pract. Nurs.* **2015**, *1*. [CrossRef]
3. Bornstein, M.H.; Arterberry, M.E.; Lamb, M.E. *Development in Infancy: A Contemporary Introduction*, 5th ed.; Psychology Press: Sussex, UK, 2013.
4. Donald, K.; Wilmhurst, J.M. Research Newsletter: Advances in Neuroscience—The First 1000 Days. Research Newsletter. Western Cape Government, Western Cape. 2016. Available online: https://www.westerncape.gov.za/assets/departments/health/research_newsletter_30-11-2016.pdf (accessed on 10 June 2018).
5. Center on the Developing Child of Harvard University. *From Best Practices to Breakthrough Impacts a Science-Based Approach to Building a More Promising Future for Young Children and Families*; Harvard University: Cambridge, MA, USA, 2016; Available online: https://developingchild.harvard.edu/wp-content/uploads/2016/05/From_Best_Practices_to_Breakthrough_Impacts-3.pdf (accessed on 3 October 2019).
6. Mezmur, B.D. Foreword. In *South African Child Gauge*; Jamieson, L., Berry, L., Lake, L., Eds.; Available online: http://www.ci.uct.ac.za/sites/default/files/image_tool/images/367/Child_Gauge/South_Afrcan_Child_Gauge_2017/Child_Gauge_2017_lowres.pdf (accessed on 10 June 2018).
7. Bhardwaj, S.; Sambu, W.; Jamieson, L. *Setting an Ambitious Agenda for Children: The Sustainable Development Goals*; The Children's Institute, University of Cape Town: Cape Town, South Africa, 2017; Available online: http://www.ci.uct.ac.za/sites/default/files/image_tool/images/367/Child_Gauge/SouthAfrican_Child_Gauge_2017/Child_Gauge_2017_lowres.pdf (accessed on 10 June 2018).
8. Mputle, L.D.P. *Nurturing Care during the First 1000 Days of Life: A Systematic Review*; Masters of Social Work in Child Protection; North-West University: Potchefstroom, South Africa, 2019.
9. Moore, T.; Arefadib, N.; Deery, A.; Keyes, M.; West, S. *The First Thousand Days: An Evidence Paper*; Melbourne: Murdoch Children's Research Institute: Parkville, Australia, 2017.
10. Thanjan, S. Report on the First Round of the First 1000 Days Roadshows Conducted in the Cape Town Metro between April–September 2016. 2017. Available online: http://www.knowledgeco-op.uct.ac.za/sites/default/files/image_tool/images/155/356_First%201000%20Days%20roadshow_DOHreport.pdf (accessed on 12 September 2019).
11. Western Cape Government. First 1000 Days Campaign. 2017. Available online: https://www.westerncape.gov.za/general-publication/first-1-000-days-campaign. (accessed on 2 March 2018).
12. Western Cape Government. First 1000 Days: Grow, Love and Play. 2019. Available online: https://www.westerncape.gov.za/first-1000-days/ (accessed on 2 March 2019).

13. Department of Basic Education. Policy on Learner Attendance (General Notice 361 of 2010). 2010. Available online: https://www.education.gov.za/Portals/0/Documents/Policies/Policy%20on%20Learner%20Attendance%202010.pdf?ver=2010-07-20-012020-000 (accessed on 2 March 2018).
14. Attendance Works. Reducing Chronic Absence Starting in the Early Grades: An Essential Ingredient for Promoting Success in School. 2011. Available online: https://sites.ed.gov/underservedyouth/files/2017/01/MS3-Absences-Add-Up-Toolkit-for-City-Leaders.pdf (accessed on 6 September 2018).
15. Henderson, T.; Hill, C.; Norton, K. The Connection between Missing School and Health: A review of Chronic Absenteeism and Student Health in Oregon. 2014. Available online: https://www.attendanceworks.org/wp-content/uploads/2017/08/Chronic-Absence-and-Health-Review-10.8.14-FINAL-REVISED.pdf (accessed on 16 October 2019).
16. Sahin, S.; Arseven, Z.; Kiliç, A. Causes of Student Absenteeism and School Dropouts. *Int. J. Instr.* **2016**, *9*, 195–210. [CrossRef]
17. Community Agency for Social Enquiry (CASE) & Joint Education Trust (JET). Learner Absenteeism in the South African Schooling System. 2007. Available online: http://us-cdn.creamermedia.co.za/assets/articles/attachments/12552_learner_absenteeism_report,_2008.pdf (accessed on 2 March 2018).
18. Ogburn, J. Study Finds New Program Reduces Absenteeism. 2017. Available online: https://sanford.duke.edu/articles/study-finds-new-program-reduces-absenteeism-primary-schools (accessed on 3 April 2018).
19. South Africa Department of Basic Education. *Notice 2433: Age Requirements for Admission to an Ordinary Public School*; South Africa Department of Basic Education: Pretoria, South Africa, 1998.
20. Embury Institute for Higher Education. Available online: https://www.embury.ac.za/foundation-phase-teacher/ (accessed on 26 July 2018).
21. Hoadley, U. Building strong foundations: Improving the quality of early education. *S. Afr. Child Gauge* **2013**, *2*, 72–77.
22. UNICEF. School Readiness: A Conceptual Framework. 2012. Available online: https://www.unicef.org/earlychildhood/files/Child2Child_ConceptualFramework_FINAL(1).pdf (accessed on 17 October 2019).
23. Pretorius, E.; Jackson, M.; McKay, V.; Murray, S.; Spaull, N. *Teaching Reading (and Writing) in the Foundation Phase: A Concept Note*; ReSEP Projects; Research on Socio-Economic Policy: Stellenbosch, South Africa, 2016.
24. Van Zyl, E. The Relationship between School Readiness and School Performance in Grade 1 and Grade 4. *S. Afr. J. Child. Educ.* **2011**, *1*, 82–94.
25. Maalouf-Manasseh, Z.; Oot, L.; Sethuraman, K. Giving Children the Best Start in Life: Integrating Nutrition and Early Childhood Development Programming within the First 1000 Days. Technical Brief; Food and Nutrition Technical Assistance III Project. 2016. Available online: https://pdfs.semanticscholar.org/7f33/01507c5f7f34d9ad89f3a5486983a86ea41a.pdf (accessed on 2 July 2018).
26. Finnegan, L. *Licit and Illicit Drug Use during Pregnancy: Maternal, Neonatal and Early Childhood Consequences*; Canadian Centre on Substance Abuse: Ottawa, ON, Canada, 2013; Available online: https://csuch-cemusc.ccsa.ca/sites/default/files/2019-04/CCSA-Drug-Use-during-Pregnancy-Report-2013-en.pdf (accessed on 26 July 2018).
27. Addiction Centre. Pregnant Women and Alcohol: Drinking While Pregnant. 2019. Available online: https://www.addictioncenter.com/addiction/pregnant-women-alcohol/ (accessed on 28 September 2019).
28. Berk, L.E. *Child Development*, 9th ed.; Pearson Education: Boston, MA, USA, 2013.
29. Adnams, C. *Research Newsletter: Alcohol in Pregnancy and the Developing Child: What Can Be Done?* Research Newsletter; Western Cape Government: Western Cape, South Africa, 2016. Available online: https://www.westerncape.gov.za/assets/departments/health/research_newsletter_30-11-2016.pdf (accessed on 10 June 2018).
30. Kellerman, T. Secondary Disabilities in FASD. Available online: http://www.come-over.to/FAS/fasconf.htm (accessed on 10 April 2018).
31. Center on the Developing Child of Harvard University. Brain Architecture. Available online: https://developingchild.harvard.edu/science/key-concepts/brain-architecture/ (accessed on 25 February 2018).
32. Thompson, R.A. Stress and child development. *Future Child.* **2014**, *24*, 41–59. [CrossRef]
33. Berg, A. *Research Newsletter: Parent-Infant Attachment*; Research Newsletter; Western Cape Government: Western Cape, South Africa, 2016. Available online: https://www.westerncape.gov.za/assets/departments/health/research_newsletter_30-11-2016.pdf (accessed on 10 June 2018).
34. Newman, L.; Sivaratnam, C.; Komiti, A. Attachment and early brain development–neuroprotective interventions in infant–caregiver therapy. *Transl. Dev. Psychiatry* **2015**, *3*, 28647. [CrossRef]
35. Jamieson, L.; Richter, L.; Cavoukian, R. Striving for the sustainable development goals: What do children need to thrive? *Child Gauge* **2017**, *2*, 201733.
36. Ebrahim, H.; Seleti, J.; Dawes, A. Learning begins at birth: Improving access to early learning. *Early Child. Res. Q.* **2013**, *21*, 153–157.
37. Hesse-Biber, S.N. *The Practice of Qualitative Research*, 3rd ed.; Sage Publications Ltd.: Thousand Oaks, CA, USA, 2017; p. 38.
38. Brynard, D.J.; Hanekom, S.X.; Brynard, P.A. *Introduction to Research*, 3rd ed.; Van Schaik Publishers: Pretoria, South Africa, 2014.
39. Ivankova, N.V.; Creswell, J.W.; Clark, V.L.P. Foundations and approaches to mixed methods research. In *First Steps in Research*, 2nd ed.; Maree, K., Ed.; Van Schaik: Pretoria, South Africa, 2016; pp. 305–336.
40. Lambert, V.A.; Lambert, C.E. Qualitative descriptive research: An acceptable design. *Pac. Rim Int. J. Nurs. Res.* **2012**, *16*, 255–256.
41. Marshall, C.; Rossman, G.B. *Designing Qualitative Research*, 6th ed.; Sage Publications Ltd.: Thousand Oaks, CA, USA, 2016.

42. Patton, M.Q. *Qualitative Research & Evaluation Methods: Integrating Theory and Practice*, 4th ed.; Sage Publications: Thousand Oaks, CA, USA, 2014.
43. Khula Development Group. Available online: http://www.khuladg.co.za/index.php/programs (accessed on 21 July 2018).
44. South Africa Western Cape Government Community Safety. Policing Needs and Priorities (PNP) 2017/2018 Report for the Paarl-East Police Precinct. 2017. Available online: https://www.westerncape.gov.za/assets/paarl_east_pnp_report_final.pdf (accessed on 24 September 2019).
45. Violence Prevention through Urban Upgrading (VPUU). Safe Node Area: Paarl-East. 2016. Available online: http://vpuu.org.za/safe-node-area/paarl-east/ (accessed on 6 February 2021).
46. Wagner, C.; Kawulich, B.; Garner, M. *Doing Social Research: A Global Context*; McGraw-Hill Education Ltd.: Berkshire, UK, 2012.
47. Braun, V.; Clarke, V. Using thematic analysis in psychology. *Qual. Res. Psychol.* **2006**, *3*, 77–101. [CrossRef]
48. Clarke, V.; Braun, V. Teaching thematic analysis: Overcoming challenges and developing strategies for effective learning. *Psychologist* **2013**, *26*, 120–123.
49. Babbie, E.R.; Mouton, J. *The Practice of Social Research*; Oxford University Press Southern Africa: Cape Town, South Africa, 2001.
50. Biswas, C.; Amato, P.; Dorling Kindersley, I. *The Pregnancy Encyclopaedia: All Your Questions Answered*; DK Publishing: New York, NY, USA, 2016.
51. The Royal Australian and New Zealand College of Obstetricians and Gynaecologist. Pre-Eclampsia and High Blood Pressure during Pregnancy. 2017. Available online: https://ranzcog.edu.au/RANZCOG_SITE/media/RANZCOG-MEDIA/Women%27s%20Health/Patient%20information/Pre-eclampsia-and-High-Blood-Pressure-During-Pregnancy.pdf?ext=.pdf (accessed on 24 August 2019).
52. World Health Organization. WHO Recommendation on Tuberculosis Testing in Pregnancy. 2016. Available online: https://extranet.who.int/rhl/topics/preconception-pregnancy-childbirth-and-postpartum-care/antenatal-care/who-recommendation-tuberculosis-testing-pregnancy (accessed on 1 September 2019).
53. Statistics South Africa. Demographic and Health Survey. 2017. Available online: https://www.statssa.gov.za/publications/Report%2003-00-09/Report%2003-00-092016.pdf (accessed on 22 September 2019).
54. Ankin Law. Even Mild Oxygen Deprivation at Birth Can Have Lasting Effects. Available online: https://ankinlaw.com/oxygen-deprivation-at-birth/#:~{}:text=According%20to%20research%20studies%2C%20even,learning%20disabilities%2C%20and%20behavioral%20problems (accessed on 29 August 2019).
55. Birth Injury Guide. Oxygen Deprivation. Available online: https://www.birthinjuryguide.org/infant-brain-damage/causes/lack-of-oxygen-at-birth-causes-long-term-effects-for-babies/ (accessed on 29 August 2019).
56. Murkoff, H. *What to Expect When You're Expecting*; Workman Publishing: New York, NY, USA, 2016.
57. Perinatal Mental Health Project. About Us. Available online: https://pmhp.za.org/about-us/ (accessed on 30 August 2019).
58. American Pregnancy Association. Depression during Pregnancy. Available online: https://americanpregnancy.org/pregnancy-health/depression-during-pregnancy/ (accessed on 30 September 2019).
59. Marroun, H.; Zou, R.; Muetzel, R.L.; Jaddoe, V.W.; Verhulst, F.C.; White, T.; Tiemeier, H. Prenatal exposure to maternal and paternal depressive symptoms and white matter microstructure in children. *Depress. Anxiety* **2018**, *35*, 321–329. [CrossRef] [PubMed]
60. American College of Obstetricians and Gynaecologists. Postpartum Depression. 2013. Available online: https://www.acog.org/en/Patients/FAQs/Postpartum-Depression (accessed on 24 September 2019).
61. American Psychiatric Association. What Is Postpartum Depression? Available online: https://www.psychiatry.org/patients-families/postpartum-depression/what-is-postpartum-depression (accessed on 24 September 2019).
62. Mayo Clinic. Postpartum Depression. 2018. Available online: https://www.mayoclinic.org/diseases-conditions/postpartum-depression/symptoms-causes/syc-20376617 (accessed on 27 September 2019).
63. Prado, E.L.; Dewey, K.G. Nutrition and brain development in early life. *Nutr. Rev.* **2014**, *72*, 267–284. [CrossRef] [PubMed]
64. UNICEF. Nutrition's Lifelong Impact. Available online: https://www.unicef.org/nutrition/index_lifelong-impact.html (accessed on 1 September 2019).
65. World Health Organization. Management of Substance Abuse. Available online: https://www.who.int/substance_abuse/activities/pregnancy_substance_use/en/ (accessed on 7 September 2019).
66. Irner, T.B. Substance exposure in utero and developmental consequences in adolescence: A systematic review. *Child Neuropsychol.* **2012**, *18*, 521–549. [CrossRef] [PubMed]
67. Olivier, L.; Viljoen, D.; Curfs, L. Fetal alcohol spectrum disorders: Prevalence rates in South Africa: The new millennium. *S. Afr. Med. J.* **2016**, *106*, 103–106. [CrossRef]
68. UNICEF. First 1000 Days the Critical Window to Ensure that Children Survive and Thrive. 2017. Available online: https://www.unicef.org/southafrica/sites/unicef.org.southafrica/files/2019-03/ZAF-First-1000-days-brief-2017.pdf (accessed on 8 April 2018).
69. McEvoy, C.T.; Spindel, E.R. Pulmonary effects of maternal smoking on the fetus and child: Effects on lung development, respiratory morbidities, and lifelong lung health. *Paediatr. Respir. Rev.* **2017**, *21*, 27–33. [CrossRef] [PubMed]

70. South Africa Department of Health. Improving Antenatal Care. Available online: https://www.google.com/search?client=firefox-b-d&q=www.health.gov.za%252Findex.php%252Fshortcodes%252F2015-03-29-10-42-47%252F2015-04-30-08-18-10%252F2015-04-30-08-24-27%253Fdownload%253D2002%253Aleaflet-improving-antenatal-care-in-south-africa%26usg%3DAOvVaw3yiYekpR8afbHRZKmHi+Linda%2C+1bm1y (accessed on 19 September 2019).
71. World Health Organization. *Global Strategy for Infant and Young Child Feeding*; World Health Organization: Geneva, Switzerland, 2003.
72. Department of Health. Nutrition Guidelines for Early Childhood Development Centres. Available online: https://ilifalabantwana.co.za/wp-content/uploads/2016/12/Nutrition-guidelines-for-ECD-centres_Draft-2_30-September-2016.pdf (accessed on 29 September 2019).
73. Australian Government. Infant Feeding Guidelines. 2013. Available online: https://www.eatforhealth.gov.au/sites/default/files/files/the_guidelines/n56b_infant_feeding_summary_130808.pdf (accessed on 14 September 2019).
74. UNICEF; WHO; World Bank. Levels and Trends in Child Malnutrition, 2018. Joint Child Malnutrition Estimates: Key Findings of the 2018 Edition. Available online: https://www.google.com/url?sa=t&rct=j&q=&esrc=s&source=web&cd=5&ved=2ahUKEwiVyb_7yvXkAhWnThUIHbRGDgwQFjAEegQIBRAC&url=https%3A%2F%2Fdata.unicef.org%2Fwp-content%2Fuploads%2F2018%2F05%2FJME-2018-brochure-.pdf&usg=AOvVaw3QEb_l6x53enmewSTXg8eu (accessed on 19 September 2019).
75. Nurullah, A.S. Received and provided social support: A review of current evidence and future directions. *Am. Health Stud.* **2012**, *27*, 173–188.
76. C. S. Mott Children's Hospital. Partner Support During Pregnancy. Available online: https://www.mottchildren.org/health-library/abp7352 (accessed on 15 September 2019).
77. Allen, S.M.; Daly, K.J. *The Effects of Father Involvement: An Updated Research Summary of the Evidence*; University of Guelph's Centre for Families, Work & Well-Being: Guelph, ON, Canada, 2007; Available online: http://www.ecdip.org/docs/pdf/IF%20Father%20Res%20Summary%20(KD).pdf (accessed on 16 September 2019).
78. Scorgie, F.; Blaauw, D.; Dooms, T.; Coovadia, A.; Black, V.; Chersich, M. "I get hungry all the time": Experiences of poverty and pregnancy in an urban healthcare setting in South Africa. *Glob. Health* **2015**, *11*, 37. [CrossRef]
79. Higgens, S. The Psychology of Dealing with an Unplanned Pregnancy, 2018. PsychCentral. Available online: https://psychcentral.com/blog/the-psychology-of-dealing-with-an-unplanned-pregnancy/ (accessed on 22 September 2019).
80. Faisal-Cury, A.; Menezes, P.R.; Quayle, J.; Matijasevich, A. Unplanned pregnancy and risk of maternal depression: Secondary data analysis from a prospective pregnancy cohort. *Psychol. Health Med.* **2017**, *22*, 65–74. [CrossRef] [PubMed]
81. National Health Service. Attachment and Bonding during Pregnancy. 2019. Available online: https://www.nhsinform.scot/ready-steady-baby/pregnancy/relationships-and-wellbeing-in-pregnancy/attachment-and-bonding-during-pregnancy (accessed on 23 September 2019).
82. Wheatley, S. Why Bonding During Pregnancy Matters. 2018. PsychReg. Available online: https://www.nhsinform.scot/ready-steady-baby/pregnancy/relationships-and-well-being-in-pregnancy/attachment-and-bonding-during-pregnancy (accessed on 8 September 2019).
83. Van der Walt, M.M.; Coetzee, H.; Lubbe, W.; Moss, S.J. Effect of prenatal stimulation programmes for enhancing postnatal bonding in primigravida mothers from the Western Cape. *Afr. J. Nurs. Midwifery* **2016**, *18*, 27–46. [CrossRef]
84. Stoppard, M. *Bonding with Your Bump: The First Book on How to Begin Parenting in Pregnancy*; Dorling Kindersley Ltd.: London, UK, 2008.
85. Center on the Developing Child of Harvard University. Serve and Return. Available online: https://developingchild.harvard.edu/science/key-concepts/serve-and-return/ (accessed on 1 October 2019).
86. Louw, D.A.; Louw, A.E. *Child and Adolescent Development*, 2nd ed.; Psychology Publications: Bloemfontein, South Africa, 2014.
87. Zastrow, C.; Kirst-Ashman, K. *Understanding Human Behavior and the Social Environment*, 9th ed.; Cengage Learning: Boston, MA, USA, 2013.
88. Rosa, E.M.; Tudge, J. Urie Bronfenbrenner's theory of human development: Its evolution from ecology to bioecology. *J. Fam. Theory Rev.* **2013**, *5*, 243–258. [CrossRef]
89. Beckley, P. *The New Early Years Foundation Stage: Changes, Challenges and Reflections*, 1st ed.; McGraw-Hill Education: London, UK, 2013.

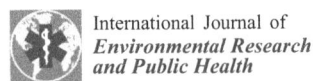

Project Report

The Routines-Based Model Internationally Implemented

R. A. McWilliam [1,*], Tânia Boavida [2,†], Kerry Bull [3], Margarita Cañadas [4], Ai-Wen Hwang [5], Natalia Józefacka [6], Hong Huay Lim [7], Marisú Pedernera [8], Tamara Sergnese [9] and Julia Woodward [10]

1. Department of Special Education and Multiple Abilities, The University of Alabama, Tuscaloosa, AL 35405, USA
2. Department of Social and Organizational Psychology, ISCTE—University Institute of Lisbon, Avenida das Forças Armadas, 1649-026 Lisbon, Portugal
3. Noah's Ark Inc., Melbourne 3442, Australia; Kerry.bull@noahsarkinc.org.au
4. Occupational Sciences, Speech Therapy, Evolutionary and Educational Psychology, Catholic University of Valencia, 46023 Valencia, Spain; margarita.canadas@ucv.es
5. Graduate Institute of Early Intervention, Chang Gung University, Tao-Yuan City 33302, Taiwan; awhwang@mail.cgu.edu.tw
6. Institute of Psychology, Pedagogical University in Krakow, 30-084 Kraków, Poland; nmjozefacka@gmail.com
7. Rophi Consultancy, Singapore 329563, Singapore; honghuaylim@gmail.com
8. Telethon Paraguay Foundation, Asunción 2420, Paraguay; marisupedernerag@gmail.com
9. The Regional Municipality of York, Newmarket, ON L3Y 6Z1, Canada; tamara.sergnese@york.ca
10. New Zealand Ministry of Education, 1666 Auckland, New Zealand; julia.woodward@education.govt.nz
* Correspondence: theramgroup0@gmail.com
† This author is deceased.

Received: 16 August 2020; Accepted: 23 October 2020; Published: 10 November 2020

Abstract: Professionals from 10 countries are implementing practices from the Routines-Based Model, which has three main components: needs assessment and intervention planning, a consultative approach, and a method for running classrooms. Its hallmark practices are the Routines-Based Interview, support-based visits with families, and a focus on child engagement. Implementers were interested in actual practices for putting philosophy and theory into action in their systems and cultures. We describe implementation challenges and successes and conclude that (a) models have to be adaptable, (b) some principles and practices are indeed universal, (c) we can shape excellent practices for international use, and (d) leadership is vital.

Keywords: routines; intervention planning; collaborative consultation; international; implementation

1. Introduction

In Minga Guazú, in the hot eastern side of Paraguay, where many of the families in early intervention (birth–6 years of age) are indigenous Guaraní, a young occupational therapist (OT) welcomes a family to the early intervention center. The center is for children with physical disabilities. This OT has been trained in the Routines-Based Model (RBM) and, today, she will talk to the family about 2 or 3 of the 12 goals on the child's and family's intervention plan.

Meanwhile, in Lisbon, a physical therapist (PT) is going on a home visit. The family has 10 goals, and this PT will talk to the family about, perhaps, 3 of these goals. In one of them, she will ask the family whether they would like to show her what they have been doing, and she will guide them through some strategies that, together, they have decided might help the child participate meaningfully in breakfast time.

In Cieszyn, Poland, workers are still hammering nails, as a dorm on a university campus is being remodeled to become a preschool ("kindergarten" in Polish parlance) following the Engagement Classroom Model. This model demonstration site will show how you can run a classroom to promote child engagement.

In this article, we discuss the Routines-Based Model—how it became of interest internationally, what practices implementers adopted, what challenges they faced, what successes they had, and our conclusions about what has to happen to improve early intervention around the world.

2. The Model

McWilliam and colleagues developed the Routines-Based Model over many years [1,2]. The model has three main components: needs assessment and intervention planning, a consultative approach, and a method for running classrooms. The model focuses on children's functioning in everyday routines and on family needs, strengths, and capacities. Figure 1 shows the flow of major components of the model.

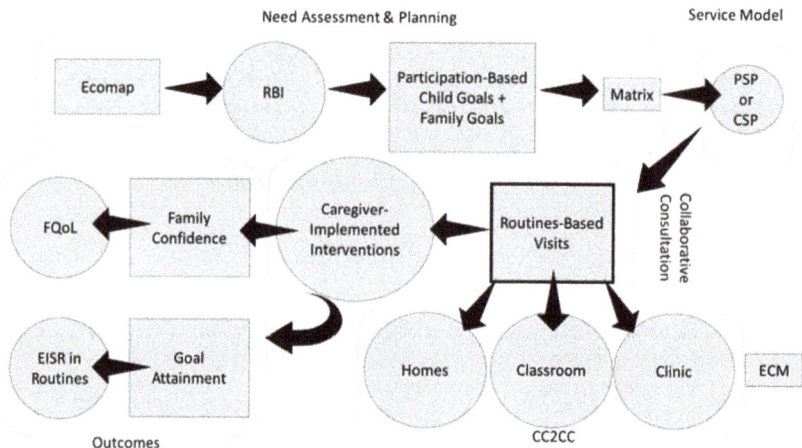

Figure 1. Flow of the Routines-Based Model. RBI: Routines-Based Interview, PSP: primary service provider, CSP: comprehensive service provider, FQoL: family quality of life, EISR: Engagement, Independence, and Social Relationships, ECM: Engagement Classroom Model, CC2CC: collaborative consultation to children's classrooms.

2.1. Needs Assessment and Intervention Plan Development

In the RBM, nothing good can happen unless we have a list of goals meaningful to the family and other caregivers spending time with the child [3]. To develop an intervention plan, which goes by different names in different countries, we conduct an ecomap and a Routines-Based Interview (RBI), from which the family chooses functional goals and family goals. This RBI is the assessment of needs upon which the entire goal plan rests.

Ecomap. The ecomap is a picture of the family's ecology [4]. The professional draws the ecomap by asking the family questions about the frequency of their contact with friends, extended family, and neighbors and how much they like the professionals and agencies they work with. Along with formal supports, it identifies the family's informal supports, which is most important. Most early intervention services do no find out about the informal supports the family might be able to count on for support before resorting to formal supports.

Routines-Based Interview. The Routines-Based Interview (RBI) is the best known component of the RBM, but it is only one of the components [5]. An early interventionist interviews the family about the details of child and family functioning in daily routines, and the family chooses functional child goals/outcomes and family goals. In New Zealand [6], they try to avoid "interview," because some people thought it was a formal 2-h bombardment of the family with questions [7]. From an implementation and branding perspective, however, we encourage implementers to keep using the Routines-Based Interview because of its name recognition.

Functional goals. Goals for child functioning are written to emphasize the child's participation in routines, such as "Jared will participate in breakfast time, hanging out time, and outside time by using single words" [8]. Furthermore, we write the goals with criteria for acquisition, generalization, and maintenance, such as "We will know he can do this when he uses five different single words, in two of these three times of day in one day, over four consecutive days."

Family goals. As a result of the RBI, the family chooses goals for themselves and siblings of the child but not of adults not present at the RBI. The most common goal is time for oneself, such as "Diane will have two hours for herself every two weeks, for 10 consecutive weeks."

2.2. Consultative Approach to Early Intervention

A principle of the RBM is that the intervention occurs between visits, so the point of visits with caregivers is to build their capacity to meet child and family needs when the professional is gone (i.e., during all the other hours of the week).

Family consultation. Family consultation involves the professional, usually a home visitor in the U.S. and other countries, working with the family to identify (a) why a child is not doing something, (b) what might be a viable solution, and (c) whether the strategy worked. This involves the professional asking many questions to find out what has being going on so far before making a suggestion [9–11]. He or she also asks the family whether they would like to try it out during the session and whether they think it is feasible.

Collaborative consultation to children's classrooms (CC2CC). Similarly, when professionals see "a child" in child care or preschool, they actually go to visit the teaching staff. Again, they jointly decide why a child is not doing something, what the strategy might be, and whether it has worked. This practice is based on seven years of research on "integrated therapy" [10].

2.3. Engagement Classroom Model

The RBM includes procedures for running classrooms to promote child engagement, which we have dubbed the Engagement Classroom Model [12]. Implementers focus on five components:

1. Conducting an RBI to establish functional, routines-based goals;
2. Incidental teaching to address all goals in all routines, by following the child's lead and eliciting higher-order functioning;
3. Integrated therapy, meaning specialists work with teachers in the classroom and never pull the child out;
4. Zone defense schedule to arrange the room in zones, to organize the adults, and to decrease non-engagement time during transitions between activities;
5. Incorporating Reggio Emilia concepts to promote children's exploration, to encourage creativity in art, and to make the environment "provocative" and beautiful.

2.4. How the Model Became of Interest, Internationally

The profile of implementation of the RBM, globally, is shown in Table 1. Each country has had its experiences with the exploration stage of implementation, the installation stage, the extent of implementation, systemic or cultural barriers or enhancers, and leadership.

Table 1. Stages of Implementation by Locations.

Location	Exploration/Introduction	Installation/Implementation Planning	Extent of Implementation	Systemic/Cultural Barriers or Enhancers	Leadership
Australia	Presentations at national conference	Systematic planning at Melbourne/Canberra agency	1 large agency in Melbourne and Canberra; sole trainer in Perth. Limited to RBI.	National Disability Insurance Scheme poses challenges; system already implementing PSP (key worker).	Agency head and key employees in Melbourne/Canberra. Individual PT in Perth. Both closely affiliated with national professional assoc. for early childhood intervention.
Canada	Presentations at Ontario mental health/early intervention conference	Systematic planning in York Region	Full model being implemented with dedicated coach.	Separate staff for home-based services from itinerant services, with different funding sources.	Regional leaders committed resources to certification of trainers.
New Zealand	Presentations followed by more intensive training sessions, primarily on RBI	Commitment by the Ministry of Education to implement the model	Whole model implemented but lapse in fidelity measures.	Coaches initially assigned, then withdrawn, now reinstated.	Initially, one of four regions, then national leadership.
Paraguay	Spanish leader in RBM implementation introduced large rehab agency to the model	After visits from the purveyor, the agency committed to implementation and sent a staff member to study with the purveyor	Implementing the RBI, without fidelity checks, and routines-based clinic visits. Planning home visits.	Rehab center philosophy, historically. Many families are rural, extremely poor, with domestic violence.	Leaders of the agency have invested in the model. Currently, one coach carries the load.
Poland	Shared platform at international conference led to presentation at university conference	Decision to found a preschool classroom using the Engagement Classroom Model (ECM)	Classroom built to accommodate the ECM, which includes RBI.	Highly therapy-focused approach to EI 0–6. Heavy governmental involvement in curriculum.	Owner, directors, faculty member, and coach all part of tight-knit group making decisions with the purveyor
Portugal	Purveyor had been teaching classes in Porto for years. Students wrote grant to study engagement	National professional organization wrote manual based largely on RBM and offered training	Whole model is endorsed, although fidelity of implementation is unknown.	Two key players in implementation have died within one year. Difficult to achieve national consensus on approach to EI. First country outside U.S. to adopt practices.	Historically, very senior faculty member, then his acolytes and their students pushed implementation. Three leaders remain who could energize implementation.

Table 1. Cont.

Location	Exploration/Introduction	Installation/Implementation Planning	Extent of Implementation	Systemic/Cultural Barriers or Enhancers	Leadership
Singapore	One developmental pediatrician invited purveyor to present. Other agencies became interested	Three agencies showed interest in in-depth implementation and developed separate plans	Different agencies have committed to different amounts of the model.	Service historically have been in group sessions with therapists. Caregivers are often domestic workers. Culturally, education is formal, not play based.	In each of the three major agencies, leaders have pushed for continued professional development
Spain	Purveyor asked to consult and present in Valencia and for national audience	University-affiliated EI program adopted RBI. ECM not as successful	Training now occurring in some states, primarily on RBI. Confederation of agencies endorsed the model.	Confusion between the "family-centered model" and RBM has slowed implementation. Historically, EI provided in centers.	University faculty have led the charge, establishing model demonstration projects, conducting research, providing training to master's students, and training programs.
Taiwan	Purveyor asked to make long presentations	Core group, primarily of PTs, interested in adopting and studying practices	Interest began with routines-based visits, then Engagement Classroom Model. One model demonstration preschool opened in Taichung.	Services have traditionally been hospital based. Demonstration preschool very different from most preschools.	Taiwanese professional org. for EI involved, researcher has led the way, PT leaders critical, core group of 7 trained in the RBI.
USA	The model was developed here and has increasingly become known through workshops, presentations, and certification institutes	Implementation plans have been developed in Multnomah County, OR; Maine, Missouri, Alabama, Colorado, Montana, etc.	Currently, Maine is the flagship implementer. Multnomah County, Alabama, and Mississippi are currently being trained to implement the full model.	History of year-by-year planning for personnel development has not led to a culture of implementation. Loathing of endorsing a model has resulted in stunted practice development. Culture of going after the latest bright, shiny object has meant little multi-year commitment.	Key individuals can be identified in each of the strong implementation sites. Always, the top person needs to be on board, if not the leader. Often, someone just under the leader is the flag bearer. Those flag bearers are more successful when they have co-conspirators.

RBI: Routines-Based Interview, PSP: the primary service provider, EI: early intervention.

When we talk about global implementation, we need to remember that U.S. implementation counts too. The RBM is implemented, to one extent or another, in many places in the U.S. The RBI specifically or the RBM as a whole are the most frequently cited strategies for improving federal child or family outcomes in state systemic improvement plans (SSIPs) [13]. Some states, such as Alabama, Maine, and Mississippi, have adopted the model and are at different stages of implementation. Other states—four that we know of—were strong implementers but have waned in recent years, which is a lesson in implementation, specifically sustainability. Siskin Children's Institute, where McWilliam used to work, still demonstrates most of both the home- and community-based components of the model as well as the Engagement Classroom Model, under the leadership of Deidra Love (director of the home- and community-based early intervention program) and Julie Mickel (director of the classroom programs), respectively. Community-based components are visits to children's child care centers or preschools. In addition, the Multnomah Early Childhood Program (MECP) in Portland, Oregon, is adopting the needs assessment, intervention planning, and home- and community-based practices in a large metropolitan environment, under the leadership of Cami Stevenson (assistant administrator). MECP is the mothership demonstration site of the model.

Implementation data have come from leaders in each of the implementation countries. [FIRST AUTHOR] has collected data from individual states and ECTA. Key informants from U.S. states and other countries have been participants in the action research involved in this implementation science. These key informants are the authors and their colleagues. Data collection has ranged from anecdotal reports to checklist data on individual practitioners.

The first non-U.S. country to show an interest in implementation of the RBM was Portugal, because McWilliam had been working intensively with the University of Porto (under the leadership of Professor Joaquim Bairrão, psychology professor) [14,15]. Eventually, the national association for early intervention adopted the model, wrote a manual, and provided sporadic training around the country [16]. Meanwhile, students McWilliam had worked with, such as Cecília Aguiar and Tânia Boavida (faculty members at ISCTE), began their own leadership in Lisbon.

Spain followed suit, when Marga Cañadas (director of an early intervention program at the Catholic University of Valencia, UCV) became an indefatigable ambassador for the approach. Within countries, the spread of the model is something that we try to keep track of. In Spain, for example, implementation sites are gradually growing and, even within *comunidades autónomas* (states) such as Castilla-La Mancha, officials are documenting the extent to which the RBM is being adopted. Currently, Pau García Grau, also on the faculty of UCV, is training professionals there on the RBI, and Catalina Morales Murillo (on faculty at La Universidad de la Rioja) has also trained Manchegos and Manchegas in RBM practices. Some Canadians were interested, in particular Kamal Haffar, who worked to spread the word in Ontario. In Taiwan, Ai-Wen Hwang went about conducting research on the model in Taiwan, and she has produced the only randomized control trial on the RBM [17]. This study showed that the RBM (called Routines-Based Early Intervention then) group had a faster progress rate in self-care functions and independence in social functions in the first 3 months of intervention and at the 6 month follow up than the traditional home-visiting group. Traditional home visiting was not more effective on any outcomes measured.

In Singapore, Lim Hong Huay led Project ECHO, which used the model for classroom practices. In New Zealand, Julia Woodward and colleagues at the Ministry of Education decided that all children and families receiving early intervention through their system would receive practices under the RBM. In Australia, a program in Victoria and Canberra, Noah's Ark, under the leadership of John Forster and his lieutenant, Kerry Bull, implemented the model. Meanwhile, in Western Australia, Denise Luscombe was also using many of the model's practices in her training and consultation to others in the Perth area. Through connections Cañadas had made, a large agency serving children with physical disabilities, Teletón Paraguay, adopted the model. This agency is one of a number in Oritel, a federation of Teletones, meaning that we might have the opportunity for implementation throughout Central and South America. The most recent implementer has been an agency in Silesia, in Poland, which has constructed classrooms expressly designed to implement the Engagement Classroom Model, under the leadership of Krystian Kroczek, Lucyna Legierska, Sylwia Wrona, and, formerly, Natalia Józefacka.

2.5. Why International Implementers Were Interested

International implementers were interested, first, because the model provides actual practices for implementing a family-centered approach. As professionals around the world began to hear and think about family-centered practices, they were intrigued and motivated [18,19]. However, they needed to know what to do. The perspectives and experiences reported here come from the reports of key informants—the leaders and implementers in these different countries: they are represented in the authors. For example, Portuguese early interventionists had difficulty implementing family-centered practices; they could not figure out how to implement these practices with the families they were working with. The RBM provided concrete professional practices in assessment, intervention planning, making decisions about services, and providing services in a family-centered way. Taiwanese experts were interested in the implementation stages of the RBM, which provided a guide and tools for early interventionists to follow. In Paraguay, they were interested in identifying families' informal and formal supports, their concerns about their child's functioning, and how to build the family's capacity to improve child functioning.

In New Zealand, similarly, the Ministry of Education wanted practical tools and a step-by-step process to implement family-centered principles. In particular, in New Zealand, the Ministry's early intervention leaders wanted a way to strengthen how they worked with their indigenous Māori people to fulfill their Treaty of Waitangi obligations: to promote partnership, protection, and participation and *Tino Rangatiratanga*—Māori control over Māori affairs. They also wanted to reduce reliance on professionals, to target support at families' day-to-day needs, to ensure everyone was clear that it is *between* visits that the intervention occurs, and to motivate adults around the child with useful intervention plans, rather than having plans sitting in filing cabinets not being implemented.

Experts in Spain saw the need for a different approach when, in 15 *comunidades autónomas*, an average of 75% of the visit (range = 51–95%) was reported to be in direct service to the child [20,21]. Spanish implementers said the model gave methods to put into everyday practice each of the DEC recommended practices [21]. This is noteworthy, because the RBM was developed before these recommended practices were chosen but perhaps it provides some informal validation for the model.

Second, as the International Classification of Functioning, Disability, and Health (ICF) hones its methods for using subsets of the ICF for Youth and Children (ICF-CY), the RBM has proceeded to develop functional profiles [22–24]. In the *Measure of Engagement, Independence and Social Relationships Manual*, the alignment of ICF-CY and the Measure of Engagement, Independence, and Social Relationships (MEISR) is presented [25]. Implementers have found that the model has resulted in more professional attention to the child's engagement, independence, and social relationships within routines—our definition of functioning. Polish implementers were attracted by the practice of following the child's lead (i.e., incidental teaching) and the precision of the zone defense schedule, in terms of every adult in the classroom having a role at every time of day [26]. For Singaporeans, one appeal of the RBM was to move services towards a more social-inclusion approach to early intervention service delivery. Five of the 10 early childhood intervention service providers in Singapore are using selected components of the RBM. One agency has developed an implementation plan for the whole model, and another is embarking on training RBI coaches with a view to their training the staff in the RBI.

Third, many of our tools are available in languages other than English. The most common translations are into Spanish, Portuguese, traditional Chinese, and Polish. Other languages for some tools are Arabic and Slovene. Professionals have found the translations of *Routines-Based Early Intervention* [9] (Chinese, Portuguese, Korean), *Engagement of Every Child in the Preschool Classroom* [12] (Chinese), and *Working With Families of Young Children With Disabilities* [27] (Portuguese, Korean) particularly helpful.

2.6. Adopted Practices

What are the most commonly implemented practices from the RBM? Many implementers, such as MECP, have adopted the whole model, albeit with adaptations. In McWilliam's experience, southern Europeans love tools. Not surprisingly, therefore, in Spain, implementers use the numerous performance-based checklists defining the major practices of the model, the MEISR [25], the Families in Natural Environments Scale of Service Evaluation (FINESSE) [28–30], and the Scale for Teachers' Assessment of Routines Engagement (STARE); Casey and McWilliam, 2007). Now, owing to García-Grau's landmark dissertation study, the Families in Early Intervention Quality of Life (FEIQoL) scale [31] is increasingly used. One characteristic of successful model adoption is when adopters consider the model their own [32]. Noah's Ark, Teletón Paraguay, and Singaporean agencies have developed their own model, incorporating parts of the RBM that fit their cultural and organizational contexts. In Singapore, four of the organizations implementing RBM practices are part of the Thye Hua Kwan (THK) Early Intervention Program for Infants and Children (EIPIC) centers, with the others being the AWWA Ltd., Singapore. Early Intervention Centre, SPD's (SPD was formerly known as the Society for the Physically Disabled) Building Bridges EIPIC centers, Fei Yue Community Services EIPIC centers, and Rainbow Centre Early Intervention Programme. SPD is the agency with an implementation plan, and AWWA is the one pursuing certification of coaches.

2.7. RBI Plus

The RBM has a cohesive set of practices for developing a functional, family-chosen set of goals. All implementers have chosen to adopt the Routines-Based Interview (RBI), which is accompanied by an ecomap (depicting a family's informal, intermediate, and formal supports), participation-based goals for children, and family goals for siblings and parents [33]. These three practices constitute the RBI Plus. The RBI is a needs assessment and typically results in 10–12 goals/outcomes. This long, meaty list of family-chosen goals is one of the hallmarks of the model.

Since 2009, Portugal has had legislation establishing the National Early Childhood Intervention System, but it does not define specific procedures. In 2016, the national association for early intervention produced a manual, which contained much of the RBM but also other practices, which has diluted the effect of the RBM [34]. This mixing of models is a two-edged sword: it purports to bring the best of different models together but it might diminish the effects of any one model.

Implementers in Taiwan began with RBI Plus and moved on to the Engagement Classroom Model. New Zealand adopted the intervention planning practices and Routines-Based Home Visits and they are working towards the primary service provider (PSP) (called a keyworker in Australia and New Zealand) [35], CC2CC, and the Engagement Classroom Model (ECM). In one of the Singapore agencies, the ecomap and RBI are the most widely adopted components of the RBM.

In Australia, Noah's Ark adopted the RBI to fully understand the family environment, conduct a functional assessment of child and family needs, and develop clear, specific, measurable goals that directly address the family's priorities and help children develop skills relevant to everyday life. Noah's Ark implemented the RBI by sending a staff member to be certified by Robin McWilliam, having that staff member and colleagues develop an implementation plan for 150 staff working with over 2000 families. McWilliam provided a 4 day boot camp in Melbourne to train 18 additional trainers.

2.8. Family and Collaborative Consultation

A second set of practices that implementers often choose are those related to a consultative approach. In particular, York Region, in Ontario, Canada, for example, felt the RBM would assist them in moving from an expert model to a collaborative approach with caregivers, ensuring the family were the primary decision makers. International adopters of the model also implement *family consultation*, which is the collaborative-consultation method we have developed, giving families opportunity to be partners in selecting strategies for them to use with their children [36]. When professionals visit classrooms, within the RBM, they work with teachers, using collaborative consultation, rather than working directly with children. In both support-based home visits and collaborative consultation to children's classrooms (CC2CC), caregivers might demonstrate what they or the child does, or the early interventionist might demonstrate a strategy the caregiver is interested in.

2.9. Engagement Classroom Model

A less commonly implemented set of practices is the Engagement Classroom Model (ECM), although the Słonezna Kraina and the University of Silesia at Katowice (Cieszyn campus) are implementing the ECM [12]. It includes the RBI, integrated therapy, incidental teaching, the zone defense schedule, and Reggio Emilia features. One of our American sites, MECP in Portland, is working with Head Start programs and other preschools where suspension and expulsion of children with disabilities occurs at a high rate. Implementation of the ECM would reduce, if not eliminate, suspension and expulsion, because the practices include ways to keep children engaged and include effective behavior management strategies for those occasions when prevention of behavior problems has not worked.

Taiwanese implementers are using goal-attainment scaling (GAS), the Teaching Styles Rating Scale (TSRS) [37,38], the STARE [30], and the Vanderbilt Ecological Congruence of Teaching Opportunities in Routines (VECTOR) [39] to determine the interaction of the STARE and VECTOR with the TSRS.

Across implementation sites, therefore, RBI Plus (the needs assessment and intervention-planning practices), our consultative-service-delivery approach, and the ECM have been implemented. This constitutes the whole model, but the whole model is not implemented by any one program. Plans are under way to add ECM to MECP in Portland, which would make that site the most comprehensive adopter of the RBM.

3. Implementation Challenges

Implementation of new practices can be exciting but it involves change. We highlight here seven areas that have been the most challenging in international implementation of the RBM. A common implementation challenge, from the perspective of the purveyor, is professionals' claiming they are implementing a model when, in fact, they are not. Their claims are usually based on an honest belief they are doing what they understand to be the practices in the model.

3.1. Natural Environments

In Spain, Marga Cañadas and McWilliam tried for 4 years to persuade early intervention programs to leave their clinics ("centers") and go into homes and communities to implement the RBM. The two main reasons for the attachment to centers were control and money. In their rooms in their centers, professionals are in control of the session. In their centers, they can see eight clients a day, whereas, visiting natural environments, they would be able to see only four or five children and families. When it was clear professionals could not be budged out of their clinics, McWilliam made a huge concession and developed procedures for routines-based clinic visits. By the same means that home visits can be performed in a clinical fashion, clinic visits can be performed in a family-centered fashion, with obvious limitations. Taiwan [40] and Paraguay have also found it difficult to use the model in natural environments. Poland would also find it difficult, but they are focusing on the Engagement Classroom Model rather than the home- and community-based practices in the model.

What about our "churches"? In working on international implementation, we came across the phenomenon of the importance of the building [2]. When agencies erect or modify buildings to house their early intervention programs, they are proud of them and want to get the most out of them. You can sense an almost religious devotion to the building. McWilliam first realized this at the Asunción center of Teletón Paraguay-the flagship center. It is a beautiful, modern, spacious building, with a remarkable curved wood-slat ceiling over the therapeutic swimming pool. Why would they not use this lovely space?

3.2. Primary Service Provider

A second challenge in implementing the RBM is the use of a primary service provider (PSP), rather than having a host of different providers from different disciplines working with the child [35,41]. Many early intervention cultures, worldwide, are very discipline driven, with a view that more is better. In Poland, for example, sensory integration therapists are separate from occupational therapists, and, in most other countries, psychologists play a much bigger role in early intervention than they do in the U.S. In Spain, they have psychometricians, a discipline that does not even exist in some other countries. In Paraguay, they have "early intervention professionals" who are different from teachers, therapists, and so on. So, when implementers try to organize a PSP approach, they meet much resistance. When a primary service provider cannot be used, one provider serves as the *comprehensive* service provider, attending to all child and family needs [42].

3.3. Relinquishing Control to Families

A central tenet of the RBM is that families make meaningful decisions [2]. For example, they decide on the functional needs of (goals for) the child and family, they decide on what to work on between visits, and they decide on what to focus on, in each visit. For many international implementers (and American implementers), giving families this amount of control is unusual and therefore uncomfortable. The medical or psychological model, which is common across the globe, places much control in the professional's hands.

In Singapore, a cultural challenge is that many middle-class families have a "foreign domestic helper" in the home. This young woman from Indonesia or Malaysia might care for the child for 8–14 h a day, yet she has little decision-making power. The parents participate in the needs assessment (i.e., the RBI), yet they might know little about their child's functioning in everyday routines. Furthermore, the domestic helper would be the person caring for the child, yet she has little say in the needs or the goals. The RBM has been described as a paradigm shift in disability services in Singapore, which, before the model, had adopted the special-education and medical-therapeutic approach. The model challenges teachers and therapists to listen reflectively and to use motivational interviewing techniques. It also challenges social workers in early intervention services to improve their child development knowledge and collaborate effectively as a team with therapists and teachers. In Singapore, social workers play a prominent role, as in Europe psychologists do. In the U.S., these disciplines are less frequently represented in early intervention programs.

In Taiwan, families and professionals alike are used to professionals giving suggestions, especially on the first visit, such as a visit to the doctor. Furthermore, the time it takes to conduct an RBI is considered a barrier in Taiwan, as it is elsewhere. In some situations, professionals (and families) think professionals should provide suggestions on the first visit: in the RBM, we do not provide suggestions during the RBI or until the family has chosen goals. Recently, the Taiwan government and early intervention professionals have promoted family-centered approaches and the ECM [40].

In Paraguay, the biggest challenges have been (a) abandoning a clinical approach and moving to a family-centered approach (including a flattening of the hierarchy between professional and family) and (b) broadening professionals' scope beyond their formal training. In many countries outside the U.S., both professionals and families expect the former to tell the latter what to do.

3.4. Lack of Follow through

In implementation planning, we encourage adopters to realize that, after intensive training, they need to keep monitoring and supporting professionals. In Portugal, for example, teams were well trained initially but poorly supervised afterwards. In New Zealand, supervision and ongoing professional development varied across early intervention sites. In Australia (Noah's Ark), the most significant challenge has been in supporting newly inducted team leaders and subsequent key workers in reaching fidelity to the model in a timely way. York Region, Ontario, listed resources required for ongoing training as a challenge.

3.5. Organization and Reorganization

The geographic and administrative organization of services-especially change in organization-can wreak havoc on implementation of the RBM. For example, Portuguese early intervention is overseen by three ministries, which is extremely challenging. Mississippi moved from nine regions to three. A change like that requires much energy and time, distracting from implementation. In New Zealand, the national practice support network, which had been active early in implementation, was disestablished, reducing the amount and quality of communication among districts.

3.6. Checklists

Implementation of the model over time requires people to observe and provide feedback—actual training and maintenance. This presents a challenge in terms of who is available and of scheduling. In Poland and New Zealand, for example, they are concerned about who will have the time to make all the checklist-based observations. Implementers, such as York Region and our Portland, OR, site, have found it difficult to find the time to ensure interobserver agreement.

3.7. You Are Doing It Wrong

Popular on the internet are articles about what we are doing wrong, from parenting to cutting cucumbers to facing the future. With the RBM, some experts and practitioners believe that they are using the model when they are not. We see this challenge all over the place. This phenomenon is known as the Dunning–Kruger effect, where implementers with little knowledge of the details of the model have much confidence in their ability to execute the practices (see Figure 2) [43]. It is particularly difficult because the believers see no reason to change, and it is bad for the model: people see bad practices and hear they are part of the RBM. We often have to be clear about what does *not* constitute the RBM.

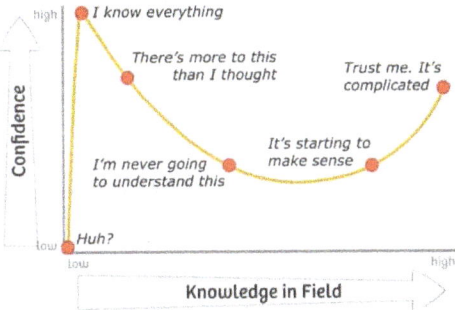

Figure 2. The Dunning–Kruger effect [44]. Reproduced with permission from Stanford Brown, retrieved from https://stanfordbrown.com.au/finance-101-the-dunning-kruger-effect/.

In Spain, we have been concerned that professionals obtain some of the increasingly available materials and tools and use them with no training. For example, professionals have been known, not only in Spain, to conduct an ecomap and then file it away, never to use it in supporting the family.

In general, change is often difficult. For some professionals, the change is welcome: they get to do what they instinctively would do or they have a structure for what they were doing. For others, it is simply a change, and accommodating to new ways of doing things is inherently difficult. For yet others, the focus on child functioning in routines and the empowerment of families is not what they believe early intervention should be about. For them, the change is the hardest. It does not help when some families want the expert approach [45].

4. Implementation Successes

International implementers of the RBM report successes in a number of outcomes.

4.1. Professionals Feeling Useful

When professionals use the RBM, they feel more useful than before they adopted the model. They feel they make a difference in the areas of child and family functioning that matter to families. Before, they were focused on what they or their assessment procedures identified as deficits in child development. With the RBM, they focus on children's meaningful participation in everyday routines and on things that families care about. In Portugal, we actually saw improved goals, in terms of functionality and measurability, improved team functioning, and more collaborative consultation [46]. Similarly, in New Zealand and Ontario, goals became more functional and not arbitrary. In Singapore, professionals report parents' finding goals now easier to understand, leading to better "family engagement." Professionals also find the goals more functional and meaningful in the lives of children and families and more easily attained, which has led to greater work satisfaction.

In Taiwan, 218 professionals attended training on the RBM. The outcomes were based on McWilliam's 12 mental shifts (www.naturalenvironemnts.blogspot.com) and 10 mistakes in early intervention [47]. Professionals with less experience shifted their mindsets more than did those with more experience ($p < 0.05$) [48]. Those who had ever attended any presentations on the RBM or who had read anything about the model were more aware of the practices at pretest ($p < 0.05$) compared to those who had not. Those who received job-embedded professional development were more likely to have shifted mindsets compared to those who received other forms of professional development ($r = 0.56$–0.82). High interrater agreement on the mental-shifts scale was reported.

In Paraguay and Singapore, professionals report listening more to families' concerns and needs; constructing interventions in partnership with families, building on their strengths; collaborating more with each other; seeing progress using goal-attainment scaling. In Singapore, the RBI, specifically, resulted in parent engagement and empowerment as well as professionals' feeling empowered to understand and empathize with families. Paraguayan, Australian, and New Zealand professionals have found the model works well in aligning early intervention with indigenous ways of perceiving the family system (whānau in Māori). In Paraguay, implementers are using a smiley-face version of goal-attainment scaling with Guaraní families who do not read.

In New Zealand, the well-being of staff improved, because they did not have to have all the answers. In addition, professional support has become more purposeful and focused. Our colleagues in New Zealand also reported an outcome we have seen in different parts of the world, including the U.S.: Principles of the model have been adopted in other areas of the agency's or district's work.

In Poland and Singapore, they have begun to see the value of really listening to parents, rather than simply giving them instructions. Furthermore, they have seen a shift in professionals' mentality towards supporting families rather than "repairing" children. York Region reports child care staff and families more engaged and feeling they are an integral part of the team.

4.2. Families Feeling Confident

Across implementation sites, families feel confident about meeting children's and families' needs (e.g., in Ontario and Singapore). We now have an instrument assessing this confidence. In Paraguay, families are more empowered and confident, can identify their formal and informal supports, and now have their own needs addressed, rather than professionals' priorities for the child. In New Zealand, some families are running transition (to school) meetings, which did not happen before the RBM was implemented.

Noah's Ark (Australia) conducted semi-structured telephone interviews with 14 families participating in the RBI bootcamp training. The families said it was cathartic, beneficial, and relaxing. They highlighted the positive impact of having a professional who was warm, caring, and personable really listen to them. Many parents indicated that developing functional goals was the most valuable part of the process. Parents commented that the two-hour interview was long, but that it went by quickly. Similar results were seen in Singapore. Not all parents were thrilled about every part of the RBI, but the interviewers were new to the RBI with fidelity, and we have not matched comments to the fidelity checks. In association with The University of Alabama, Noah's Ark has been studying the impact of the RBI on goal functionality and found that, now, goals are largely participation based, observable, and functional.

4.3. Children Functioning in Routines

When professionals implement the model, children function well in routines [49]. Although routines vary somewhat across cultures, families generally want their children to participate meaningfully in the different times of day. In Portugal, professionals report that implementation has led to higher family engagement, higher implementation by families of strategies, better family well-being, families' feeling more competent, and quicker development in children. Results from Taiwan show the ECM has positive effects on child functioning [48]. Implementers such as York Region have seen children making progress based on what is important-building on engagement, independence, and social relationships rather than developmental skills in isolation that might not promote inclusion in their community.

Implementation successes, therefore, have been that professionals feel useful, families feel confident, and children are functioning in their routines. In Singapore, as an example, implementation of the RBM has brought about a paradigm shift in early intervention towards more family centeredness and a focus on functionality. It has paved the road to actualizing developmentally appropriate practices and inclusion principles.

5. Conclusions

The remarkable extent of implementation of the RBM, globally but not universally, can point to four general conclusions: models must be adaptable, some principles and practices are indeed universal, some experts do think globally about practices, and leadership is needed for successful implementation. Finally, we use our experiences with global implementation of the RBM to propose framework for the relationships among evidence, public policy, and adoption of best practices.

5.1. Models Have to Be Adaptable

Some implementers have looked for ways to work with different cultures and countries. Baumann and colleagues [50] conducted a systematic review of the literature for four evidence-based parent-training interventions, involving 610 articles. Only eight reported a cultural adaptation, and only two tested the efficacy with rigorous research methods. In addition to needing more implementation studies, we need to include cultural adaptations, especially for models used internationally. Practices developed in one country inevitably have to be adapted for implementation in other countries. With the current rigid approach to implementation fidelity, we can expect little international replication. Seeking the balance is the key.

Obsession with evidence is an American preoccupation, and the RBM is no exception [51–53]. One of our tenets in the model is to eschew non-evidence-based practices, which means we have to discard bogus practices overseas (which abound) and in the U.S. [54].

However adaptable a model is to local customs and preferences, implementers might still move on to other models. Many implementers have trouble with sticking with a model over a 5 year implementation plan and having the courage to stay away from other bright shiny objects that come along and divert attention and resources from the model.

5.2. Some Principles and Practices Are Indeed Universal

The principles undergirding the RBM appear to be universal: we want children to function well in their natural routines, we want families to have the confidence to teach their children through their natural parenting, we want professionals to build caregivers' capacity, and we want supervisors and trainers to use observation and feedback. Practitioners and administrators no longer want to hear about rhetoric, theory, advocacy, and esoteric research, such as "recommended practices" [21] or a "family-centered model" [55]: They want to hear about specific, evidence-based ways of doing things.

With respect to natural environments, specifically, when professionals concentrate on *what* happens during the visit more than *where* it occurs, they can truly build the caregiver's capacity and end up with more intervention for the child than a hands-on approach. If purveyors insist on supports being provided in natural environments, they will not be implemented at scale overseas. Portugal, however, did pass legislation and provided training, so early interventionists do make home and community visits.

5.3. Promoting a Global Perspective on Excellent Practices

Some American-developed models are designed to address American contexts and are difficult to implement outside the U.S. Early intervention in the U.S. can be considered somewhat ethnocentric. Many professionals assume the early intervention landscape internationally is like the U.S. one. However, U.S. perspectives can be international: for example, the headquarters of the International Society on Early Intervention is in Seattle, because that's where its founder and president, Michael Guralnick, works. Further, the scholarly journal *Infants and Young Children* under the editorship of Mary Beth Bruder, deliberately publishes international research and perspectives and even has an international editor (self-disclosure: it is McWilliam).

Many practitioners overseas and in the U.S. are impressed with entertrainment, but we need to focus on specific practices and models. *Entertrainment* is a portmanteau of entertainment and training and refers to an appealing presentation with few practical strategies and no provision for follow-up observation and feedback (i.e., real training). Implementation can only happen if implementers commit to serious, long-term, job-embedded professional development [56].

5.4. Leadership

The purveyor must be in control and has to relinquish control. The purveyor (in this case, Robin McWilliam) has to be the arbiter of what constitutes fidelity to the model [57]. The purveyor has to protect and promote this fidelity for two reasons. One is that any evidence on which the model is based involved specific practices, so deviation can render the practice no longer evidence based. The second reason is a branding and credibility one: If people are saying they are using a model or its practices, when in fact they are not, any success or failure of their efforts will not really reflect the model.

Local leadership is the key [58]. In every successful implementation of the RBM, one or more local leaders have gone through the stages of implementation to explore options, decide on the RBM as a solution to needs they saw, shepherded the initial implementation, and planned for full implementation. Some of our sites are well into implementation and others are near the beginning, but the role of key players, many of whom are authors of this article, cannot be underestimated.

Because this model was developed in the U.S., one might think the implementation over the past 15 years has been one way. Actually, as we have mentioned a number of times, to make it truly a global model, we have had to make modifications. Implementers from different countries have learned from each other. For example, Marisú Pedernera, the bright young linchpin for the Paraguayan implementation, corresponds with a colleague in Taiwan, with Cami Stevenson in Portland, Oregon, and with colleagues in Spain. Many implementers and other international professionals interested in the RBM are members of The RAM Group, a community of practice dedicated to the exchange of information about the model (www.ramgroup.info).

5.5. Framework Regarding Evidence, Policy, and Implementation

The role of the government, through policies or legislation, in early intervention varies greatly. In most countries, its primary concern has been the provision of services, ensuring services are available to young children with disabilities. Not all governments have been involved with the quality of services. The United States has provisions built in, such as the requirement that services be provided in natural or least restrictive environments. Different state systems of early intervention or preschool special education have varying levels of interest in the quality of services. Some, such as Alabama and Maine, have invested heavily in improving and maintaining high quality services. Outside the U.S., Portuguese law deals with the establishment of the system for managing early intervention, with a nod to quality by requiring the International Classification of Functioning, Health, and Disability be used in assessment [22,59]. In Australia, the government has established the National Disability Insurance Scheme, ostensibly to provide consumer choice, yet the scheme challenges family-centered practices and promotes a multidisciplinary approach to early childhood intervention [60].

As shown in Figure 3, the provision of services comes largely from the impetus of government policies and from legislation. To some extent, we have seen that the face value of RBM practices and the theories underpinning it have had some impact on systems. Those systems concerned about the quality of services have invested in training on, for example, the RBM. New Zealand's Ministry of Education adopted the RBI initially in one region, then spread it to the other three regions, and now uses other aspects of the RBM. They, like Australia, had a leg up because they were already using keyworkers, who are like primary service providers in the RBM. We see that the common sense of the RBM, the family-centered principles, and the theories about child functioning have had more impact on impact by agencies and governmental agencies than has the empirical evidence. However, the RBM's face value has credibility because of its basis in evidence-based practices.

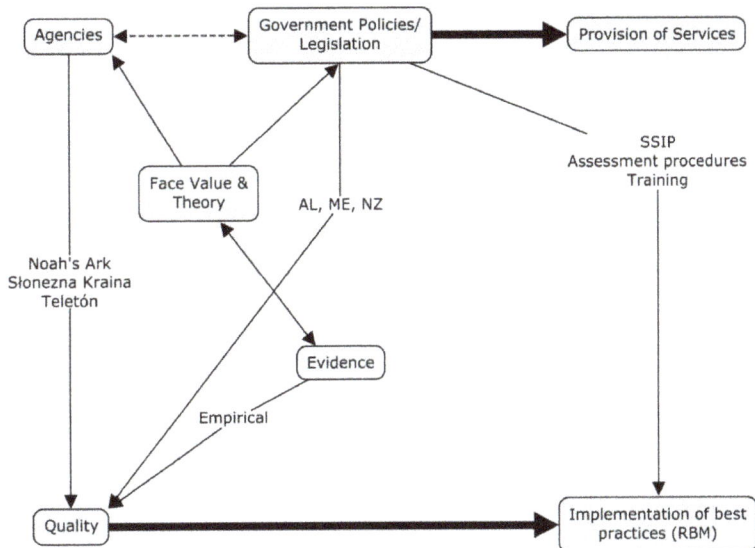

Figure 3. Relationships among government, evidence, and implementation. AL: Alabama: ME: Maine, NZ: New Zealand. RBM: Routines-Based Interview.

Agencies in various international implementation sites have had a key role. To some extent, they might influence governmental agencies, and, certainly, they are influenced by the governments (i.e., they usually exist within the constraints of governmental regulations). In Australia, we have see Noah's Ark, in Melbourne and Canberra, embrace high-quality supports to children and families-not only with the RBM but also other philosophically and empirically sound models. They have been vocal in warning the National Disability Insurance Scheme about challenges to quality. In Poland, the implementation site for the Engagement Classroom Model, Słonezna Kraina, repudiated the traditional Polish concepts of quality early intervention approaches and boldly adopted the RBM. Teletón Paraguay, similarly, broke with cultural traditions to reimagine quality, moving from a rehabilitation approach to a functional, family-centered approach. These agencies and others were influenced primarily by the logic and values of the RBM.

An interest in quality, therefore, has been the driving force behind implementation of best practices. Circling back to governmental input, we have seen that some actions by governmental agencies have enhanced implementation of the RBM. For example, in the U.S., 24% of the states have included practices from the RBM in their state systemic improvement plans, which are required, annually [61]. In these improvement plans, most often states have included the RBI in their assessment procedures. Finally, governmental agencies have invested in training in the RBM. For example, various U.S. states such as Alabama, Kentucky, Maine, Mississippi, Montana, and Nebraska have funded professional development in the RBM. Outside the U.S., governmental investment has been restricted largely to New Zealand. In Spain, some states (comunidades autónomas), such as Castilla la Mancha, have funded training in the model.

The interaction among governmental interest, research, and implementation is, therefore, a complicated and fascinating one. Pragmatists would like to find the perfect solution. Descriptivists, however, are content with admiring the phenomenon.

We end with three inferences. First, working with implementers in a caring, respectful, and honest way leads to appropriate modifications of the model. Second, sustaining an innovation is harder than implementing it: things change (funding mechanism, geographical organization, leadership), and carrying out the innovation with fidelity to the model is shaken. Third, some practices are good for young children with disabilities and their families, wherever they are. These practices might be that early intervention and parenting should help children participate in their lives meaningfully, that early intervention should support families to be the caregivers they want to be, and that early intervention professionals should know what they are doing. International implementation of the RBM has, therefore, provided a prototype for how to work across cultures, countries, and customs.

Author Contributions: Conceptualization, R.A.M.; methodology, R.A.M.; writing—original draft preparation, R.A.M.; investigation, resources and writing—review and editing: R.A.M., T.B., K.B., M.C., A.-W.H., N.J., H.H.L., M.P., T.S., J.W.; visualization, R.A.M.; supervision, R.A.M.; project administration, R.A.M. All authors have read and agreed to the published version of the manuscript.

Funding: This research received no external funding.

Acknowledgments: We acknowledge, with gratitude, contributions from Stacey Hodgson, Becky Hoo, Iris Lin, Low Hwee San, Agatha Tan, Tan Peng Chian, Sze Wee Tan, and Marla Teicher.

Conflicts of Interest: Authors declare no conflict of interest.

References

1. McWilliam, R.A.; Trivette, C.M.; Dunst, C.J. Behavior engagement as a measure of the efficacy of early intervention. *Anal. Int. Dev. Disabil.* **1985**, *5*, 59–71. [CrossRef]
2. McWilliam, R.A. Metanoia in early intervention: Transformation to a family-centered approach. *Rev. Latinoam. Educ. Inclusiva* **2016**, *10*, 155–173.
3. Idol, L.; Nevin, A.; Paolucci-Whitcomb, P. *Collaborative Consultation*, 2nd ed.; PRO-ED: Austin, TX, USA, 1994.
4. Jung, L.A. Identifying families' supports and other resources. In *Working with Families of Young Children with Special Needs*; McWilliam, R.A., Ed.; Brookes Publishing: Baltimore, MD, USA, 2010; pp. 9–26.

5. McWilliam, R.A. The Routines-Based Model for supporting speech and langauge. *Logop. Foniatr. Audiol.* **2016**, *36*, 178–184. [CrossRef]
6. Locke, E.; Latham, G. Goal-setting theory. In *Organizational Behavior 1: Essential Theories of Motivation and Leadership*; Miner, J.B., Ed.; Routledge: New York, NY, USA, 1994; pp. 159–183.
7. Woods, J.J.; Lindeman, D.P. Gathering and giving information with families. *Infants Young Child.* **2008**, *21*, 272–284. [CrossRef]
8. Fleming, J.L.; Sawyer, L.B.; Campbell, P.H. Early intervention providers' perspectives about implementing participation-based practices. *Top. Early Child. Spec. Educ.* **2011**, *30*, 233–244. [CrossRef]
9. McWilliam, R.A. *Routines-Based Early Intervention*; Brookes Publishing Co.: Baltimore, MD, USA, 2010.
10. McWilliam, R.A. Integration of therapy and consultative special education: A continuum in early intervention. *Infants Young Child.* **1995**, *7*, 29–38. [CrossRef]
11. McWilliam, R.A.; Wolery, M.; Odom, S.L. Instructional perspectives in inclusive preschool classrooms. In *Early Childhood Inclusion: Focus on Change*; Guralnick, M.J., Ed.; Brookes Publishing: Baltimore, MD, USA, 2001; pp. 503–530.
12. McWilliam, R.A.; Casey, A.M. *Engagement of Every Child in the Preschool Classroom*; Paul H. Brookes Co.: Baltimore, MD, USA, 2008.
13. Early Childhood Technical Assistance Center. Idea Part C Profiles. 2014. Available online: https://osep.grads360.org/#program/idea-part-c-profiles (accessed on 17 July 2020).
14. Grande, C.; Pinto, A.I. Estilos interactivos de educadoras do Ensino Especial em contexto de educação-de-infância. *Psicol. Teor. Pesqui.* **2009**, *25*, 547–559. [CrossRef]
15. Pessanha, M.; Pinto, A.I.; Barros, S. Influência da qualidade dos contextos familiar e de creche no envolvimento e no desenvolvimento da criança. *Psicologia* **2009**, *23*, 55–71. [CrossRef]
16. Serrano, A.M.; Pereira, A.P.; Carvalho, M.L. Oportunidades de aprendizagem para a criança nos seus contextos de vida: Família e comunidade/Child's learning opportunities in natural environments: Family and community. *Psicol. Rev. Assoc. Port. Psicol.* **2003**, *17*, 65–80.
17. Hwang, A.-W.; Chao, M.; Liu, S. A randomized controlled trial of routines-based early intervention for children with or at risk for developmental delay. *Res. Dev. Disabil.* **2013**, *34*, 3112–3123. [CrossRef]
18. Dunst, C.J.; Johanson, C.; Trivette, C.M.; Hamby, D.W. Family-oriented early intervention policies and practices: Family-centered or not? *Except. Child.* **1991**, *58*, 115–126. [CrossRef] [PubMed]
19. McWilliam, R.A. *Family-Centered Intervention Planning: A Routines-Based Approach*; Communication Skill Builders: Tucson, AZ, USA, 1992.
20. Cabrerizo de Diago, R.; López Pisón, P.; Navarro Callau, L. *La Realidad Actual de la Atención Temprana en España*; Real Patronato sobre Discapacidad: Madrid, Spain, 2012.
21. Division for Early Childhood. DEC Recommended Practices in Early Intervention/Early Childhood Special Education. 2014. Available online: http://www.dec-sped.org/recommendedpractices (accessed on 16 July 2020).
22. World Health Organization. *International Classification of Functioning, Disability, and Health: Children & Youth Version: ICF-CY*; World Health Organization: Geneva, Switzerland, 2007.
23. Hwang, A.-W.; Liao, H.-F.; Granlund, M.; Simeonsson, R.J.; Kang, L.-J.; Pan, Y.-L. Linkage of ICF-CY codes with environmental factors in studies of developmental outcomes of infants and toddlers with or at risk for motor delays. *Disabil. Rehabil.* **2013**, *36*, 89–104. [CrossRef] [PubMed]
24. Pan, Y.-L.; Hwang, A.-W.; Simeonsson, R.J.; Lu, L.; Liao, H.-F. Utility of the early delay and disabilities code set for exploring the linkage between ICF-CY and assessment reports for children with developmental delay. *Infants Young Child.* **2019**, *32*, 215–227. [CrossRef]
25. McWilliam, R.A.; Younggren, N. *Measure of Engagement, Independece, and Social Relationships (MEISR™), Research Edition, Manual*; Paul H. Brookes Publishing Co.: Baltimore, MD, USA, 2019.
26. Casey, A.M.; McWilliam, R.A. The impact of checklist-based training on teachers' use of the zone defense schedule. *J. Appl. Behav. Anal.* **2011**, *44*, 397–401. [CrossRef]
27. McWilliam, R.A. (Ed.) *Working with Families of Young Children with Special Needs*; Guilford Press: New York, NY, USA, 2010.
28. McWilliam, R.A. Families in Natural Environments Scale of Service Evaluation (FINESSE). In *Routines-Based Early Intervention: Supporting Young Children and Their Families*; McWilliam, R.A., Ed.; Paul H. Brookes Publishing Co.: Baltimore, MD, USA, 2010; pp. 212–220.

29. McWilliam, R.A. *Families in Natural Environments Scale of Service Evaluation (FINESSE II)*; University of North Carolina: Chapel Hill, NC, USA, 2000.
30. Casey, A.M.; McWilliam, R.A. The STARE: Data collection without the scare. *Young Except. Child.* **2007**, *11*, 2–15. [CrossRef]
31. McWilliam, R.A.; García Grau, P. *Families in Early Intervention Quality of Life*; The University of Alabama: Tuscaloosa, AL, USA, 2017.
32. Evidence-Based Intervention (EBI) Work Group. Theories of change and adoption of innovations: The evolving evidence-based intervention and practice movement in school psychology. *Psychol. Sch.* **2005**, *42*, 475–494. [CrossRef]
33. McWilliam, R.A. Assessing families' needs with the routines-based interview. In *Working with Families of Young Children with Special Needs*; McWilliam, R.A., Ed.; Guilford: New York, NY, USA, 2010; pp. 27–59.
34. Associação Nacional de Intervenção Precoce. *Práticas Recomendadas em Intervenção Precoce na Infância: Um Guia para Profissionais*; Associação Nacional de Intervenção Precoce: Coimbra, Portugal, 2018.
35. McWilliam, R.A. The primary-service-provider model for home- and community-based services. *Psicol. Rev. Assoc. Port. Psicol.* **2003**, *17*, 115–135.
36. Woods, J.J.; Wilcox, M.J.; Friedman, M.; Murch, T. Collaborative consultation in natural environments: Strategies to enhance family-centered supports and services. *Lang. Speech Hear. Serv. Sch.* **2011**, *42*, 379–392. [CrossRef]
37. McWilliam, R.A.; Scarborough, A.A.; Kim, H. Adult interactions and child engagement. *Early Educ. Dev.* **2003**, *14*, 7–27. [CrossRef]
38. McWilliam, R.A.; Scarborough, A.A.; Bagby, J.H.; Sweeney, A.L. *Teaching Styles Rating Scale*. Frank Porter Graham Child Development Center; University of North Carolina at Chapel Hill: Chapel Hill, NC, USA, 1998.
39. Casey, A.M.; Freund, P.J.; McWilliam, R.A. *Vanderbilt Ecological Congruence of Teaching Opportunities in Routines (VECTOR) Classroom Version*; Vanderbilt Center for Child Development: Nashville, TN, USA, 2004.
40. Liao, H.-F.; Wu, P.-F. Early childhood inclusion in Taiwan. *InfantsYoung Child.* **2017**, *30*, 320–327. [CrossRef]
41. Shelden, M.L.; Rush, D.D. *The Early Intervention Teaming Handbook: The Primary Service Provider Approach*; Paul H. Brookes: Baltimore, MD, USA, 2013.
42. McWilliam, R.A.; Garcia Grau, P. Towards Implementation of an early intervention model by a Paraguayan organization. *Educação* **2020**, *43*, e35700. [CrossRef]
43. Dunning, D. The Dunning-Kruger effect: On being ignorant of one's own ignorance. In *Advances in Experimental Social Psychology*; Olson, J.M., Zanna, M.P., Eds.; Academic Press: Cambridge, MA, USA, 2011; Volume 44, pp. 247–296. [CrossRef]
44. Dargahwala, I. The Dunning Kruger Effect. 2019. Available online: https://dev.to/theiyd/the-dunning-kruger-effect-3cj2 (accessed on 15 July 2020).
45. McWilliam, R.A.; Casey, A.M. *More is Not Always Better: Research Findings*; Presented at the International Conferene on Early Childhood (Division for Early Childhood of the Council for Exceptional Children), Chicago, IL, USA, 2004; Division for Early Childhood of the Council for Exceptional Children: Los Angeles, CA, USA, 2004.
46. Boavida, T.; Aguiar, C.; McWilliam, R.A.; Correia, N. Effects of an in-service training program using the routines-based interview. *Top. Early Child. Spec. Educ.* **2016**, *36*, 67–77. [CrossRef]
47. McWilliam, R.A. The top 10 mistakes in early intervention—And the solutions. *Zero Three* **2011**, *31*, 11.
48. Hwang, A.-W. *The Long-Term Effectiveness of Implementing a Participation-Based Early Intervention Program for Children with Developmental Delay: A Cluster-Randomized Controlled Trial*; Final Report (Project NO.: MOST-105-2314-B-182-012-); Unpublished Report; Ministry of Science and Technology: Taipei, Taiwan, 2017.
49. Garcia Grau, P.; McWilliam, R.A.; Martínez-Rico, G.; Grau Sevilla, M.D. Factorial structure and internal consistency of a Spanish version of the Family Quality of Life (FaQoL) Scale. *Appl. Res. Qual. Life* **2018**, *13*, 385–398. [CrossRef]
50. Baumann, A.A.; Powell, B.J.; Kohl, P.L.; Tabak, R.G.; Penalba, V.; Proctor, E.K.; Domenech-Rodriguez, M.M.; Cabassa, L.J. Cultural adaptation and implementation of evidence-based parent-training: A systematic review and critique of guiding evidence. *Child. Youth Serv. Rev.* **2015**, *53*, 113–120. [CrossRef] [PubMed]
51. Dunst, C.J.; Trivette, C.M. Using research evidence to inform and evaluate early childhood intervention practices. *Top. Early Child. Spec. Educ.* **2008**, *29*, 40–52. [CrossRef]

52. Odom, S.L. The tie that binds evidence-based practice, implementation science, and outcomes for children. *Top. Early Child. Spec. Educ.* **2009**, *29*, 53–61. [CrossRef]
53. Cook, B.G.; Cook, S.C. *Thinking and Communicating Clearly about Evidence-Based Practices in Special Education*; Division for Research, Council for Exceptional Children: Reston, VA, USA, 2011.
54. McWilliam, R.A. Controversial practices: The need for a reacculturation of early intervention fields. *Top. Early Child. Spec. Educ.* **1999**, *19*, 177–188. [CrossRef]
55. Dalmau, M.; Balcells-Balcells, A.; Giné, C.; Cañadas, M.; Casas, O.; Salat, Y.; Farré, V.; Calaf, N. How to implement the family-centered model in early intervention. *An. Psicol.* **2017**, *33*, 641–651.
56. Dunst, C.J.; Trivette, C.M. Let's be PALS: An evidence-based approach to professional development. *Infants Young Child.* **2009**, *22*, 164–176. [CrossRef]
57. Halle, T.; Metz, A.; Martinez-Beck, I. *Applying Implementation Science in Early Childhood Programs and Systems*; Paul H. Brookes Publishing Company: Baltimore, MD, USA, 2013.
58. Ploeg, J.; Davies, B.; Edwards, N.; Gifford, W.; Miller, P.E. Factors influencing best-practice guideline implementation: Lessons learned from administrators, nursing staff, and project leaders. *Worldviews Evid. Based Nurs.* **2007**, *4*, 210–219. [CrossRef] [PubMed]
59. Pinto, A.I.; Grande, C.; Aguiar, C.; de Almeida, I.C.; Felgueiras, I.; Pimentel, J.S.; Serrano, A.M.; Carvalho, L.; Brandão, M.T.; Boavida, T.; et al. Early childhood intervention in Portugal: An overview based on the developmental systems model. *Infants Young Child.* **2012**, *25*, 310–322. [CrossRef]
60. Marchbank, A.M. The National Disability Insurance Scheme: Administrators' Perspectives of Agency Transition to 'User Pay' for Early Intervention Service Delivery. *Australas. J. Early Child.* **2017**, *42*, 46–53. [CrossRef]
61. Early Childhood Technical Assistance Center. SSIP Phase III, Year 3 Analysis: Data. 2019. Available online: https://ectacenter.org/topics/ssip/ssip_p3.asp (accessed on 18 July 2020).

Publisher's Note: MDPI stays neutral with regard to jurisdictional claims in published maps and institutional affiliations.

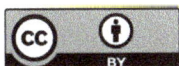

© 2020 by the authors. Licensee MDPI, Basel, Switzerland. This article is an open access article distributed under the terms and conditions of the Creative Commons Attribution (CC BY) license (http://creativecommons.org/licenses/by/4.0/).

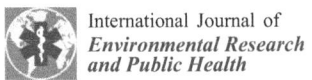

Review

Promoting Developmental Potential in Early Childhood: A Global Framework for Health and Education

Verónica Schiariti [1,*], Rune J. Simeonsson [2,3] and Karen Hall [2]

1. Division of Medical Sciences, University of Victoria, Victoria, BC V8W 2Y2, Canada
2. School Psychology Program, School of Education, University of North Carolina, Chapel Hill, NC 27599, USA; rjsimeon@email.unc.edu (R.J.S.); karench@live.unc.edu (K.H.)
3. School of Education and Communication, Jönköping University, SE-551 11 Jönköping, Sweden
* Correspondence: vschiariti@uvic.ca; Tel.: +1-250-472-5500

Abstract: In the early years of life, children's interactions with the physical and social environment-including families, schools and communities—play a defining role in developmental trajectories with long-term implications for their health, well-being and earning potential as they become adults. Importantly, failing to reach their developmental potential contributes to global cycles of poverty, inequality, and social exclusion. Guided by a rights-based approach, this narrative review synthesizes selected studies and global initiatives promoting early child development and proposes a universal intervention framework of child-environment interactions to optimize children's developmental functioning and trajectories.

Keywords: early child development; ICF; education; health; inequality; rights; functioning; potential; intervention; disability

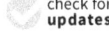

Citation: Schiariti, V.; Simeonsson, R.J.; Hall, K. Promoting Developmental Potential in Early Childhood: A Global Framework for Health and Education. *Int. J. Environ. Res. Public Health* **2021**, *18*, 2007. https://doi.org/10.3390/ijerph18042007

Academic Editor: Mirja Hirvensalo

Received: 26 December 2020
Accepted: 16 February 2021
Published: 19 February 2021

Publisher's Note: MDPI stays neutral with regard to jurisdictional claims in published maps and institutional affiliations.

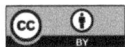

Copyright: © 2021 by the authors. Licensee MDPI, Basel, Switzerland. This article is an open access article distributed under the terms and conditions of the Creative Commons Attribution (CC BY) license (https://creativecommons.org/licenses/by/4.0/).

1. Introduction

Access to health and education services, are essential factors for optimal development, functioning and well-being of the child, factors paralleling the development, functioning and well-being of family, community, and society. Limited or deprived access to health services and education significantly challenges the development of children, as well as the development of families and communities, restricting their developmental potential for school and work. The extent to which developmental outcomes of child, family or community is favorable is defined by the realization of basic human rights of access to health and education services. Recognition of the parallel between the development of the child and the development of families and communities has served as the basis for national and global initiatives in health and education in recent decades exemplified by Education for All, the Millennium Development Goals (MDG), and the Sustainable Development Goals (SDG) [1,2]. Implementation of each of these initiatives over the last three decades has been associated with variable progress in addressing the enduring cycles of poverty, infant mortality, malnutrition, illiteracy, and inequalities in access to health care and education of children. However, risks for delay and disability and unmet potential in early development of young children are still pervasive, particularly in low- and middle-income countries [3].

The Declaration of Human Rights in the middle of the 20th century formalized the recognition of basic human rights of access to health and education and provided a standard for referencing the association of inequalities of those rights with limited development of nation states. Recognition of the extent of those inequalities and their disproportionate impact on children and their development was formalized decades later with the United Nations Convention of the Rights of the Child—UNCRC [4]. Although all of the articles of UNCRC define conditions for reducing inequalities and promoting children's developmental potential, the rights to health and nutrition (Article 24), education (Articles 28 and 29), and articles ensuring that those rights are realized without discrimination of gender, ethnicity, disability and other identities (Articles 2 and 23) are particularly germane to the priorities defined by the MDG and the SDG. This perspective builds on documentation of the status of children, their health and development through comprehensive surveys on national, regional, and global levels. The surveys established the prevalence of child and maternal health conditions and the environmental factors that placed children's development at significant risk for delay and disability. In higher income countries, documentation of risk factors to children's health and development led to more effective medical care and improved services for children with chronic conditions. In middle- and lower income countries, such documentation served as the basis for population-based program of disease prevention development of primary care.

Although, documentation of child-environment developmental risk factors has made a great contribution to our understanding of modifiable risk factors, there is a need for a universal framework promoting early child development in low-, middle- and higher-income countries across the health and education sectors, that could guide assessments and interventions as the children grow and develop globally. Therefore, the aims of this paper were to:

(1) Synthesized selected studies identifying children at risk for developmental delay or loss of developmental potential.
(2) Describe key global initiatives to illustrate the impact of environmental factors on children's developmental potential around the world.
(3) Propose a global framework of child-environment interaction guiding assessment and intervention for health and education.

Synthesis of Studies and Core Themes of This Paper

Guided by a rights-based approach, this narrative review synthesizes selected studies and global initiatives promoting early child development. Selection for inclusion consisted of the most relevant initiatives to the areas listed in the introduction, decided by consensus, and published in English from 2001 to 2020. Specifically, we synthesized Initiatives addressing environmental factors influencing children's development, as well as prevalence and estimates of children at risk for developmental delay or loss of developmental potential in low-, middle- and high-income countries. Limitations of this approach are addressed in the paper.

Subsequently, a universal intervention framework of child-environment interactions is proposed for optimizing children's developmental functioning and progress drawing on the International Classification of Functioning, Disability and Health for Children and Youth (ICF-CY) [5,6]. Finally, we highlight the importance of adopting a global framework guiding assessments and evaluations of children's development across sectors. As such, the content of this study is organized in three themes as follows:

(a) A global initiative to promote early child development.
(b) A dimensional framework of child functioning and development.
(c) Promotion of children's development: assessment and intervention in health and education.

2. A Global Initiative to Promote Early Child Development

Although initiatives at country levels and programs at global levels by UNICEF, World Health Organization (WHO) and various non-governmental organizations (NGOs) over the last three decades have contributed to significant reductions in the scope and nature of childhood mortality and morbidity, challenges to the healthy development of young children remain pervasive, particularly in low- and middle-income countries, where the largest proportion of children in the world are found. In contrast to earlier population-based studies focusing on specific child or maternal conditions, more recent research is increasingly recognizing the significant role of inadequate or deprived physical and social environments associated with poor developmental outcomes. Increased recognition of the significance of environmental factors is evident in the review by Black et al. [7] of research publications since 2000 indicating that the number of publications on stimulation (n = 1121), micronutrients (n = 936) and nutrition-related issues (n = 508) were 2 to 8 times more frequent than studies of specific conditions such as malaria (n = 255), abuse and neglect (n = 298) or maternal depression (n = 139). This increased research focus on the physical and social environment is consistent with the broader agenda of the MDG and the SDGs. This perspective is in keeping with the challenge of documenting equitable early development as proposed by Barros [2], "entailing that every girl and boy should have the same opportunities to fully develop their potential, which is only achievable if they have good nutrition, good health, and a rich and stimulating home environment" (p. e873).

Indicators defining the child's loss of potential and limited opportunities have increasingly become representative of the focus of studies estimating risk for developmental delay, disability or disorders complementing other markers of developmental morbidity. Representative of this perspective is the study by Grantham-McGregor et al. [8] examining developmental potential of children in the context of the first and second MDGs, namely eradicating hunger and poverty and the completion of primary schooling by children globally, respectively. A comprehensive analysis was made of data on children under five in developing countries drawing on the indicators of stunting, available in 126 of these countries, and poverty, available in 88 of the countries. Of the 559 million children under five living in the developing countries, 22% were found to live in poverty, 28% were stunted and 39% were identified as stunted, living in poverty or both. This latter group served as the estimate of disadvantaged children defined in terms of risk for loss of developmental potential. The prevalence estimates for each of the indicators varied widely across regions of the world, with the percent of children living in poverty being lowest in Central and Eastern Europe at 4% and highest in Sub-Saharan Africa at 46%. The range of corresponding values for stunting were 14% for Latin America and the Caribbean and 39% for South Asia. The widest range was found for the combined indicators defining disadvantaged children, with 18% found in Central and Eastern Europe and 61% in Sub-Saharan Africa. The prevalence of lost developmental potential of disadvantaged children was supported by country-specific findings linking stunting and poverty to fewer years of education and limited learning per year of schooling with implications for deficits of income in adulthood.

The estimates of disadvantaged children based on 2004 data by Grantham-McGregor et al. [8] were updated and new estimates were generated for 2010 data in a study by Lu et al. in 2016 [9]. The study used essentially the same approach in the identification of children under five years of age manifesting stunting or exposed to poverty. Recalculating estimates of 2004 data for 141 of the developing countries with improved analytic methods indicated a higher prevalence (51%) of disadvantaged children than the 39% reported in 2007. However, a comparison of estimates based on analysis of data for the 141 countries at two time points, revealed a reduction in the prevalence of disadvantaged children from 51% in 2004 to 43% in 2010. The reduction in the prevalence of children at risk for poor development was attributed largely to reduction in stunting and poverty in South Asia including India and China. Similar to the findings of the Grantham-McGregor et al. [8] study, prevalence estimates varied widely across regions of the world, with the percent of children living in extreme poverty being lowest in Middle East and North Africa at 3% and highest in Sub-Saharan Africa at 54%. The range of corresponding values for stunting were 16% for Latin America and the Caribbean and 47% for South Asia. As in the 2007 study, the widest range was found for the combined indicators defining disadvantaged children, with 21% found in Latin America and the Caribbean and 70% in Sub-Saharan Africa. Lu et al. [9] conclude that findings reflect progress in global efforts to reduce the risk for poor development of young children, but the developmental potential of disadvantaged children continues to be significantly limited in developing countries, particularly in Sub-Saharan Africa. Challenges remain to promote children's development by reducing stunting and poverty through improved health and increased access to education, reinforcing the premise by Rippoin et al. that "increasing the educational level of their population will lead to better nourished populations, and the ability to improve gross domestic product (GDP)" [10].

The above studies have documented the scope of risk to developmental potential of young children using proxy variables of stunting and living in poverty. In more recent research, surveys such as the UNICEF Multiple Indicator Cluster Survey (MICS) encompass a range of variables more directly linked to developmental aspects of the young child in the Early Child Development Index (ECDI) of relevance in documenting progress to achieving the SDGs. Accessing data from a study of 35 countries, Manu et al. [11] conducted a secondary analysis of literacy-numeracy skills of 100,012 three to five-year-old children. A literacy-numeracy index was derived from the ECDI based on naming 10 letters of the alphabet, knowing four simple words and names and symbols for the numbers 1-10. The index was used to define an outcome variable, classifying children dichotomously as on-track or not on-track. Other variables of interest were availability of children's books in the home, urban or rural residence, and demographic variables of child age and gender, maternal education and a home wealth index. Analyses revealed that just over half (51.8%) of the children had one book in their home and less than a third (29.9%) met the criteria of being on track for literacy-numeracy. The facilitating role of the home environment was evident in the fact that having a book in the home almost doubled the likelihood of a child meeting the criteria for literacy-numeracy, after adjusting for maternal education, wealth index and demographic variables.

The broader aspects of development as assessed by the ECDI also served as the basis for a study by Gil et al. [12] to document the prevalence of children at developmental risk in low and middle-income countries. In this study, data were available from the administration of the MICS and Demographic and Health Surveys between 2010 to 2016 to families of 330,613 children, ages 3 to 5 years, in 63 low and middle-income countries. In addition to the EDCI, data was also obtained on contextual variables of rural/urban residence, maternal education, child gender and wealth inequality indicators. As in the previous survey studies of children in low and middle-income countries, large variability was found for prevalence of developmental risk between and within world regions as well as between countries. The prevalence of suspected developmental delay by region, based on the ECDI, ranged from a low of 10.1% for Europe and Central Asia and a high of 41.4% for West and Central Africa. Within the West and Central Africa region, the variability ranged from 24.9% for Ghana to 67.3% for Chad. The role of country income on prevalence of suspected developmental delay based on EDCI values yielded parallel findings with a prevalence of 41.2% for low-income countries and only 9.7% for high income countries. Prevalence estimates of suspected delay by assessed domains across all countries was lowest for physical development (3.5%), followed by learning (9.2%) and social-emotional development (24.0%).

Although the issue of promoting early child development as a global initiative is appropriately focused within the framework of inequalities faced by children in low and middle-income countries as illustrated above, initiatives of the SDGs are universal, applying to countries defined by higher incomes as well. Thus, the nature of developmental problems faced by young children, and how those problems are defined and surveyed in highly developed countries do differ, but the focus is the same, that of identifying children at a population level at risk for developmental delay or loss of developmental potential. Estimating the prevalence of children at developmental risk in higher income countries may involve several different surveys as is the case in the U.S. [13]. The National Survey of Children's Health (NSCH) generates prevalence estimates of 20 specified health conditions, as well as the status of overweight/obesity, risk for developmental delay and having a specified health care need. Based on data of a nationally representative sample of U.S. children 0–17 years of age (N = 91,642), Bethell et al. reported the prevalence of children with a chronic condition to be 43%, an estimate was increased to 54.1% with the inclusion of children with the status of overweight or obesity and risk for developmental delay [14]. Based on screener data to identify children with special health care needs such as needs for medication, additional health, mental health, or educational services, 19.2 % of the children were documented to have special health care needs. The National Health

Interview Survey (NHIS) is also administered to nationally representative samples of households with 3–17 year-old children to estimate the prevalence of one of ten diagnosed disabilities (attention deficit hyperactivity disorder [ADHD], autism spectrum disorder [ASD], blindness, cerebral palsy, hearing loss, learning disabilities, intellectual disabilities, seizures, stuttering or stammering and other developmental delay). In a comparative analysis of data from the 2009–2011 to the 2015–2017 administrations of the NHIS, Zablotsky et al. [15] reported an increased prevalence of any diagnosed disability from 16.2% to 17.8%. Among children 3–5 years of age, developmental problems were reflected in prevalence estimates of 10.55% for any disability, 2.73% for stuttering/stammering, 3.30% for learning disabilities, 2.13% for ADHD and 4.67% for other developmental delays.

Reporting on NHIS data for the period 2006 to 2010, Schieve et al. found the prevalence of diagnostic conditions in children 3–17 years of age to be, learning disabilities [LD] (7.8%), ADHD (7.9%), other developmental disabilities [ODD] (4.3%), ASD (0.09) and intellectual disability [ID] (0.07%) [16]. As some children were identified with more than one diagnosed condition, Schieve et al. (2012) derived prevalence on the basis of assignment of children to one of four mutually exclusive groups. This resulted in decreased prevalence estimates as follows, ASD only (0.9%), ID without ASD (0.5%), ADHD without ASD or ID (7.3%), and LD and ODD without ADHD, ASD or ID (5.0%).

As referenced above in the study by Bethell et al. [14], estimates of loss or delay of developmental potential has also been estimated on a functional basis of identifying special health care needs of children. Children with special health care needs were defined by McPherson et al. as children 0–17 years of age "who have or are at increased risk for a chronic physical, developmental, behavioral or emotional condition and who also require health and related services of a type or amount beyond the required of children generally" [17]. Prevalence estimates for children with special health care needs are derived from the inclusion of a screener in the administration of the National Survey of Children with Special Health Care Needs (NS-CSHCN), combined with the National Survey of Children's Health (NSCH) in 2016. The five screener items are "(1) need for or use of prescription medications, (2) above-routine use of medical, mental health, or educational services compared with other children, (3) daily activity limitations, (4) need or use of specialized therapies; and (5) need or use of treatment or counseling for emotional developmental or behavioral conditions" [18]. Use of the screener in the NS-CSHCN, the NSCH and the Medical Panels Survey have yielded prevalence estimates of children with special health care needs ranging from 12.8% to 19.3% [13]. A consistent finding of the prevalence estimates derived in these US studies is the role social determinants of poverty and limited parental education, a role shared with risks to development in low and middle-income countries.

3. A Dimensional Framework of Child Functioning and Development

Epidemiological studies on the nature and extent of developmental problems of young children globally [3,8,9] reveals that using indicators such as being disadvantaged, at risk for developmental delay and/or experience loss of developmental potential may account for prevalence estimates ranging from 19% to 51% in countries across income levels. Prevalence estimates vary based on the nature of the indicator, from proxy variables of stunting, poverty status, wealth inequalities to caregiver report of the child's medical condition, health care needs or social and academic skills. Of note is the large variability of children's risk of poor development between world regions and low and middle-income countries within regions, ranging from 7% to 73% [9]. The role of environmental factors on children's poor development is evident in the variability of prevalence of risk paralleling variability in the status of economic development of countries. Perhaps the strongest reflection of the role of the home and community environment placing children at developmental risk is high level of suspected developmental delay in literacy-numeracy, across the seven world regions, ranging from 56.3% to 87% [12]. Although the studies utilized different indicators to document developmental risk, the findings provide a consistent picture of problems and delays of development in up to half of all children 3 to 5 years of age growing up in low and middle-income countries. Lower, but comparable prevalence estimates of developmental delay and elevated health care needs in higher income countries supports the premise that developmental risk is a universal concern for young children with implications for policy and practice in the form of SDGs as well as regional and national initiatives.

The gradual decline in the prevalence of children at developmental risk in recent decades with estimates declining from about half to slightly less than 40% of the population in low and middle-income countries [9] has been documented even in the context of variability in how developmental risk was identified. Variability in prevalence estimates may reflect the conceptualization of developmental risk as well as the specific way in how the target problem was defined and cases identified. Different terms defining the population of interest such as "loss of developmental potential " [8], "disadvantaged children" [9], or "risk for developmental delay" [12] reflect different conceptual and assessment criteria and may thus account for some of the variability of prevalence estimates. However, there is correspondence of these overall prevalence estimates supporting the premise of common, underlying factors of developmental risk. When a more specific definition such as "literacy-numeracy delay" [11] with an associated Literacy-Numeracy Index (LNI) was used in a survey of 35 low and middle-income countries, mean prevalence estimate of children not meeting the criteria for being on-track of LNI was 70.1%, with large variability across countries, ranging from a low of 10.1% to 94.3%.

Although the succession of prevalence estimates over recent decades provides overall documentation of the scope of children at developmental risk, differences in the identification of risk yields different implications for policy and practice. In part, differences in the identification of risk may reflect trends in moving from the use of proxy indicators (e.g., stunting and poverty), subgroup designations (e.g., disadvantaged children) to more specific dimensions of developmental delay (e.g., social-emotional development; literacy-numeracy development). Comprehensive initiatives for children have been listed in term of goals in the MDG and SDG as the basis for defining earlier studies, but an integrated, conceptualization of the developing child within limiting or facilitating environments has been lacking in defining the focus of studies. The importance of a conceptual framework integrating components of child development within a life-course perspective to promote early development of children in low and middle-income countries has been advanced by Black et al. [7]. Central to their approach is the promotion of the child's developmental potential across the life-course through the provision of nurturing care for health, nutrition, security and safety, responsive caregiving, and early education. Implementation of such an approach recognizes the facilitating role of the systems and policy environment and the caregiving environment of family and community.

Within the ongoing commitment to advance the SDGs for children, a conceptual framework is needed that captures the dimensions of the child's interaction with the environment defined by the SDG 4 target indicators for early childhood development 4.2, 4.2.1 and 4.2.2. Specifically, the emphasis of the target indicators on children's access to, and participation in, nurturing and learning environments to ensure their rights to health, learning and well-being requires a conceptual framework integrating dimensions of the child's developmental interactions with the environment. Central to that framework is a view of early development as the product of the child's ongoing interactions with the physical, social, and attitudinal environments. The significance of these interactions in defining developmental trajectories and different outcomes of children has been defined in the transactional model of Sameroff and Fiese [19] in which reciprocal child-environment interactions account for developmental change. A similar approach has been proposed by Batorowicz et al. [20] emphasizing transactions as the important feature for interventions for young children. Drawing on the transactional approach, elements of the child-environment interaction need to be defined in dimensional terms of characteristics of the child, of the environment and of the interactions of the child with the environment. To that end, the ICF-CY [4] offers a dimensional taxonomy and accompanying codes of body functions

(8 chapters), body structures (8 chapters), environmental factors (5 chapters), and activities and participation (9 chapters), well suited to document the characteristics of the child, the environment and child-environment interactions, respectively.

Drawing on the findings of the above prevalence studies, the variable or variables defining children's developmental risk or loss of developmental potential can be identified as elements of the child's interaction with the environment as shown in Figure 1. Approaching prevalence studies within a framework incorporating the ICF-CY may be useful in several ways [6] in that it promotes focusing on developmental risk in interactional terms rather than solely as characteristics intrinsic to the child. As a universal classification, the ICF-CY codes offer a common language integrating data collection and analysis in health and education sectors that may differ across countries. Further, the codes address the need to assess child, environment and interaction variables in a standard manner across time, for example, in specific contexts such as special education services in Portugal [21] and in broader applications for documenting intervention outcomes in low-and middle-income countries [22].

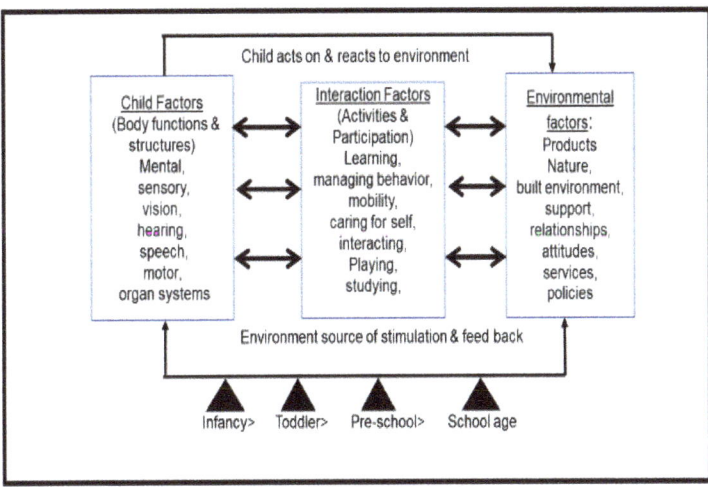

Figure 1. Interactional framework—modeling child-environment interaction within International Classification of Functioning, Disability and Health for Children and Youth (ICF-CY) domains.

4. Promoting Children's Development: Assessment and Intervention in Health and Education

Within an interactional framework, assessment, intervention, and evaluation activities should target key developmental indicators, in order to identify and address the specific delays in functioning an individual child may be experiencing. Each of these activities can significantly influence the developmental progress of children who are experiencing delays in development. The timing of assessment and intervention is critical.

Disparities in development can be enhanced or remediated based on the child's interactions within their environment. Risk factors are barriers and adverse influences on the development of the child. Protective factors are beneficial facilitating development. Exposure to risk and protective factors have cumulative effects [23] that occur when a child is exposed to the same factor repeatedly or different factors with fewer occurrences. Children who have accumulated more risk therefore need more protective factors to promote development. Greater protective factors are associated with better outcomes for children [24]. For example, children who experience multiple risk factors such as poverty, malnutrition, delayed motor development, and delayed speech are impacted by all of the factors cumulatively. Early assessment and intervention practices are key for children facing increased risk, as they allow a mechanism to also increase protective factors during a critical time for child development. A time where gaps in delay can more easily be lessened. Evaluation of assessment and intervention practices allows for more target progress.

Assessment provides information about the level of current functioning, strengths, and deficits, which can then be used to drive the individual goals of an intervention. There are many key issues to consider when planning for developmental assessment. Assessment practices begin with instrument selection. An assessment plan should include gathering baseline information as well as measures to monitor progress. Instrument selection should be culturally relevant, valid, and reliable within the population context. When choosing an instrument, stakeholders should consider the benefits and risks of using a measure.

Although there is a range of developmental assessment measures, particularly in higher income countries, their applicability for use in low-resource countries is limited. Semrud-Clikeman et al. [25] compiled a comprehensive review of neurodevelopmental assessments and screeners for clinicians to determine the best instrument for their goals. In this review, the authors defined the additional considerations needed in order to choose an appropriate assessment tool in the context of low- and middle-income countries. Stakeholders need to determine whether they will use a formal assessment tool, an adapted version of a formal assessment tool, or a locally developed test. Administering a formal assessment tool allows for standardized data to be collected, with scores comparable to a norm reference group. This data provides a clear picture of how an individual child is performing in various domains, it also provides norm referenced scoring which is useful for determining delay. Using formal assessment tools are useful when they are assessing children who are represented in the norm referenced sample.

When assessing children who are in a different cultural context than where the assessment was developed, an approach that has been taken has been to develop an adaptation of the measure for the local context. To avoid overidentification due to cultural bias, and changes in reliability and validity, children should be assessed using data pre- and post- intervention to determine the change in functioning rather than focusing solely on norm referenced data to define delay. Developing local tests can be useful to determine a child's developmental functioning in the context of their community environment, which may have distinct priorities that shape the developmental trajectory of a child. Though Semrud-Clikeman et al. [25] provide a framework for thinking through the context of a developmental assessment, the bulk of their review provides a matrix of assessments for various neuropsychological domains with specific information about adaptations, training requirements, and test-specific information for practitioners. Their seminal work can be used as a guide for practitioners to begin choosing a specific measure within context of culture, disease, and area of development.

The lack of standardized measures suitable for use in assessment of young children in low-resource countries has been identified by Bhavnani [26] as a significant impediment for population-based screening and for assessing dimensions of child functioning for planning and monitoring interventions. The use of existing tools and measures is often not an option for a number of reasons. From a practical standpoint, the use of standardized, proprietary measures may not be feasible because of cost and the requirement for highly trained professionals to administer them. Lack of standardization with a reference population, concerns about cultural fit, specificity of content and mode of administration are additional constraints on developmental assessment of young children. Recognizing these constraints for valid developmental assessment, particularly of children in rural contexts, a gamified tool was developed to assess cognitive development using tablet technology that could be administered by non-specialists. Specifically, the Developmental Assessment on an E-Platform (DEEP) tool, uses games and narratives on tablets to assess cognitive development of three-year old children across six domains: response inhibition, divided attention, visual form perception, visual integration, reasoning and memory. The cognitive domains were assessed on the basis of the child's play of nine interactive games such as hidden objects, odd one out, jigsaw and location recall. In a phased testing of alpha and beta versions of the DEEP, the tool generated metrics that reflected individual differences in accuracy and completion of cognitive skills. In a subsequent proof of concept study, Mukherjee et al. [27] administered the DEEP to 200 three-year old children in a rural district in India to test the utility of derived scores to predict children's performance on a standardized tool, the Bayley Scales of Infant Development-III. Results indicated that DEEP scores were predictive of, and positively correlated with cognitive performance on the BSID-III. The potential utility of the DEEP for developmental assessment of children in low-resource countries is supported by the fact that it yielded reliable data in the context of a developmentally homogeneous study population (mean BSID-III cognitive score of 8), and physical limitations with one-third characterized by stunting and one-fourth being underweight.

Optimal intervention occurs as early as possible, recognizing that disparities in early childhood have long lasting consequences. These consequences can be mediated by early intervention programs in which long-term effects have been noted related to cognitive development, as well as behavioral and emotional development in children [28]. In higher income countries, early intervention focuses increasingly on preparing for educational readiness through programs such as preschool, head start, or home visit interventions. In low- and middle-income countries, additional consequences of health and environmental factors, such as increased risk for malnutrition or infection and disease, may require the creation of different types of intervention feasible in low-resource settings.

Interventions to facilitate improved developmental outcomes for children may involve implementing community-based programs or processes that promote children's development in low- and middle-income countries. Interventions may target the child directly or aim to involve the interactions between the child and their environment. Eickmann et al. [29] described a community-based intervention program implemented in Brazil in which the intervention program was designed to improve cognitive and motor development by targeting the interaction between the child and their mother. Mothers were trained to implement simple interactions that promote motor and cognitive development within the home environment. Children who received the intervention showed significant improvements in both cognitive and motor development. Children who showed greater initial delays made larger overall gains from the intervention. Children who received the intervention maintained their developmental progress when measured 12–18 months later, while children who did not receive the intervention showed scoring decline.

The intervention included a workshop component as well as home visits. The intervention was designed to increase the mother's skill through demonstration, practice, skill building, and reinforcement in the home environment. The intervention was intensive, with three workshops and ten home visits occurring over a period of five months. This study highlighted several key factors for optimal intervention, including early assessment leading to targeted intervention for children most at risk. The study also promoted a process that changed the social and environmental interactions of children to increase stimulation.

In upper middle- and high-income countries, intervention priorities may shift toward the developmental risk factors present in the population served to also include school readiness behaviors as part of developmental outcomes. In the U.S., children with developmental delays or other disabilities can begin receiving early intervention services beginning at birth, and eventually provided through the public-school system beginning at age three. Elbaum [30] investigated the developmental outcomes of children with delays ($n = 17,828$) who participated in preschool special education. Children received services to support the development of communication, cognitive, adaptive, motor, and social development. Using the Battelle Developmental Inventory, Second Edition (BDI-2), children were categorized into severity of delay (no delay, mild/moderate delay, and severe delay). Children with a mild or moderate delay (24.2% of the sample, upon entry) made significant gains, with over half (57.6%) exiting the preschool program functioning at age level development. Of the children with a severe delay (60% of sample, upon entry), developmental gains were made as well with 23% exiting the program meeting age level developmental expectations.

Children with more complex delays (including delays across multiple measured categories) showed higher level of risk upon entry and less age expected developmental progress upon exiting the program [30]. This outcome speaks to the importance of considering the complex nature of supporting children with multiple areas of delay or children with special healthcare needs, as their developmental needs are unique. These groups of children benefit from early developmental intervention, but may not experience the same immediate gains in developmental progression as children with fewer domain areas of delay or children without special healthcare needs.

Early childhood interventions in Turkey [31] and Austria [32] have structures similar to those in the U.S., beginning at birth with early intervention services which transition to school-based services around 36 months. Early intervention programs in each of these countries are structured by legislation and public policy. They also illustrate similar challenges in cohesiveness across sectors. For example, integrating health and nutrition programs into early intervention services require an integration of intervention from multiple stakeholders. These three countries also face challenges of public awareness of intervention programs as well as limitations with diagnostic requirement for services and lack of opportunities for inclusive programing with typically developing children.

A specific example of an early intervention program implemented in the context of a school-based service, is the Tools of Mind (Tools) program. Recognizing the importance of environmental interactions in intervention, Diamond et al. [33] investigated the impact of Tools on individual and environmental factors in Canadian kindergarten classrooms. The Tools curriculum is designed to teach strategies to support executive functioning skills by teaching contextually based attentional control and self-control strategies. The authors built on previous studies of the Tools intervention to further investigate the impact of the intervention on the environment by measuring the child's prosocial behavior, academic performance, classroom stress, and teacher burnout. Results of the study, as measured by standardized academic assessment tools and teacher surveys, indicated the contextually based Tools intervention resulted in individual and environmental impacts. Children who were enrolled in a classroom where the teacher used Tools had improved self-regulation skills and performed better academically. Environmental impacts in the classroom included less bullying, increased helping behavior of students, and increased enthusiasm, and decreased burnout among teachers.

In defining replicable strategies of intervention for low-income countries, Engle et al. [34] examined the effectiveness of cross sector programs to optimize the health and the environment of children through intervention. Factors associated with effective intervention included: direct services provide to children, early intervention- especially to those most disadvantaged, and longer or more intensive exposure to the intervention. Additionally, structure and establishing processes were associated with program quality. Though early intervention provides significant benefits strategies to minimize environmental, health, and social risks are also key. This can be challenging as it requires investments beyond direct child intervention, and into other sectors of public policy, research, and governmental programming working together to support comprehensive early child development interventions.

Evaluation of implemented interventions should be considered at both the systemic and individual level. Promoting optimal functioning for children requires the facilitation and coordination of assessment, intervention, and evaluation efforts. Evaluation should include systemic indicators as well as individual indicators. Framed within the lens of transactional theory, Black and Dewy [35] emphasized the importance of integrated interventions, while also magnifying challenges in evaluation. Integrated interventions across health and education target a child's developmental needs across sectors (i.e., early child development and nutrition). Integrating nutrition programs into early education programs intuitively makes sense, as better nutrition is linked to cognitive development and functioning. Research is needed to demonstrate that nutrition and early child development programs are more effective than early education programs alone [35]. This perspective is elaborated by Lipina and Posner's [36] comprehensive review demonstrating the relationship of cognitive, linguistic and behavioral development with nutrition and underlying development of brain networks. Within this perspective, interventions, particularly for children in poverty need to address the associated risk factors of malnutrition, inadequate housing, and limited access to health care, support and early education.

Given the importance of integrated interventions to promote children's developmental potential, meaningful evaluation becomes a key priority. Systematic efforts to evaluate interventions that combine cross-sector programs are challenging in that they require multiple stakeholders to coordinate, organize, and monitor programming. In providing combined health and educational services emphasizing child-environment interactions, there is a need for collaborative initiatives across sectors serving young children, particularly children at risk and with disabilities. Studies focused on child-environment interactions in the educational or health settings. For example, Sanches-Ferreira M et al. [20] described special needs assessment in the Portuguese educational system. Interestingly, the authors' findings support the need for an expanded focus on person-environment interactions, considering students' participation in different domains of life—besides learning—as well as the impact of environmental barriers over students' participation. In addition, they highlight the need for training programs centered on a biopsychosocial understanding of human functioning, the establishment of a transdisciplinary collaborative culture and the use of dynamic assessment tools to equip professionals with appropriate conditions to use the ICF-CY within an interactive perspective. Moreover, Batorowicz et al. [19] proposed a model for research and clinical practice that directs researchers and practitioners working in rehabilitation of young children toward interventions that address the mechanisms of child-environment interaction and that can build capacity within both children and their social environments, including families, peers' groups and communities. In this service provision approach, the authors highlight that health is created and lived by people within the settings of their everyday life; where they learn, work, play, and love [19].

Table 1 shows the key findings of the studies included in this section applying a child-environment interaction framework. Promoting early child development, we have identified children's factors, environmental factors, and interaction factors facilitating child development and functioning in different settings (Table 1).

Table 1. Promoting early child development: a child-environment interaction framework.

Study Authors	Child Factors	Interaction Factors	Environmental Factors
Eickmann et al. 2003	Cognitive functions Motor functions	Increase play interactions between mother and child Increase maternal knowledge of development, while teaching skills Changing of maternal self-perceptions	Home environment factors Addressing limited resources Early assessment and intervention Skill reinforcement in home visits
Elbaum, 2020	Communication Cognitive functions Motor functions Psycho-social functions	Promoting and supporting developmental progress Increase ability to participate in activities typical for same aged peers	Provision of preschool special education services under Part B-619- IDEA legislation Children deemed eligible for special education services through federal guidelines

Table 1. *Cont.*

Study Authors	Child Factors	Interaction Factors	Environmental Factors
Engle et al. 2007	Sensorimotor functions Cognitive functions language development Psycho-social functions Physical functions	Parenting/parent-child interactions Provision of nutrition and education) Early, intense intervention programing Enhanced, coordinated intervention Families partnering in intervention	Center based programing Optimal environment: early childhood programs with structure and established processes Environmental risks- toxins Infectious risks: HIV/AIDS, malaria Social risks- maternal depression, experiencing violence, abuse, or neglect
Diamond et al. 2019	Cognitive functions Executive function) Psycho-social functions	Teacher/Child interactions Peer interactions Play based intervention environmentally embedded in kindergarten classroom	School based programming, embedded in kindergarten curriculum Protective factors- proactively teaching executive functioning skills in generalizable context Addressing social risks- bullying, loneliness
Black and Dewey, 2014	Cognitive functions Executive function) Psycho-social functions	Learning through enrichment experiences Responsive interactions with caregivers Providing structure and encouragement	Addressing barriers associated with poverty Integrated interventions that include nutrition and early child development
Semrud-Clikeman, 2017	Neurodevelopmental functions Attention/memory functions Visual-motor, and motor functions	Provision of appropriate developmental assessment within the country of interest Child's experiences and world view	Assessment in language of origin Context of assessment administration Assessment tasks matching culturally developed abilities
Mukherjee et al. 2020	Cognitive functions Physical functions	Cognitive assessment of development of 3-year old children with gamified measure Performance predictive of standardize measure of development	Low-cost technology Tablet with games Utility in rural context

5. Contribution to the Field of Early Child Development

This narrative review highlights the pivotal studies supporting the role of environmental factors and interaction factors influencing child development, developmental potential, and functioning trajectories globally (Table 1). In addition, the selected studies show the gaps related to the lack of comprehensive and collaborative frameworks of assessment and service provision in early child development across sectors. Hence, guided by the ICF-CY, we propose an intervention framework of child-environment interactions to optimize children's developmental functioning and trajectories at a population level (Figure 1). The proposed interactional framework can guide the identification of key developmental indicators for assessments, interventions, and evaluations. Moreover, the universal adoption of the ICF-CY and pediatric ICF-based tools as guiding frameworks for comprehensive assessment of children's development and optimal functioning across health and education, promotes professional training on integrated assessments, evaluations, and interventions, fosters collaborative service provision across sectors, and facilitate communication among multiple stakeholders [6,37–39]. Systematic efforts to use a common language in assessments and interventions across sectors will facilitate continuity of care, coordination, organization, and monitoring of programs throughout the children's developmental trajectories.

Limitations

Despite the wide scope of this narrative review of global initiatives reporting on children, families and environmental factors impacting early child development, it is important to note some limitations. The main limitation relates to the authors' personal preferences and areas of expertise which could have influenced the selection of studies reviewed in this paper. Moreover, we included studies published in English, therefore, we might have missed important information published in other languages.

6. Conclusions

The goals of assessment to promote children's developmental trajectories are to gather accurate data about the child's level of functioning across domains of cognitive, communicative, motor, social and adaptive development. Such assessment provides the basis for identifying areas of strength and if delays exist- while also considering the cultural context of the child and communicating the assessment findings to specify targeted intervention. Given the significant need, but limited availability of developmental measures appropriates for low and middle-income countries, an important priority in the continuing implementation of SDG is the development of measures that assess proximal aspects of child functioning that can complete more distal, proxy measures of development such as poverty and stunting. The ECDI and the literacy-numeracy index, and the development of the DEEP represent measures appropriate for assessing developmental functioning of young children in low-resource countries. The integration of multiple sectors, although challenging yields potential benefits to the evaluation process. To this end, Black and Dewey recommend designing evaluative processes with multiple integrated interventions in mind, examining population factors, and then promoting capacity among care providers to support evaluation from a theory-based perspective [35].

This narrative review advances the importance of adopting a universal child-environment interaction framework in initiatives to promote the early development of children around the world. Using the ICF-CY as a guiding framework, assessments and interventions can be planned and delivered considering dynamic child-environment interactions, facilitating communication across sectors, and facilitating continuity of care in the changing environment—home, school, community—where children grow, develop, and play.

Future Direction

For children to realize their developmental potential, there is a priority to ensure equitable access to appropriate screening, assessment, and intervention. As countries vary in terms of environmental, societal, and economic challenges, it is important to consider country contexts when developing and evaluating assessment and intervention initiatives. Considering low cost and sustainable options for assessment and intervention can reduce financial barriers. Incorporating technology into early intervention and assessment practices can decrease barriers imposed by distance and increase access to trained professionals. Incorporating mechanisms for identifying culturally appropriate assessment practices increases accuracy of identification of need while reducing the potential for overidentification of delays. Capitalizing on the expertise of interdisciplinary teams can also support stakeholders across sectors to ensure continuity and proper administration of interventions. Adoption of a common language to report outcomes can facilitate comparison of outcomes and interventions across sectors, programs, and countries. Continued work is needed globally to support children's developmental trajectories toward positive outcomes. This is especially true as countries adapt assessment and intervention practices in the face of evolving environmental impacts of poverty, natural disasters, pandemics, societal and economic changes to prevent the loss of developmental potential of all children.

Author Contributions: Conceptualization and methodology, V.S. and R.J.S.; writing—original draft preparation, K.H., R.J.S. and V.S.; search, summary, and interpretation of resources, K.H., R.J.S. and V.S.; review and editing, K.H., R.J.S. and V.S. All authors have read and agreed to the published version of the manuscript.

Funding: This research received no external funding.

Institutional Review Board Statement: This narrative review did not require ethics review.

Informed Consent Statement: This narrative review did not require informed consent.

Data Availability Statement: Data sharing is not applicable to this article as no new data were created in this study. The data supporting our proposed framework are available within the article.

Conflicts of Interest: The authors declare no conflict of interest.

References

1. Raikes, A.; Devercelli, A.E.; Kutaka, T.S. Global goals and country action: Promoting quality in early childhood care and education. *Child. Educ.* **2015**, *91*, 238–242. [CrossRef]
2. Barros, A.J.D. Early childhood development: A new challenge for the SDG era. *Lancet* **2016**, *4*, e873–e874. [CrossRef]
3. McCoy, D.C.; Peet, E.D.; Ezzati, M.; Danael, G.; Black, M.M.; Sudfeld, C.R.; Fawzi, W.; Fink, G. Early childhood developmental status in low and middle-income countries: National, regional and global prevalence estimates using predictive modeling. *PLoS Med.* **2016**, *13*, e1002034. [CrossRef]
4. United Nations Office of the High Commissioner for Human Rights. *Convention on the Rights of the Child 1989*. Available online: www.unhchr.ch/html/menu3/b/kcrc.htm (accessed on 29 January 2021).
5. World Health Organization. *International Classification of Functioning, Disability and Health: Children & Youth Version (ICF-CY)*; World Health Organization: Geneva, Switzerland, 2007.
6. Simeonsson, R.J. ICF-CY: A universal tool for documentation of disability. *J Policy Pract. Intellect. Disabil.* **2009**, *6*, 70–72. [CrossRef]
7. Black, M.M.; Walker, S.P.; Fernald, L.C.H.; Andersen, C.T.; DiGirolamo, A.M.; Lu, C.; McCoy, D.C. Advancing early childhood development: From science to scale. *Lancet* **2017**, *389*, 77–90. [CrossRef]
8. Grantham-McGregor, S.; Cheung, Y.B.; Cueto, S.; Glewwe, P.; Richter, L.; Strupp, B. International Child Development Steering Group. Developmental potential in the first 5 years for children in developing countries. *Lancet* **2007**, *369*, 60–70. [CrossRef]
9. Lu, C.; Black, M.M.; Richter, L.M. Risk of poor development in young children in low-income and middle-income countries: An estimation and analysis at the global, regional and country level. *Lancet Glob. Health* **2016**, *4*, e916–e922. [CrossRef]
10. Rippin, H.L.; Hutchinson, J.; Greenwood, D.C.; Jewell, J.; Breda, J.J.; Martin, A.; Rippin, D.M.; Schindler, K.; Rust, P.; Fagt, S.; et al. Inequalities in education and national income are associated with poorer diet: Pooled analysis of individual participant data across 12 European countries. *PLoS ONE* **2020**, *15*, e0232547. [CrossRef]
11. Manu, A.; Ewerling, F.; Barros, A.J.D.; Victora, C.G. Association between availability of children's book and the literacy-numeracy skills of children aged 36 to 59 months: Secondary analysis of the UNICEF Multiple-Indicator cluster surveys covering 35 countries. *J. Glob. Health* **2019**, *9*, 1–11. [CrossRef]
12. Gil, J.D.C.; Ewerling, F.; Ferreira, L.Z.; Barros, A.J.D. Early childhood suspected developmental delay in 63 low-and middle-income countries: Large within- and between-country inequalities documented using national health surveys. *J. Glob. Health* **2020**, *10*, 1–10. [CrossRef]
13. Bethell, C.D.; Read, D.; Blumberg, S.J.; Newacheck, P.W. What is the prevalence of children with special health care needs? Toward an understanding of variations in findings and methods across three national surveys. *Matern. Child Health J.* **2008**, *12*, 1–14. [CrossRef] [PubMed]
14. Bethell, C.D.; Kogan, M.D.; Strickland, B.B.; Schor, E.L.; Robertson, J.; Newacheck, P.W. A national and state profile of leading health problems and health care quality for US children: Key insurance disparities and across-state variations. *Acad. Pediatrics* **2011**, *11* (Suppl. 3), S22–S33. [CrossRef] [PubMed]
15. Zablotsky, B.; Black, L.I.; Maenner, M.J.; Schieve, L.A.; Danielson, M.L.; Bitsko, R.H.; Blumberg, S.J.; Kogan, M.D.; Boyle, C.A. Prevalence and Trends of Developmental Disabilities among Children in the United States 2009–2017. *Pediatrics* **2019**, *144*. [CrossRef]
16. Schieve, L.A.; Gonzalez, V.; Boulet, S.L.; Visser, S.N.; Rice, C.E.; VanNaarden, B.K.; Boyle, C.A. Concurrent medical conditions and health care use and needs among children with learning and behavioral developmental disabilities, National Health Interview Survey, 2006–2010. *Res. Dev. Disabil.* **2012**, *33*, 467–476. [CrossRef]
17. McPherson, M.; Arango, P.; Fox, H.; Lauver, C.; McManus, M.; Newacheck, P.W.; Perrin, J.M.; Shonkoff, J.P.; Strickland, B. A new definition of children with special health care needs. *Pediatrics* **1998**, *102*, 137–140. [CrossRef] [PubMed]

18. Akobirshoev, I.; Parish, S.; Mitra, M.; Dembo, R. Impact of medical home on health care of children with and without special health care needs: Update from the 2016 National Survey of Children's Health. *Matern. Child Health J.* **2019**. [CrossRef]
19. Sameroff, A.J.; Fiese, B.H. Models of development and developmental risk. In *Handbook of Infant Mental Health*, 2nd ed.; Zeanah, C.H., Ed.; Guilford: New York, NY, USA, 2000.
20. Batorowicz, B.; King, G.; Mishra, L.; Missiuna, C. An integrated model of social environment and social context for pediatric rehabilitation. *Disabil. Rehabil.* **2015**, *38*, 1204–1215. [CrossRef]
21. Sanches-Ferreira, M.; Silveira-Maia, M.; Alves, S.; Simeonsson, R.J. The use of the ICF-CY for supporting inclusive practices in education: Portuguese and Armenian experiences. In *Using the ICF-CY in Education and Care: International Perspectives*; Castro, S., Palikara, S., Eds.; Routledge: London, UK, 2017.
22. Magnusson, D.; Sweeney, F.; Landry, M. Provision of rehabilitation services for children with disabilities living in low- and middle-income countries: A scoping review. *Disabil. Rehabil.* **2019**, *41*, 861–898. [CrossRef]
23. Maggi, S.; Irwin, L.J.; Siddiqi, A.; Hertzman, C. The social determinants of early child development: An overview. *J. Paediatr. Child Health* **2010**, *46*, 627–635. [CrossRef]
24. Masten, A.S. Ordinary magic: Resilience processes in development. *Am. Psychol.* **2001**, *56*, 227. [CrossRef]
25. Semrud-Clikeman, M.; Romero, R.A.; Prado, E.L.; Shapiro, E.G.; Bangirana, P.; John, C.C. Selecting measures for the neurodevelopmental assessment of children in low-and middle-income countries. *Child Neuropsychol.* **2017**, *23*, 761–802. [CrossRef] [PubMed]
26. Bhavnani, S.; Mukherjee, D.; Dasgupta, J.; Verma, D.; Parameshwaran, D.; Divan, G.; Sharma, K.K.; Thiagarajan, T.; Patel, V. Development, feasibility and acceptability of a gamified cognitive Developmental assessment on an E-Platform (DEEP) in rural Indian preschoolers-pilot study. *Glob. Health Action* **2019**, *12*, 1548005. [CrossRef]
27. Mukherjee, D.; Bhavnani, S.; Swaminathan, A.; Verma, D.; Parameshwaran, D.; Divan, G.; Dasgupta, J.; Sharma, K.; Thiagarajan, T.C.; Patel, V. Proof of concept of a gamified Developmental assessment on an E-Platform (DEEP) tool to measure cognitive development in rural Indian preschool children. *Front. Psychol.* **2020**, *11*, 1202. [CrossRef]
28. Karoly, L.A.; Kilburn, M.R.; Cannon, J.S. Early childhood interventions: Proven results, future promise. *Rand Corp.* **2006**, 4–7, 60.
29. Eickmann, S.H.; Guerra, M.Q.; Lima, M.C.; Huttly, S.R.; Worth, A.A. Improved cognitive and motor development in a community-based intervention of psychosocial stimulation in northeast Brazil. *Dev. Med. Child Neurol.* **2003**, *45*, 536–541. [CrossRef] [PubMed]
30. Elbaum, B. Developmental Outcomes of Preschool Special Education. *Infants Young Child.* **2020**, *33*, 3–20. [CrossRef]
31. Diken, I.H.; Bayhan, P.; Turan, F.; Sipal, R.F.; Sucuoglu, B.; Ceber-Bakkaloglu, H.; Gunel, M.K.; Kara, O.K. Early childhood intervention and early childhood special education in Turkey within the scope of the developmental system approach. *Infants Young Child.* **2012**, *25*, 346–353. [CrossRef]
32. Pretis, M. Early childhood intervention and inclusion in Austria. *Infants Young Child.* **2016**, *29*, 188–194. [CrossRef]
33. Diamond, A.; Lee, C.; Senften, P.; Lam, A.; Abbott, D. Randomized control trial of Tools of the Mind: Marked benefits to kindergarten children and their teachers. *PLoS ONE* **2019**, *14*, e0222447. [CrossRef]
34. Engle, P.L.; Black, M.M.; Behrman, J.R.; De Mello, M.C.; Gertler, P.J.; Kapiriri, L.; Martorell, R.; Young, M.E.; International Child Development Steering Group. Strategies to avoid the loss of developmental potential in more than 200 million children in the developing world. *Lancet* **2007**, *369*, 229–242. [CrossRef]
35. Black, M.M.; Dewey, K.G. Promoting equity through integrated early child development and nutrition interventions. *Ann. N. Y. Acad. Sci.* **2014**, *1308*, 1–10. [CrossRef] [PubMed]
36. Lipina, S.J.; Posner, M.I. The impact of poverty on the development of brain networks. *Front. Hum. Neurosci.* **2012**, *6*, 238. [CrossRef]
37. Schiariti, V.; Mahdi, S.; Bolte, S. International Classification of Functioning, Disability and Health Core Sets for Cerebral Palsy, Autism Spectrum Disorder, and Attention-Deficit-Hyperactivity Disorder. *Dev. Med. Child Neurol.* **2018**, *60*, 933–941. [CrossRef] [PubMed]
38. Schiariti, V.; Longo, E.; Shoshmin, A.; Kozhushko, L.; Besstrashnova, Y.; Król, M.; Campos, T.N.C.; Ferreira, H.N.C.; Verissimo, C.; Shaba, D.; et al. Implementation of the International Classification of Functioning, Disability, and Health (ICF) Core Sets for Children and Youth with Cerebral Palsy: Global Initiatives Promoting Optimal Functioning. *Int. J. Environ. Res. Public Health* **2018**, *15*, 1899. [CrossRef] [PubMed]
39. Ferreira, H.N.C.; Schiariti, V.; Regalado, I.C.R.; Sousa, K.G.; Pereira, S.A.; Fechine, C.P.N.D.S.; Longo, E. Functioning and Disability Profile of Children with Microcephaly Associated with Congenital Zika Virus Infection. *Int. J. Environ. Res. Public Health* **2018**, *15*, 1107. [CrossRef]

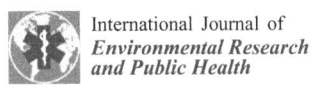

Protocol

Go Zika Go: A Feasibility Protocol of a Modified Ride-on Car Intervention for Children with Congenital Zika Syndrome in Brazil

Egmar Longo [1,*], Ana Carolina De Campos [2], Amanda Spinola Barreto [3], Dinara Laiana de Lima Nascimento Coutinho [3], Monique Leite Galvão Coelho [4], Carolina Corsi [2], Karolinne Souza Monteiro [1,3] and Samuel Wood Logan [5]

1. Postgraduate Program in Rehabilitation Sciences and Postgraduate Program in Collective Health, Federal University of Rio Grande do Norte—Faculty of Health Sciences of Trairi (UFRN-FACISA), Santa Cruz 59200-000, Brazil; smkarolinne@gmail.com
2. Department of Physical Therapy, Federal University of São Carlos, São Carlos 13565-905, Brazil; accampos@ufscar.br (A.C.D.C.); carol.corsi7@gmail.com (C.C.)
3. Postgraduate Program in Rehabilitation Sciences, Federal University of Rio Grande do Norte—Faculty of Health Sciences of Trairi (UFRN-FACISA), Santa Cruz 59200-000, Brazil; amandaspinola@gmail.com (A.S.B.); dinaralaiana@hotmail.com (D.L.d.L.N.C.)
4. Postgraduate Program in Collective Health, Federal University of Rio Grande do Norte—Faculty of Health Sciences of Trairi (UFRN-FACISA), Santa Cruz 59200-000, Brazil; monique.masso@gmail.com
5. College of Public Health and Human Sciences, Oregon State University, Corvallis, OR 97331, USA; sam.logan@oregonstate.edu
* Correspondence: egmarlongo@yahoo.es; Tel.: +55-8432912411

Received: 15 August 2020; Accepted: 10 September 2020; Published: 21 September 2020

Abstract: Children with congenital Zika syndrome (CZS) present severe motor disability and can benefit from early powered mobility. The Go Zika Go project uses modified ride-on toy cars, which may advance the body functions, activities, and participation of children. This paper describes the study protocol aiming to assess the feasibility of a modified ride-on car intervention for children with CZS in Brazil. A mixed-methods design with a multiple 1-week baseline, 3-month intervention, and 1-month follow-up will be implemented. Modified ride-on car training sessions will be conducted three times a week at the participants' home or in the clinic. The primary outcome will be a narrative description of study feasibility (photovoice method, focus groups, parent feasibility questionnaire and assessment of learning powered mobility). Secondary outcomes will be switch activation, driving sessions journal, social-cognitive interactions, mobility (pediatric evaluation of disability inventory computer adaptive test), goal attainment scaling (GAS), and participation (young children's participation and environment measure). Go Zika Go is expected to be viable and to improve function, activity, and participation of children with CZS, providing a low-cost, evidence-based rehabilitation option that will be relevant to early child development in a global perspective.

Keywords: congenital Zika syndrome; user participation; mobility; intervention

1. Introduction

Congenital Zika syndrome (CZS) became a global concern after the Zika virus outbreak in 2015, which mainly affected Brazil [1]. The situation is more serious in the Northeast region, which concentrates the majority of cases, and is marked by strong social problems, scarcity of investments in the training of human resources and in the provision of health services [2]. Children with CZS have severe motor disability, the majority of them compatible with Gross Motor Function Classification System (GMFCS) classification V (i.e., no prognosis for independent mobility) [3].

Only one study evaluated the profile of functioning of children with CZS in Brazil, demonstrating that activity and participation were highly impacted, and that societal attitude was the main barrier to participation [4]. To date, only one preliminary study has been published on the rehabilitation of children with CZS between 3 and 9 months of age. The results indicated that the intervention program based on the principles of Goals-Activity-Motor Enrichment (GAME) improved mothers' assessment of their babies' performance, and satisfaction with the performance of functional priorities and the perception of an enriched home environment [5].

As CZS is a completely new condition, rehabilitation approaches more commonly used are based on recommendations for cerebral palsy (CP). Even for CP, evidence-based interventions are more easily available for children with mild to moderate motor impairment, and interventions are limited for children with severe motor impairment [2,6]. Young children with typical development exhibit gains in cognitive development, communication, and social skills after starting independent walking [7–9]. Young children with motor disabilities are often not able to take part in self-initiated mobility, and are more likely to experience cognitive and developmental delays, as well as less social interactions with caregivers and peers [10,11].

For young children with disabilities, early powered mobility may advance the body function, activity, and participation, in contrast to other interventions within pediatric rehabilitation which are often focused exclusively on one physical skill (body structure domain) in isolation of other therapeutic goals within a stagnant clinical environment (ex. treadmill training). Research indicates positive results of powered mobility interventions for young children with functional impairments [11,12] since battery-operated ride-on cars are easily modified and are considered as an option of increasing interest for motorized mobility for children with disabilities.

Globally, there are very few commercially available motorized wheelchairs for young children with disabilities and existing options are extremely expensive (>USD 17,000 for a base model) [13]. Environmental inaccessibility and device characteristics inhibits motorized wheelchair use [12–15].

The low cost of modified cars (<USD 400) can minimize some of the barriers previously reported, such as an inaccessible physical environment, financial impact, and peculiarities of motorized wheelchairs readily available commercially. The modifications are fundamental and include the use of large and easy-to-press actuators generally positioned on the steering wheel; in addition to the requirements to provide stability in the seat using common materials, such as polyvinyl chloride (PVC) pipe, swimming kickboards, and Velcro.

Several studies have showed the results of a powered mobility intervention with modified ride-on car on the behavior and development of young children with disabilities, including CP. Although none of the children in these studies were formally referred to use powered mobility devices due to their young age or diagnosis, all demonstrated the ability to independently press the activation switch, enjoyed driving sessions, and some experienced increased self-care mobility [16], social skills [16,17], as well as increased peer interaction on the playground [18], and during an inclusive playgroup [19]. The limitations of previous work includes a heavy reliance on low-evidence level research designs (i.e., case reports and case series); the inclusion of participants with varying disabilities in the same sample; and the reporting of a wide variety and often very low adherence rates to recommended use guidelines. These limitations have hindered the interpretation and generalization of study results and will be addressed in the current protocol.

Although participation-based interventions are a promising strategy not only to improve participation but also body functions [20], there are no evidenced-based practices to guide clinical recommendations of early powered mobility device use, including modified ride-on cars, for young children with disabilities, including CZS. The current protocol will address this gap in knowledge and will have a direct and immediate impact on clinical practice. From a global health standpoint, the results may provide an evidence-based rehabilitation option that will be relevant to early child development in low resource contexts. The objective of this study is to determine the feasibility of a powered mobility intervention for young children with CZS with severe motor impairment including acceptability and effectiveness. The specific aims are:

I. To evaluate the acceptability of a modified ride-on car intervention for young children with CZS and their families.
II. To determine the effect of a modified ride-on car intervention on the (a) mobility and social function, and (b) participation of young children with CZS and their families.
III. To understand the barriers and facilitators of a modified ride-on car intervention for young children with CZS and their families.

2. Materials and Methods

2.1. Design

This is a feasibility trial of a mixed-methods case series, prospectively registered, with 3-month intervention and 1-month follow-up. The follow-up will aim to assess preliminary learning retention and implications of modified ride-on car training sessions [16]. This prospective study will provide important information about the feasibility, assistive effectiveness, and rehabilitative effectiveness of the first intervention focusing on powered mobility for children with CZS in Brazil. The procedures and timeline of the study are included in Figure 1 and Table 1.

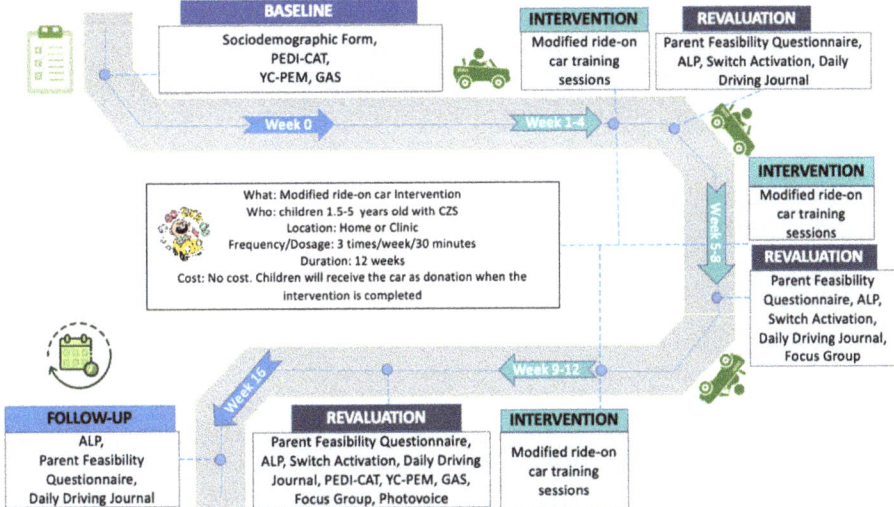

Figure 1. Go Zika Go timeline and procedure intervention for children with congenital Zika syndrome (CZS) between 1.5–5 years age.

Table 1. Study design schedule.

Assessment Tools	Enrolment	Baseline	Intervention	Revaluation			Follow up
Time Point	Week 0	Week 0	Weeks 1–12	Week 4	Week 8	Week 12	Week 16
Eligibility screening	X						
Informed consent	X						
Modified ride-on car training sessions			X				
Sociodemographic Form		X					
PEDI-CAT		X				X	
YC-PEM		X				X	
GAS		X			X	X	
PFQ				X	X	X	X
ALP				X	X	X	X
Switch Activation				X	X	X	
Daily Driving Journal				X	X	X	X
Focus Group					X	X	
Photovoice						X	

PEDI-CAT: Pediatric Evaluation of Disability Inventory–Computer Adaptive-test; YC-PEM: Young Children's Participation and Environment Measure; GAS: Goal Attainment Scaling; PFQ: Parents Feasibility Questionnaire; ALP: Assessment of Learning Powered Mobility.

2.2. Participants

Inclusion criteria: (a) Diagnosis of CZS, (b) GMFCS [21], level IV or V, (c) aged between 1.5 and 5 years, (d) no previous experience with powered mobility.

Exclusion criteria include the presence of uncontrolled seizures and musculoskeletal deformities that prevent adaptation of the seating support in the device.

2.3. Sample Size Estimation

In this feasibility study, we will recruit 10 children with CZS. This small sample will provide data on the feasibility of the protocol, thus helping determine the sample size for a larger randomized trial using powered mobility in children with CZS. Given the lack of previous studies measuring the outcomes of interest for this study, the sample size was estimated according to recommendations of the minimum sample for pilot studies [22].

2.4. Settings and Locations Where the Data Will Be Collected

The scenario of CZS in Brazil is 3523 confirmed cases, with the Northeast region being the most affected, with 1907 cases. Rio Grande do Norte, where this study will occur, is one of the 9 states in the Northeast region and has 126 confirmed cases of CZS. In the national gross income ranks, it occupies the 17th position among the 34 Brazilian states. In 2010, the Human Development Index of Rio Grande do Norte was 0.684 and ranked 16th among the 27 federative units in the country.

Recruitment of participants will take place through early intervention services, pediatric clinics that provide physical and occupational services, and community-based programs that serve the study populations throughout Rio Grande do Norte (RN) state in Brazil. The recruitment will take place between January and December 2021.

2.5. Patient and Public Involvement

Parents' involvement in the design of the protocol: parents or caregivers of children diagnosed with CZS who received a rehabilitation service at Clínica Escola de Fisioterapia da Facisa—Santa Cruz, RN were asked to answer a questionnaire prepared by the researchers, with 8 questions related to intervention preferences. Initially, the parents watched a video about the Go Zika Go project and then they were interviewed by the first author (EL) at the clinic or at home. The questions included aspects of the families' interest in participating in the intervention, space available at home to use the ride-on car, ideal time for mobility training, preference for the place to perform the intervention, etc. Five parents/caregivers participated in this exploratory stage of the research. The results of this stage showed that all families were interested in participating in the intervention and stated that the training can be performed at home and/or at the clinic setting.

2.6. Outcomes Measures

2.6.1. Primary Outcome

The primary outcome of the study will be the feasibility of the protocol, including a narrative description, recruitment and retention rates, adherence and acceptability of the protocol. A mixed methods approach will be used to assess the primary outcome.

A document analysis will determine the number of parents who received information about the study by mail, the number of potential participants contacted by telephone, how many parents met the inclusion criteria and how many provided informed consent, received, and completed the intervention.

Qualitative data will be collected using the photovoice method and focus groups. Photovoice is a participatory action-research modality that uses photographs to express individuals' experiences during their daily realities [23].

Photovoice aims to record and present everyday realities using photography; promote dialogue and critical reflection of reality and know the strengths and weaknesses of the target audience; and reach decision makers [24]. Photovoice will explore families' perception of the feasibility of modified ride-on cars for children with CZS at home and in the community. In the eighth week of the intervention, the parents of children with CZS will be invited to participate in a focus group to provide information about the application of photovoice, its ethical aspects, to clarify doubts about the handling of cameras, expectations in participation and to solve personal issues that may arise. Thus, the methods will follow the Wang and Burris [25] recommendations. Disposable cameras will be offered to record the photos. Parents or caregivers who prefer not to use the camera offered by the researchers will use the cameras on their smartphones and share information by the messaging app. Guidance will be provided on how to capture quality photos, and information about the privacy of people in the scene to be photographed. Parents/caregivers will be instructed to photograph moments of the child's routine at home and in the community. To guide the capture of the photos, parents/caregivers should follow a script of questions asked by the researchers, which include: (1) How does my child feel when using the modified ride-on car? (2) Does the modified ride-on car help my child to get around at home and in the community? (3) Does the modified ride-on car help my child to play with other children? When and where is the modified ride-on car used? Participants will be instructed to capture photos that answer study questions over the next 4 weeks (the third month of intervention). It is recommended that each participant register between 20 and 30 photos [25]. After this period, digital images or printed photographs will be delivered to the research team for the preparation of the second focus group.

In the 12th week of the intervention, the second focus group will be held, where the photos will be displayed and shared with the researchers and other participants, so that the images can be discussed, allowing for a deep reflection from the creation of a proper reading of each moment, on the use of modified ride-on cars by children with CZS at home and in the community. Each participant will be asked to select the most significant pictures representing the experience of their children using the ride-on car. The showed method [26] will be used through its specific questions to facilitate assistance to participants in contextualizing the meaning of their photographs. In addition to the discussion on the contents of the photos, the following feasibility questions guide will be used: What is your perception of the intervention with modified ride-on cars? What helped or hindered your child's use of the modified ride-on cars at home and in the community? Do you think the intervention was useful for your child? All focus groups will be conducted in person by two members of the research team. The sessions will be recorded in audio and video, transcribed and analyzed thematically [27,28].

Quantitative data will be collected from feasibility questionnaires for parents and professionals. The parents feasibility questionnaire (PFQ) [29,30] includes questions related to satisfaction with the intervention, the time of use at home and in the community, the usefulness of the ride-on car, the level of comfort related to the time of its use and the need for help from others during use. PFQ will be used at the end of week 4, 8, and 12 of the intervention, and at follow-up. The assessment of learning powered mobility (ALP) [31] will be used to measure the feasibility of the intervention. This tool is able to describe the learning process' phase at the initial stages of using a powered mobility device. It also documents the child's occupational performance, thus supporting the selection of learning strategies. Phases are scored from 1 (novice) to 8 (expert) to describe occupational performance while using a powered mobility device, considering five categories: understanding of tool use, level of attention, expressions and emotions, activity and movement, and interaction and communication [31,32]. In this study, the ALP will be applied at the end of weeks 4, 8, and 12 of the intervention, and at the follow-up. In addition, a sociodemographic questionnaire will be used for all participants at the baseline.

2.6.2. Secondary Outcomes

Switch Activation

Switch activation is defined as when the switch is pressed to activate the modified ride-on car and make it "go", thereby moving in space from one place to another [30]. Switch activation may occur from the child in the modified ride-on car independently or with assistance (either physical or verbal cueing) from others. Assistance may be provided by a sibling or peer, or an adult such as a parent/caregiver or clinician. The duration of switch activation, who activated the switch, and the level of assistance, if any, provided to the child using the modified ride-on car will be coded. Total switch activation time (minutes and seconds) and percentage of time of each 10-min video will be coded and reported. Switch activation analyses will be carried out at the end of week 4, 8, and 12 of the intervention.

Inter- and intra-rater reliability (at least 85% agreement) will be established on 10% of the video recordings amongst one expert coder and two secondary coders. Training will include coding of video recordings, discussion of disagreements, and coding of additional videos until reliability is established. All videos will be coded in Datavyu.

Daily Driving Journal

Parents will record the date, duration (minutes) location, and activities during each driving session in a daily driving journal. The researcher will collect the daily driving journal at the end of the study. The daily driving journal for entries of week 4, 8, and 12 of the intervention, and in the follow-up will be analyzed.

Pediatric Evaluation of Disability Inventory–Computer Adaptive-test (PEDI-CAT)

The PEDI-CAT is the computerized version of PEDI and has been translated and adapted culturally to Brazil [33]. It is answered by the children's caregiver and has an item bank divided into two domains: (1) mobility, which includes 75 items ranging from basic motor skills (e.g., sitting without support) to more difficult motor skills (e.g., running or climbing a step ladder). Additionally, this domain includes the use of walking devices; (2) cognitive/social, which includes 60 items related to interaction (e.g., follows the gaze of another person), communication (e.g., uses gestures to ask for something), everyday cognition (e.g., recognizes his/her name), and self-management (e.g., when upset response without hitting). In these domains, the four-point scores (unable, hard, a little hard, easy) are based on different levels of difficulty. The overall score is transformed in a normative score (based on age) and a continuous score that will be used in the analyses. The PEDI-CAT will be administered on the baseline and at the end of the 12th week of the intervention.

Young Children's Participation and Environment Measure (YC-PEM)

The YC-PEM, aimed to be used for children from zero to five years, explores the frequency of participation in activities, the level of involvement of participation, the parent's satisfaction with the children's current participation and the environmental supports and barriers considered to be important. Parents will report their child's participation across home, community and childcare activities. For each type of activity, parents will report on (1) frequency of attendance (i.e., how often the child attends an activity) (8-point scale, from never (0) to once or more times every day (7)); (2) level of involvement (i.e., the child's level of engagement in the activity) (5-point scale, from not very involved (1) to very involved (5)); and (3) their desire for their child's participation to change (i.e., their dissatisfaction) [yes, no]. Then, caregivers will evaluate the impact of environmental features and resources on participation (3-point scale, from usually helps/usually yes (3) to usually makes harder/usually no (1)). The YC-PEM will be administered at baseline and at the end of the 12th week of the intervention [34].

Goal Attainment Scaling (GAS)

GAS is an objective method of quantifying goal attainment. Goals are scored on a Likert-type scale from −2 (representing no positive change at all from baseline/ regression), −1 (a little less change than expected), 0 (attainment of goal at the expected level), +1 (a little more change than expected), to +2 (attainment of goal at much more than the expected level) [35]. Goals are personally relevant to the individual family (rather than standardized), with the distance between each increment representing a relatively equal amount of effort or improvement to achieve. Outcome scores on an individual's goals will be converted to an aggregate T score (regardless of the domain to which the GAS goal is aligned) which will be the unit of analysis. One to three GAS goals will be set in the baseline and at the end of the 8th week of the intervention. At the end of the 12th week of the intervention, the goals will be reviewed.

2.7. Intervention

Modified ride-on car training sessions will be conducted three times a week at the participants' home or in the clinic, according to family preference. A therapist will guide the sessions at both locations. The intervention session will include the following: (1) environment setup (e.g., instructing families) (5 min); (2) natural play as a warm up activity (5 min); and (3) social training and mobility with modified ride-on cars (30 min). The focus of treatment sessions will be based on the social function goals and the expected mobility set by caregivers in the modified GAS after the pretest [36]. The 30-minute driving session will involve the participants learning cause–effect concepts by driving the modified ride-on car (i.e., pressing the switch for moving and releasing it for stopping). The dose of the intervention will be adjusted considering the opinion of the parents who participated in a previous interview and the results of a recent study, where the average time of interventions was 24 to 30 min [37]. The therapist and caregivers then will use verbal and physical cueing to encourage children to drive and explore the surrounding environment [17,38]. All sessions will be video- and audio-recorded. Figure 2 shows a modified ride-on car and a child with CZS.

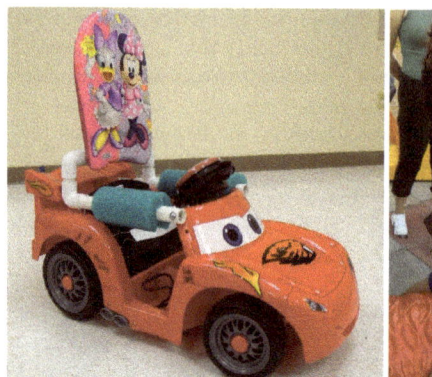
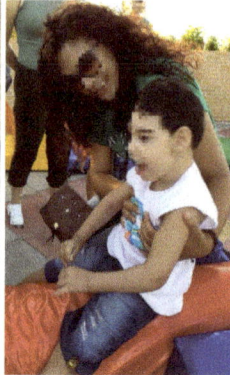

Figure 2. Modified ride-on car and a child with CZS.

2.8. Modified Ride-On Cars

Ride-on cars will be modified with a joystick for activation. Joystick control will allow omni-directional turning and proportional speed-control. The vast majority of research with modified ride-on cars has installed a large, easy-to-press, all-or-nothing activation switch that does not provide turning nor speed control. These steering and speed modifications will enhance the ability for young children with CZS to explore the environment and use the device within the home and community. Joystick activation ensures that children are provided with an opportunity to use an activation method that is consistent with future joystick-driven device options, such as motorized wheelchairs. Ride-on cars will be modified with optimal seating support using readily available, low-cost materials based on each child's individual needs. Ride-on car models will be selected based on their design and structure to provide seating support.

2.9. Statistical Analysis

Quantitative data will be imported into the Statistical Package for Social Science (SPSS) 22.0 for analysis and reported using descriptive statistics (absolute and relative frequencies, measures of central tendency and measures of variability). For numerical data, the Wilcoxon test will be used when there are two measurements, while the Friedman test will be used when there are more than two measurements. For categorical data, the Chi-Square test will be used. All the analyses will consider a confidence interval of 95% (CI95%) and a statistical significance of $p < 0.05$. Adverse events will be categorized. The percentage of scheduled and completed treatment sessions will be compared.

The feasibility results will be presented qualitatively. The researchers will analyze the audio transcripts of the focus group, Photovoice and additional questions through the thematic analysis to identify and validate the significant themes and patterns from the discussion with the parents. The ATLAS.ti software will be used to code, group and present the data, based on the results.

2.10. Ethics

This study was approved by the Research Ethics Committee of the Faculty of Health Sciences of Trairi (FACISA), of the Federal University of Rio Grande do Norte (UFRN), under opinion 3.980.703/2020 and CAAE 29582020.8.0000.5568. Written informed consent will be obtained from parent or guardian prior to data collection. The trial was prospectively registered at the Brazilian Registry of Clinical Trials (ReBEC) (RBR-2Y2Z8P). The study follows the Consolidated Standards of Reporting Trials (CONSORT) to pilot or feasibility trial.

2.11. Knowledge Translation (KT) and Dissemination

End of grant KT and Integrated KT strategies will be used [39]. An appropriate KT planning template will be used to maximize the scope of the findings, while acknowledging the nature of feasibility studies. Traditional knowledge diffusion strategies will be used as End of grant KT, such as conference presentations and papers publications. A media engagement strategy will disseminate the results in partnership with Nossa Casa, a NOG Brazilian institution responsible for the main actions of KT in Brazil on childhood disability. The results will also be shared at the REDE's website, which is an international network aiming to build research capacity as well as preparedness regarding emerging infectious diseases in Latin America and Caribbean. A video and an infographic will be made with the results of the study in plain language, which will be distributed in services and public centers that care for children with CZS. Integrated KT will involve stakeholders, families and researchers, assuring that the outcomes meet the needs of the end users. A workshop will be organized with both activities for the dissemination of results and building capacity on modification of ride-on cars. The final results will also be transformed into a policy brief and forwarded to public services and sectors. The dissemination workshop will be hosted in collaboration with families, the local research team members and international collaborators.

3. Potential Contributions of This Study

This study will fill an important research gap and may contribute to future intervention studies, having a direct and immediate impact on clinical practice in children with CZS. This study protocol will determine the feasibility of an intervention using powered mobility for young children with CZS, who present severe motor impairments. The acceptability of the intervention for young children with CZS and their families will be described. In addition, we will assess the effects of the intervention on mobility, social function and participation of children; the barriers and facilitators of the intervention will also be analyzed.

Feasibility studies are relevant as they use rigorous methods to access processes, resources, management and effects related of the intervention of interest [40]. The feasibility assessment includes data on the acceptability of the intervention and the perceived burden of the procedures. Feasibility studies may therefore contribute resources invested in larger trials that are the most likely to generate clinically significant results [41]. In this protocol, we propose an approach of mixed methods; the primary outcomes will be qualitative, which will allow a deeper understanding in terms of feasibility. The quantitative measures will enable a complementary analysis of the feasibility and contribute to answer the specific objectives of the study. Thus, data obtained in this study will be able to guide future clinical trials on powered mobility in children with CZS and benefit these children and their families. It is expected that this innovative study will contribute evidence for the adoption of low cost environmental early child interventions in Brazil and other low-and middle-income countries around the world.

Author Contributions: Conceptualization: E.L., S.W.L., A.C.D.C.; Project Administration: E.L.; Methodology: E.L., A.C.D.C., A.S.B., D.L.d.L.N.C., M.L.G.C., C.C., K.S.M., S.W.L.; Investigation: A.S.B., D.L.d.L.N.C., M.L.G.C., K.S.M.; Writing: Original draft preparation: E.W.L., A.C.d.C., S.W.L., K.S.M.; Writing: Review and editing: E.L., A.C.D.C., A.S.B., D.L.d.L.N.C., M.L.G.C., C.C., K.S.M., S.W.L.; Funding acquisition: E.L., A.C.D.C. All authors have read and agreed to the published version of the manuscript.

Funding: This research is funded by PROPESQ/UFRN, grant number (05/2019) and REDE Brazil. This study was financed in part by the Coordenação de Aperfeiçoamento de Pessoal de Nível Superior - Brasil (CAPES) - Finance Code 001.

Acknowledgments: We acknowledge the support of Bonny Baker and Luiza Lourenço at The Global Health Network/REDe, for all the efforts made for this project to come true. We are also grateful for the families who provided valuable information regarding their preferences for the intervention. Additionally, we thank Klayton Galante Sousa and Nelci Adriana C.F. Rocha, for comments on the study design.

Conflicts of Interest: The authors declare no conflict of interest.

References

1. Campos, G.S.; Bandeira, A.C.; Sardi, S.I. Zika Virus Outbreak, Bahia, Brazil. *Emerg. Infect Dis.* **2015**, *21*, 1885–1886. Available online: http://www.ncbi.nlm.nih.gov/pubmed/26401719 (accessed on 10 July 2020). [CrossRef] [PubMed]
2. Longo, E.; Campos, A.C.; Schiariti, V. Zika Virus after Emergency Response. *Pediatr. Phys. Ther.* **2019**, *31*, 370–372. Available online: http://journals.lww.com/00001577-201910000-00017 (accessed on 25 July 2020). [CrossRef]
3. Melo, A.; Gama, G.L.; Silva Júnior, R.A.; Assunção, P.L.; Tavares, J.S.; Silva, M.B.; Costa, K.N.F.S.; Vânia, M.L.; Evangelista, M.A.; De Amorim, M.M.R. Motor function in children with congenital Zika syndrome. *Dev. Med. Child Neurol.* **2020**, *62*, 221–226. [CrossRef] [PubMed]
4. Ferreira, H.N.C.; Schiariti, V.; Regalado, I.C.R.; Sousa, K.G.; Pereira, S.A.; Fechine, C.P.N.; Costa, K.N.F.S.; Vânia, M.L.; Evangelista, M.A.; De Amorim, M.M.R. Functioning and disability profile of children with microcephaly associated with congenital Zika virus infection. *Int. J. Environ. Res. Public Health* **2018**, *15*, 1107. [CrossRef] [PubMed]
5. Brandão, M.B.; Frota, L.M.C.P.; Miranda, J.L.; Brasil, R.M.C.; Mancini, M.C. Family-Centered Early Intervention Program for Brazilian Infants with Congenital Zika Virus Syndrome: A Pilot Study. *Phys. Occup. Ther. Pediatr.* **2019**, *39*, 642–654. [CrossRef] [PubMed]
6. Longo, E.; Campos, A.C.; Palisano, R.J. Let's make pediatric physical therapy a true evidence-based field! Can we count on you? *Braz. J. Phys. Ther.* **2019**, *23*, 187–188. [CrossRef]
7. Campos, J.J.; Anderson, D.I.; Barbu-Roth, M.A.; Hubbard, E.M.; Hertenstein, M.J.; Witherington, D. Travel Broadens the Mind. *Infancy* **2000**, *1*, 149–219. [CrossRef]
8. Uchiyama, I.; Anderson, D.I.; Campos, J.J.; Witherington, D.; Frankel, C.B.; Lejeune, L.; Barbu-Roth, M. Locomotor Experience Affects Self and Emotion. *Dev. Psychol.* **2008**, *44*, 1225–1231. [CrossRef]
9. Anderson, D.I.; Campos, J.J.; Witherington, D.C.; Dahl, A.; Rivera, M.; He, M.; Uchiyama, I.; Barbu-Roth, M. The role of locomotion in psychological development. *Front. Psychol.* **2013**, *4*, 1–17. [CrossRef]
10. Pavlova, M.; Sokolov, A.; Krägeloh-Mann, I. Visual navigation in adolescents with early periventricular lesions: Knowing where, but not getting there. *Cereb. Cortex* **2007**, *17*, 363–369. [CrossRef]
11. Livingstone, R.; Field, D. Systematic review of power mobility outcomes for infants, children and adolescents with mobility limitations. *Clin. Rehabil.* **2014**, *28*, 954–964. [CrossRef] [PubMed]
12. Jones, M.A.; McEwen, I.R.; Neas, B.R. Effects of Power Wheelchairs on the Development and Function of Young Children with Severe Motor Impairments. *Pediatr. Phys. Ther.* **2012**, *24*, 131–140. [CrossRef] [PubMed]
13. Feldner, H.A.; Logan, S.W.; Galloway, J.C. Why the time is right for a radical paradigm shift in early powered mobility: The role of powered mobility technology devices, policy and stakeholders. *Disabil. Rehabil. Assist. Technol.* **2015**, *11*, 89–102. [CrossRef] [PubMed]
14. Østensjø, S.; Carlberg, E.B.; Vøllestad, N.K. The use and impact of assistive devices and other environmental modifications on everyday activities and care in young children with cerebral palsy. *Disabil. Rehabil.* **2005**, *27*, 849–861. [CrossRef]
15. Emily, B.; Mclaurin, S.; Sparling, J. Parent/Caregiver Perspectives on the Use of Power Wheelchairs. *Pediatr. Phys. Ther.* **1996**, *8*, 146–150.
16. Logan, S.W.; Huang, H.-H.; Stahlin, K.; Galloway, J.C. Modified Ride-on Car for Mobility and Socialization: Single-case study of an infant with Down syndrome. *Pediatr. Phys. Ther.* **2014**, *26*, 418–426. [CrossRef]
17. Huang, H.H.; Chen, C.L. The use of modified ride-on cars to maximize mobility and improve socialization-a group design. *Res. Dev. Disabil.* **2017**, *61*, 172–180. [CrossRef]
18. Logan, S.W.; Lobo, M.A.; Feldner, H.A.; Schreiber, M.; MacDonald, M.; Winden, H.N.; Stoner, T.; Galloway, J.C. Power-up: Exploration and play in a novel modified ride-on car for standing. *Pediatr. Phys. Ther.* **2017**, *29*, 30–37. [CrossRef]
19. Ross, S.M.; Catena, M.; Twardzik, E.; Hospodar, C.; Cook, E.; Ayyagari, A.; Inskeep, K.; Sloane, B.; MacDonald, M.; Logan, S.W. Feasibility of a Modified Ride-on Car Intervention on Play Behaviors during an Inclusive Playgroup. *Phys. Occup. Ther. Pediatr.* **2017**, *38*, 493–509. [CrossRef]

20. Anaby, D.; Avery, L.; Gorter, J.W.; Levin, M.F.; Teplicky, R.; Turner, L.; Cormier, I.; Hanes, J. Improving body functions through participation in community activities among young people with physical disabilities. *Dev. Med. Child Neurol.* **2020**, *62*, 640–646. [CrossRef]
21. Palisano, R.J.; Rosenbaum, P.; Bartlett, D.; Livingston, M.H. Content validity of the expanded and revised Gross Motor Function Classification System. *Dev. Med. Child Neurol.* **2008**, *50*, 744–750. [CrossRef] [PubMed]
22. Whitehead, A.L.; Julious, S.A.; Cooper, C.L.; Campbell, M.J. Estimating the sample size for a pilot randomised trial to minimise the overall trial sample size for the external pilot and main trial for a continuous outcome variable. *Stat Methods Med. Res.* **2016**, *25*, 1057–1073. [CrossRef] [PubMed]
23. John, S.B.M.; Hladik, E.; Romaniak, H.C.; Ausderau, K.K. Understanding health disparities for individuals with intellectual disability using photovoice. *Scand J. Occup. Ther.* **2018**, *25*, 371–381. [CrossRef] [PubMed]
24. Walker, A.; Colquitt, G.; Elliott, S.; Emter, M.; Li, L. Using participatory action research to examine barriers and facilitators to physical activity among rural adolescents with cerebral palsy. *Disabil. Rehabil.* **2019**, 1–12. [CrossRef]
25. Wang, C.; Burris, M.A. Photovoice: Concept, Methodology, and Use for Participatory Needs Assessment. *Health Educ. Behav.* **1997**, *24*, 369–387. [CrossRef]
26. Liebenberg, L. Thinking critically about photovoice: Achieving empowerment and social change. *Int. J. Qual. Methods* **2018**, *17*, 1–9. [CrossRef]
27. Hsieh, H.F.; Shannon, S.E. Three approaches to qualitative content analysis. *Qual. Health Res.* **2005**, *15*, 1277–1288. [CrossRef]
28. Merriam, S.; Greiner, R. *Qualitative Research in Practice: Examples for Discussion and Analysis*, 2nd ed.; Jossey Bass: San Francisco, CA, USA, 2019; p. 451.
29. Babik, I.; Cunha, A.B.; Moeyaert, M.; Hall, M.L.; Paul, D.A.; Mackley, A.; Lobo, M.A. Feasibility and Effectiveness of Intervention with the Playskin Lift Exoskeletal Garment for Infants at Risk. *Phys. Ther.* **2019**, *99*, 666–676. [CrossRef]
30. Logan, S.W.; Catena, M.A.; Sabet, A.; Hospodar, C.M.; Yohn, H.; Govindan, A.; Galloway, J.C. Standing Tall. *Pediatr. Phys. Ther.* **2019**, *31*, 6–13. [CrossRef]
31. Nilsson, L.; Durkin, J. Assessment of learning powered mobility use—Applying grounded theory to occupational performance. *J. Rehabil. Res. Dev.* **2014**, *51*, 963–974. [CrossRef]
32. Field, D.A.; Livingstone, R.W. Power mobility skill progression for children and adolescents: A systematic review of measures and their clinical application. *Dev. Med. Child Neurol.* **2018**, *60*, 997–1011. [CrossRef] [PubMed]
33. Mancini, M.C.; Coster, W.J.; Amaral, M.F.; Avelar, B.S.; Freitas, R.; Sampaio, R.F. New version of the pediatric evaluation of disability inventory (PEDI-CAT): Translation, cultural adaptation to Brazil and analyses of psychometric properties. *Braz. J. Phys. Ther.* **2016**, *20*, 561–570. [CrossRef] [PubMed]
34. Silva, J.; Cazeiro, A.; Campos, A.; Longo, C. Medida da Participação e do Ambiente—Crianças Pequenas (YC-PEM): Tradução e adaptação transcultural para o uso no Brasil. *Ter. Ocup. Univ. Sao Paulo.* **2020**, in press.
35. Kiresuk, T.; Smith, A.; Cardillo, J. *Goal Attainment Scaling: Applications, Theory, and Measurement*; Lawrence Erlbaum: Hillsdale, NJ, USA, 1994.
36. Krasny-Pacini, A.; Pauly, F.; Hiebel, J.; Godon, S.; Isner-Horobeti, M.E.; Chevignard, M. Feasibility of a shorter Goal Attainment Scaling method for a pediatric spasticity clinic—The 3-milestones GAS. *Ann. Phys. Rehabil. Med.* **2017**, *60*, 249–257. [CrossRef] [PubMed]
37. Logan, S.W.; Hospodar, C.M.; Bogart, K.R.; Catena, M.A.; Feldner, H.A.; Fitzgerald, J.; Schaffer, S.; Sloane, B.; Phelps, B.; Phelps, J.; et al. Real World Tracking of Modified Ride-On Car Usage in Young Children with Disabilities. *J. Mot. Learn Dev.* **2019**, *7*, 336–353. [CrossRef]
38. Ragonesi, C.B.; Chen, X.; Agrawal, S.; Galloway, J.C. Power Mobility and Socialization in Preschool. *Pediatr. Phys. Ther.* **2011**, *23*, 399–406. [CrossRef]
39. Mallidou, A.A.; Atherton, P.; Chan, L.; Frisch, N.; Glegg, S.; Scarrow, G. Core knowledge translation competencies: A scoping review. *BMC Health Serv. Res.* **2018**, *18*, 502. [CrossRef]

40. Craig, P.; Martin, A.; Browne, S.; Simpson, S.A.; Wight, D.; Robling, M.; Moore, G.; Hallingberg, B.; Segrott, J.; Turley, R.; et al. Development of guidance for feasibility studies to decide whether and how to proceed to full-scale evaluation of complex public health interventions: A systematic review. *Lancet* **2018**, *392*, S7. [CrossRef]
41. Thabane, L.; Ma, J.; Chu, R.; Cheng, J.; Ismaila, A.; Rios, L.P.; Robson, R.; Thabane, M.; Giangregorio, L.; Goldsmith, C.H. A tutorial on pilot studies: The what, why and how. *BMC Med. Res. Methodol.* **2010**, *10*, 1. [CrossRef]

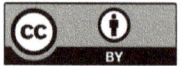

© 2020 by the authors. Licensee MDPI, Basel, Switzerland. This article is an open access article distributed under the terms and conditions of the Creative Commons Attribution (CC BY) license (http://creativecommons.org/licenses/by/4.0/).

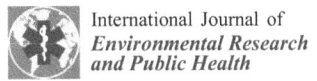

Article

Communicative Interaction with and without Eye-Gaze Technology between Children and Youths with Complex Needs and Their Communication Partners

Yu-Hsin Hsieh [1,*], Maria Borgestig [2], Deepika Gopalarao [3], Joy McGowan [4], Mats Granlund [5], Ai-Wen Hwang [6,7] and Helena Hemmingsson [1]

1. Department of Special Education, Stockholm University, Se-106 91 Stockholm, Sweden; helena.hemmingsson@specped.su.se
2. Department of Neuroscience, Uppsala University, 751 24 Uppsala, Sweden; maria.borgestig@neuro.uu.se
3. Al Noor Training Centre for Persons with Disabilities, Building No. 01, Street No. 21 Al Barsha 1, Dubai PO 8397, United Arab Emirates; deepikarao@alnoorspneeds.ae
4. Easterseals of Southeastern Pennsylvania, 3975 Conshohocken Ave., Philadelphia, PA 19131, USA; jmcgowan@easterseals-sepa.org
5. CHILD, Swedish Institute of Disability Research, School of Health and Welfare, Jönköping University, 553 18 Jönköping, Sweden; mats.granlund@ju.se
6. Graduate Institute of Early Intervention, College of Medicine, Chang-Gung University, Tao-Yuan City 33301, Taiwan; awhwang@mail.cgu.edu.tw
7. Department of Physical Medicine and Rehabilitation, Chang Gung Memorial Hospital, Linkou, 5 Fu-Xing St., Kwei-Shan, Tao-Yuan City 33301, Taiwan
* Correspondence: yu-hsin.hsieh@specped.su.se

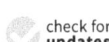

Citation: Hsieh, Y.-H.; Borgestig, M.; Gopalarao, D.; McGowan, J.; Granlund, M.; Hwang, A.-W.; Hemmingsson, H. Communicative Interaction with and without Eye-Gaze Technology between Children and Youths with Complex Needs and Their Communication Partners. *Int. J. Environ. Res. Public Health* **2021**, *18*, 5134. https://doi.org/10.3390/ijerph18105134

Academic Editor: Eunil Park

Received: 13 April 2021
Accepted: 5 May 2021
Published: 12 May 2021

Publisher's Note: MDPI stays neutral with regard to jurisdictional claims in published maps and institutional affiliations.

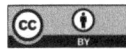

Copyright: © 2021 by the authors. Licensee MDPI, Basel, Switzerland. This article is an open access article distributed under the terms and conditions of the Creative Commons Attribution (CC BY) license (https://creativecommons.org/licenses/by/4.0/).

Abstract: Use of eye-gaze assistive technology (EGAT) provides children/youths with severe motor and speech impairments communication opportunities by using eyes to control a communication interface on a computer. However, knowledge about how using EGAT contributes to communication and influences dyadic interaction remains limited. Aim: By video-coding dyadic interaction sequences, this study investigates the impacts of employing EGAT, compared to the Non-EGAT condition on the dyadic communicative interaction. Method: Participants were six dyads with children/youths aged 4–19 years having severe physical disabilities and complex communication needs. A total of 12 film clips of dyadic communication activities with and without EGAT in natural contexts were included. Based on a systematic coding scheme, dyadic communication behaviors were coded to determine the interactional structure and communicative functions. Data were analyzed using a three-tiered method combining group and individual analysis. Results: When using EGAT, children/youths increased initiations in communicative interactions and tended to provide more information, while communication partners made fewer communicative turns, initiations, and requests compared to the Non-EGAT condition. Communication activities, eye-control skills, and communication abilities could influence dyadic interaction. Conclusion: Use of EGAT shows potential to support communicative interaction by increasing children's initiations and intelligibility, and facilitating symmetrical communication between dyads.

Keywords: complex communication needs; severe physical disabilities; eye-gaze controlled computer; communicative interaction

1. Introduction

Children and youths with complex needs, here indicating having severe physical disabilities and complex communication needs [1] such as cerebral palsy with severe motor impairments and Rett syndrome, encounter difficulties using speech for everyday communication and may be at great risk of participation restrictions in daily activities [2,3]. Without adaptations, the dysfunction of movement of children/youths with complex needs and the interplay between the impairments in cognition, motor, or other domains might hinder their communicative interaction with the environment [2–4]. Most often, these children use vocalization, eye pointing, facial expressions, or body movements to express needs or socialize; however, their idiosyncratic behaviors or communicative intentions may be subtle and difficult to be recognized or interpreted appropriately by those around them [5,6]. The lack of appropriate responses from communication partners and lack of communication access adapted to their motor impairments and speech difficulties could impede the children's motivation to communicate, hinder their communication development, and restrict participation in social life [7–9]. Therefore, their fundamental human right of communication should be addressed [10,11].

Assistive technology (AT) as a means to enhance participation has been highlighted for children with complex needs [12]. Augmentative and alternative communication (AAC), which is one type of AT designed to facilitate communicative interactions, includes unaided methods (e.g., gestures, vocalization or speech) and aided methods (e.g., low-tech communication boards or high-tech communication devices) to supplement or compensate for the impairments of verbal communication for children with complex communication needs [13]. However, previous studies found that when aided AAC resources such as communication boards were provided, most children with complex needs required considerable assistance in using the communication interfaces and preferred the use of gesture or vocalization, with which they can communicate with familiar partners quickly and easily [5,14,15]. They occasionally used aided AAC systems via eye pointing or partner-assisted scanning when they were requested to provide information or clarification in complex conversations.

In recent years, eye-gaze assistive technology (EGAT) has been demonstrated as an opportunity for children/youths with complex needs to communicate and participate in various daily activities [16–18]. This innovative technology can detect eye movements using a specialized infrared video camera mounted on a tablet/computer. This calculates the direction of eye movements within a few millimeters when a child is gazing at a screen [19]. In combination with AAC software, EGAT could help children/youths with complex needs express their opinions by using their eyes to operate an AAC interface on a tablet/computer (Figure 1). It has been shown to be a feasible and relatively intuitive way to aid their communication in school or home contexts with ongoing support from communication partners and healthcare professionals [16,20,21]. Although many research studies have demonstrated communication benefits in the adult population with severe physical disabilities, there is a need for more research to support the positive effects of using EGAT in natural contexts in the children population. Some studies indicate that children with complex needs might need long-term practice to master eye-gaze control skills [22] and to develop the communicative competency to become an efficient user of communication aids [23]. Long-term practice includes both use for extended time periods and frequent use every day. Hemmingsson and Borgestig [17] reported that these children used EGAT for only a few hours per day. Besides low exposure to technology, other factors might reduce the effectiveness of EGAT, for instance, multiple impairments (e.g., visual or cognitive impairments), eye-gaze performance [22], communication abilities, learning opportunities [24], accessibility of the devices across environments [17], and attitude, knowledge and strategies of communication partners [25]. However, one recent multicenter intervention study indicated positive effects of EGAT intervention on expressive communication skills for children/youths with complex needs [26]. The stakeholders from previous studies also revealed positive experiences as the use of EGAT gave the children an opportunity to express things on their own initiative, which could lead to more opportunities to engage in communicative interaction and participate in social life [16,24].

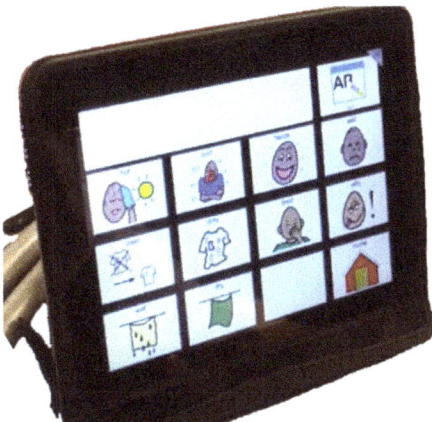

Figure 1. Example of EGAT with adapted communication page.

Communicative interaction, including interactional sequences of communicative behaviors in the persons interacting (e.g., initiation of a conversation or response), communicative functions during interaction (e.g., requesting an object or answering a question), and the means of communication (e.g., using speech or eye pointing) [27], is one of the building blocks of cognitive and social development [28]. Nevertheless, research has indicated that children/youths with complex needs show a limited range of communicative interaction as they tend to play nondirective or non-initiating roles, give more adopting responses as yes–no answers, and provide less information [5,15,27]. The communication partners usually occupy more conversational space, initiate most of the interactions and request specific responses to encourage the communicative exchanges. EGAT, which requires less physical effort and assistance from communication partners than other interfaces, could provide children/youths with complex needs with opportunities to take initiative, express opinions, and interact with others [16,24]. However, few studies have provided knowledge about how use of EGAT by the children/youths influences the communicative interaction with their communication partners.

Therefore, the central aim of this study is to investigate the impacts of employing EGAT, compared to the Non-EGAT (NEGAT) condition on communicative interaction, in terms of interactional structure and communicative functions used by children/youths with complex needs and their communication partners. The research questions posed are: Which interactional structure are shown by children/youths with complex needs and their communication partners when EGAT is or is not used? Which communicative functions are used by the dyads when EGAT is or is not used? The hypotheses are: when the children/youths use EGAT in communicative interaction, (1) children/youths initiate more frequently, in contrast to the NEGAT condition; (2) communication partners take fewer communicative turns; (3) communication partners make fewer requests or demands.

The structure of this article is organized as follows. Section 2 first describes the study design, using a systematic video-coding approach to research questions and the procedure of film clip collection. Secondly, participants and the selection of film clips based on criteria are addressed. Thirdly, a coding scheme as the outcome measure for communicative interaction is detailed. Lastly, data analysis, including video analysis and the three-tiered method of analysis, is described. Section 3 presents results based on the structure of the three-tiered method. In Section 4, study findings on communicative interaction between dyads are discussed. Section 5 concludes this study.

2. Materials and Methods

2.1. Design

This study used a within-subjects design and employed a systematic video-coding approach to investigate communicative interaction when children/youths with complex needs used EGAT to interact with their communication partners in natural contexts, comparing this to the NEGAT condition. The study was part of an international multi-center EGAT intervention project, which aimed to examine the effect of a six-month EGAT intervention on participation in activities, communication, and functional independence in everyday life of children and youths with complex needs. Further details of this project can be found in the article by Borgestig et al. [26].

To confront the methodological challenges in a small population target group, a three-tiered method proposed for research on AAC use [29] was applied. The strength of this method is to combine group, intermediate and individual analysis to validate group results and provide clinically relevant information [8,29]. The application of three-tiered method for analysis was elaborated in the later Section 2.4.3.

Procedure

This international project collected data from the AT centers in Sweden and special needs schools in Dubai and the USA [26].

To ensure consistency of data collection, the research team in Sweden provided a checklist for the research coordinators responsible for each participating organization to collect film clips in participants' natural contexts by the following instructions: (1) choose an activity that is meaningful and motivating for the children/youths to do, especially related to communication in natural routines (e.g., playing a game, performing an educational task, or the child communicating with the adult about something that had happened). The types of chosen activities are similar between the EGAT and NEGAT conditions; (2) choose a communication partner who know this child well; (3) film the activity about 5–10 min/day during three consecutive days in the contexts with a cell phone or a tablet on a stand; (4) choose a time of day when the children/youths would perform at their best; (5) try the best to film the faces, gaze direction and body movements of the child and his/her communication partner, and the computer screen with EGAT or low-tech communication devices.

After completion of data collection, these videos were sent to the research team in Sweden via the Cloud service, encrypted using Secure Sockets Layer.

2.2. Participants

2.2.1. Recruitment

The original project recruited 17 children/youths with severe physical disabilities and complex communication needs and 17 of their communication partners from the organizations in three countries (nine in Sweden, five in Dubai, and three in the USA). These children/youths were candidates for and in need of EGAT after testing other aided AAC devices that had limited functional use or were unsuccessful, and they were new to EGAT before the research started.

2.2.2. Selection of Participants and Film Clips

Fourteen of 17 dyads had completed video filming in their natural contexts. The first and second authors (Y-H.H., M.B.) conducted participant screening referring to the film instruction checklist. The inclusion criteria were: (1) the children/youths age was between 1 and 21 years old; (2) the language was English or Swedish; (3) at least two available videos of each participant and his/her communication partner showed they performed similar communicative interaction activities in the EGAT and NEGAT conditions (e.g., play or school learning); (4) the videos captured the dyadic facial expressions, gaze, body movements and gestures in addition to the computer screen or low-tech communication tools in order to observe their communicative interaction clearly; (5) the videos were informative, including activities generating dyadic communicative interaction instead of the child/youth only using EGAT to play games on a computer screen without interaction with the partner; (6) the videos showed the best ability of the child/youth in both the EGAT and NEGAT conditions, for instance, having more mouse clicks on screen using EGAT, showing longer attention/gaze towards the computer screen or longer interaction with partners, and/or demonstrating a high engagement level in that activity without a bored face. The exclusion criteria were (1) videos were too short (less than five minutes) and not informative; (2) videos failed to record the interactions between the dyads.

Eight dyads were not included due to language issues ($n = 1$), older age ($n = 1$), dissimilar tasks in the EGAT and NEGAT conditions ($n = 2$), or lack of communicative interaction ($n = 4$, where videos only showed the children conducting cause-effect games instead of communication activities). Based on the selection criteria, six children/youths and their communication partners were included. Dyads included three from Sweden, two from Dubai, and one from the USA. Each included dyad had four to 10 film clips of different lengths collected during the research period.

Following screening and after several meetings with two authors (M.B. and H.H.), the first author selected the best quality of two videos for each dyad, which showed similar activities, informative communicative interactions, and the best ability of children/youths in the EGAT and NEGAT conditions. A total of 12 videos from 47 film clips in six dyads were included, and each pair of videos in each dyad were concurrent or within two to five months. The videos ranged in length from five to 12 min, with a median length of eight minutes. The included videos with EGAT were recorded when the children/youths had accumulated three to six-month experiences of using EGAT, with four videos at three months of intervention and two at six months.

2.2.3. Ethics Approval

The project has obtained ethical approval from the ethical review boards in Sweden (Dnr 2018/1809–32), Dubai (DSREC-11/2017_10), and the USA (protocol ESSP-02) for study implementation, data transfer and data analysis.

2.3. Measures

2.3.1. Outcome Measures: Coding Scheme for Communicative Interaction

A coding scheme was used to investigate the characteristics of communicative interaction between the dyads, based on previous video-coding research on children with multiple disabilities and complex communication needs [5,14,15,27] with adaptations to fit the EGAT condition. The coding scheme applied to code all behaviors within the time frame of interaction included interactional structure, communicative functions, and modes of communication.

Interactional structure was classified as turns and moves [5,14]. Turns were determined by a succession of communicative signs with the boundary between turns a two-second gap supported by the presence of other behaviors, for example, non-verbal signals, pitch change, the listener took a turn, or the speaker came to a rest [14,15,27]. Each turn could include one or more moves. A move as defined by Pennington and McConachie comprised "single or strings of utterances/non-verbal communicative signals produced by one speaker within a conversational turn" [15], p.398. Moves included Initiation (I), opening the conversation or introducing a topic and could solicit a response; Response (R), a reply to an initiation; Response/Initiation (R/I), a reply to initiation but also requiring a response of its own; Follow-up (F), acknowledging the previous utterance; Follow-up/Initiation (F/I), acknowledging the previous move and requesting a response of its own; No Response. Table 1 displayed an example.

Table 1. Example of moves in a play activity.

Partner: "Do you think we should put on some shoes or some pants?"	(I)
Child: "Pants" (using EGAT)	(R)
Partner: "Pants! All right. What color of pants shall we do?"	(F/I)

Note. EGAT = eye-gaze assistive technology; I = Initiation; R = Response; F/I = Follow-up/Initiation.

In this study, Preparatory (P) and Operation/Navigation (ON) were added to interactional moves in consideration of the preparation act to make ready for interaction (P) [5] and when the participants spend time struggling with low-tech AAC systems or EGAT with computers (ON) [23].

Communicative functions were coded to represent the intentions and purpose of the communicative act [14,15]. Each move could contain one or more codes of communicative functions [14] if the communicative purposes in the context occurred simultaneously. The categories included Requestive (RE), request for attention, information, action or clarification; Informative (IN), comments, answers, or clarification of a previous utterance; Acknowledgment (ACK), conveying understanding to previous utterance; Confirmation/Denial (CD), affirmation or rejection; Self/shared expression (SSE), demonstration of the emotional state in individuals; and Unintelligible (U), not understandable by a listener or a coder. An example was presented in Table 2.

Table 2. Example of communicative functions in a play activity.

Partner: "Which color of shoes do you think we should wear?"	(RE)
Child: "Red!" (using EGAT)	(IN)
Partner: (Laugh)	(SSE)

Note. RE = Requestive; IN = Informative; SSE = Self/shared expression.

Modes of communication were defined as the means by which communicative functions were transmitted, including speech, vocalization, gesture, and aided AAC systems [5,14,15]. The modes were combined and coded if they appeared to signal the same communicative function. Low-tech mode (Lt) was used to indicate the individual communicated using low-tech AAC, e.g., a communication book or Bliss board, and EGAT was coded to represent that persons used eye-gaze technology for aided communication.

All categories and definitions of the codes are presented in the Appendix A Table A1.

2.3.2. Measures Related to Participant Characteristics

This study received participant information from the medical charts by research coordinators in the organizations. Motor severity levels were based on Gross Motor Function Classification System (GMFCS) with level I (ambulatory without restrictions) to V (limited ability to move around) [30], and Manual Ability Classification System (MACS), with level I (handles objects easily and successfully) to V (does not handle objects) [31]. Medical diagnosis, sensory functions (e.g., vision), severity of motor impairments and cognitive impairments of the children/youths were documented.

In addition, eye-control skills and communication abilities of the children/youths were assessed by Compass Aim test [32] and Communication Matrix [33], respectively, to describe the essential abilities related to use of EGAT. A trained AT specialist in the participating organization performed assessments before the EGAT intervention started.

Compass Aim Test

The Compass Aim test measures eye-gaze performance in computer interaction, encompassing two variables: (1) Accuracy, to measure the ability to control a mouse pointer for target selection, and (2) Time on task, to measure the required time for target selection on the screen. The test showed high test–retest reliability, good internal consistency and adequate construct validity [32].

Communication Matrix

The Communication Matrix details the earliest stage of communication behavior in children with severe and multiple disabilities, with seven levels, pre-intentional behavior (I), intentional behavior (II), unconventional communication (III), conventional communication (IV), concrete symbols (V), abstract symbols (VI) and language (VII). The primary level indicates the level at which the child/youth is operating predominantly. Total Percent is calculated using the total score of each item divided by the maximum possible score (= 160, each item scores from 0 to 2). The psychometrics showed good inter-observer reliability and adequate content validity [33].

2.4. Data Analyses

This section first described video coding analysis, followed by reliability analysis and the three-tiered method for analysis.

2.4.1. Video-Coding Analysis

The Noldus Observer XT 14.0 (Noldus Information Technology BV, Wageningen, The Netherlands) was used in video-coding analysis, which is software for behavioral research to code and visualize behaviors on a timeline accurate to the millisecond. Figure 2 shows an example of visualization in behavioral observation of moves and communicative functions on a timeline for one participant. Each video-coding was analyzed continuously, meaning the behaviors were coded whenever they appeared and were stored in the software. The software contained statistical analyses to calculate rate per minute for each specified communicative interaction behavior in dyads. Even though the software assisted the work, it took about six to eight hours for coding and rechecking each video due to the complexity of the coding scheme and the characteristics of the target group.

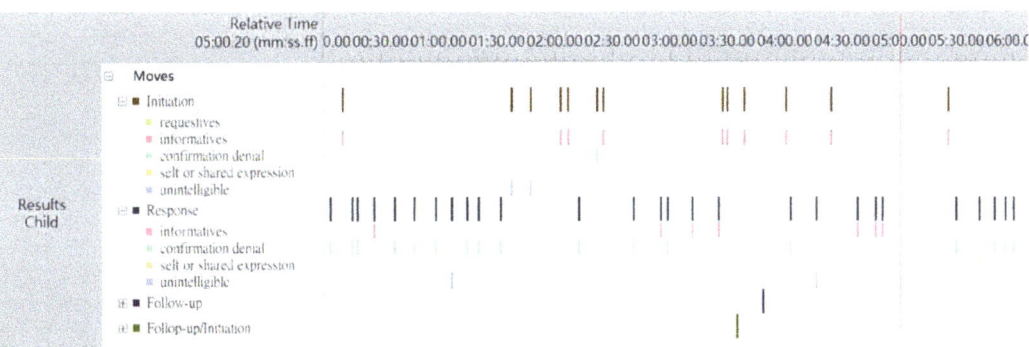

Figure 2. An example of video coding and visual analysis for moves and communicative functions. Note. It is a screen copy from the results of the Noldus Observer XT 14.0.

2.4.2. Reliability

Inter-rater reliability was determined using the kappa statistic on 10% of each video fragment (i.e., random selection of a one-minute interval) as a reliability check [34] by another rater. Due to the idiosyncratic nature of the communicative behaviors made by children/youths with complex needs, we included videos of all dyads as a reliability check since each fragment was connected with specific challenges.

The inter-rater had a background in speech-language pathology and was experienced with video-coding of communication in children with severe disabilities. Before the coding started, she received training and practiced video-coding along with the first author for 12 h online or face-to-face. Following the training, the inter-rater conducted pilot coding on two videos. Cross-examination was carried out and any discrepancies were discussed to clarify the inconsistent coding. After reaching a consensus about the definitions of each code, the inter-rater independently conducted double coding of all one-minute videos based on the coding guidelines. To avoid judgment bias due to the random selection of each video fragment, the inter-rater checked the preceding communicative behaviors before issuing a coding.

Three categories—moves, communicative functions and modes of communication—were addressed to check inter-rater reliability. Cohen's kappa was calculated to estimate the degree of consensus between raters, according to the equation [35], in which the value above 0.75 was a good agreement, between 0.4–0.75 was an acceptable agreement, and below 0.4 was low agreement [35,36]. Inter-rater reliability revealed that the average kappa values were acceptable for moves (k = 0.72 and 0.64 in EGAT and NEGAT conditions, respectively), acceptable to good for communicative functions (k = 0.85 and 0.74), and good for modes of communication (k = 0.98 and 0.89).

2.4.3. Three-Tiered Method of Analysis

To face the challenge of conducting research in this small sample and heterogeneous population and the possible occurrence of a type II error, this study utilized a three-tiered method of analysis [8,29], to firstly examine the group results of communicative interaction patterns between dyads at the general molar level, and secondly to strengthen the validity by analyzing how the communicative patterns of each dyad were congruent with or varied from the group results at the intermediate level, and lastly a further case analysis and clinical relevance at the more detailed molecular level.

Firstly, at the molar level of the group patterns, functional relationships between independent (conditions using EGAT or not) and dependent variables (communicative interaction) were examined using quantitative analysis. Rate per minute, which is the frequency divided by duration, and the proportional distribution of each communicative interaction behavior were presented using descriptive statistics (mean, standard deviation). We examined the mean differences of communicative turns in two conditions (EGAT and NEGAT) between two groups (children/youths and communication partners) using a two-way ANOVA and conducted Bonferroni post hoc analysis when the results were statistically significant. To compare the differences in frequencies of moves and communicative functions in the two conditions, parametric paired t-tests of variance was used as the data did not offend normality testing (the Shapiro–Wilk test) [37]. The significance level was set to 0.05 with two-tailed testing, and marginal significance was defined as a p value between 0.05 and 0.1 [38]. Data analyses were conducted using the Statistical Package for the Social Sciences (SPSS) version 25.0 (IBM Corporation, Armonk, NY, USA) and confirmed by a qualified statistician in the research team.

Secondly, at the intermediate level, the number of participants whose results were either congruent with or differed from the group result was counted to validate the group pattern. It was also possible to evaluate the degree to which individual variations influenced the mean value of the group in two conditions. In addition, a further analysis of the interrelationship between moves, communicative functions and modes of communication was conducted to determine how the dyads used their communicative functions in their initiations or response moves, and how they used EGAT and other modes, given that they were expressing specific communicative functions in the two conditions.

Lastly, at the molecular level, two cases who were typical or atypical of the group results were analyzed and compared to present the similarities and differences of the characteristics of communicative interaction and participant characteristics. It offered a basis for judgment of the potential factors from the environments and participant characteristics that could influence communicative interaction in dyads.

3. Results

3.1. Summary of Participant Characteristics, Communication Acitvities, and AAC Use

The participant characteristics are demonstrated in Table 3. The included children/youths aged from four to 19 years old (mean age: 11 years; gender female: male 5:1). All of them had severe motor impairments as level II-V in GMFCS and IV-V in MACS, with a diagnosis of cerebral palsy, Rett syndrome, or high spinal cord injury. Most of them except Molly had cognitive impairments based on medical records. Three children/youths (Laura, Peter, and Sarah) had visual impairments, with strabismus or refractive errors such as astigmatism and myopia. Their eye control skills to interact with computers showed varied abilities on accuracy (22–100%) and speed for target selection (3.42–18.25 s). Considering communication abilities, most children used unconventional communication predominantly to refuse, request, or socialize by means of facial expressions, gestures, or vocalization. They also showed varied emerging skills in using concrete symbols and conventional communication skills such as eye-pointing for expression, except for Molly, who had higher symbol-communication skills. The communication partners included three teachers, two mothers, and one occupational therapist.

Table 3. Participant characteristics.

Name	Age/Sex	Diagnosis/GMFCS, MACS	Vision	Compass (Accuracy (%), Time on Task (Seconds))	Communication Matrix (Primary Level, %)	Communication Partner
Jane	6 y/Female	Cerebral palsy/ V, V	Normal vision	100%, 7.41 s	Unconventional communication, 31	Teacher
Laura	16 y/Female	Cerebral palsy/ V, V	Astigmatism	36.1%, 9.76 s	Unconventional communication, 21	Teacher
Peter	19 y/Male	Cerebral palsy/ V, V	Myopia and astigmatism, with eyeglasses	22.2%, 18.25 s	Unconventional communication, 28	Teacher
Molly	4 y/Female	High spinal cord injury due to virus infection/V, V	Normal vision	100%, 3.42 s	Abstract symbols, 41	OT
Sarah	4 y/Female	Rett syndrome/ II, IV	Strabismus	33.3%, 12.44 s	Unconventional communication, 29	Mother
Anne	17 y/Female	Rett syndrome/ II, V	No vision problems with eyeglasses	39%, 12.92 s	Unconventional communication, 24	Mother

Note. GMFCS = Gross Motor Function Classification System, MACS = Manual Ability Classification System, OT = occupational therapist.

As shown in Table 4, the communication activities included unstructured play activities and mealtime and structured learning tasks (e.g., letters) in school, home or hospital contexts. The children/youths used the Tobii I-series or PCEye Mini [39] as eye-gaze devices and used Communicator 5 [39], Grid 3 [40], or Communicator with WordPower [39] as AAC software in the computers. In the NEGAT condition, they were accessed to a communication board, eye-gaze frame, or iPad with different types of AAC symbols. The numbers of symbols in the AAC system varied among the children/youths, from 3 to 50 symbols per page in EGAT and from 4 to 48 symbols per page in low-tech AAC, depending on their eye-control skills and symbol-communication abilities (Table 4).

Table 4. Video content and use of EGAT and low-tech AAC.

Name	Condition	Video Length	Activity	Context	AAC System and Content (EGAT/Low-Tech AAC) [1]
Jane	EGAT	7′32	Play dressing	Special preschool	EGAT: PCS symbols and photos, 12~20 symbols per page, total 140 symbols
Jane	NEGAT	5′38	Play "finding a teacher"	Special preschool	Communication book: PCS symbols, pictures, colored photos, 8~20 symbols/page, total 140 symbols
Laura	EGAT	10′48	Matching/ choosing letters	Special School	EGAT: 6 PCS symbols/photos per page, total 204 symbols
Laura	NEGAT	10′16	Matching/ choosing letters	Special School	Eye-gaze frame: 4 single PCS symbols/colored photos per time, total < 200 symbols
Peter	EGAT	8′04	Cognitive school task	Special School	EGAT: 4 PCS symbols/photos per page, total > 120 symbols
Peter	NEGAT	6′25	Cognitive school task	Special School	Eye-gaze frame: 4 single PCS symbols/colored photos per time, total 60 + symbols
Molly	EGAT	12′22	Pretend play using a picture book	Hospital	EGAT: Bliss symbols, 15–50 symbols/page, total 500 symbols
Molly	NEGAT	8′09	Pretend play using a picture book	Hospital	Bliss communication board: total 540 bliss symbols. Single boards with 48 colored pictures/page
Sarah	EGAT	5′29	Meal time	Home	EGAT: PCS symbols, SymbolStix, and colored photos, 3–20 symbols/page, total 51 symbols + Sono Flex
Sarah	NEGAT	5′05	Meal time	Home	Picture pocket for 10 single symbols, LITTLE step-by-step [2]
Anne	EGAT	7′55	Play games	Home	EGAT: Widgit symbols, colored photos, 7 symbols/page, total 62 symbols
Anne	NEGAT	12′00	Play games	Home	iPad: 6 symbols/page, total 100 symbols. 2–3 single colored-pictures at a time

Note. NEGAT = Non-EGAT, PCS = Picture Communication Symbols. [1] PCS [39], SymbolStix [39,40], and Widgit symbols [40] are different symbol sets with colored images. Little step-by step [41] is a speech-generating device to provide sequential messages with voice output. Sono Flex [39] is a communication app with about 6000 symbols in standard version. [2] Low tech devices received but not used in the video.

3.2. Group Results: Molar Level Analysis

Group results are presented in Table 5.

Table 5. Mean rate per minute (RPM) and mean proportion of turns, moves and communicative functions in the EGAT and NEGAT conditions.

Category Code	Children or Youths				Communication Partners			
	EGAT		NEGAT		EGAT		NEGAT	
	Mean RPM (SD)	Mean Proportion	Mean RPM (SD)	Mean Proportion	Mean RPM (SD)	Mean Proportion	Mean RPM (SD)	Mean Proportion
Turns	4.08 (1.50)	0.41	4.50 (1.68)	0.37	5.79 (1.22)	0.59	7.65 (1.91) *	0.63
Moves								
Preparation/Operation, Navigation	0.72 (0.80)	-	0.03 (0.08)	-	0.07 (0.08)	-	0.08 (0.12)	-
Initiation	1.16 (0.94) †	0.28	0.43 (0.27)	0.10	1.97 (0.92)	0.33	3.87 (1.74) *	0.49
Response	2.41 (1.43)	0.59	3.87 (1.63) *	0.86	0.73 (0.57)	0.12	0.35 (0.21)	0.04
Response/Initiation	0.09 (0.22)	0.02	0 (0.00)	0	0.52 (0.53)	0.09	0.21 (0.19)	0.03
Follow up	0.38 (0.43)	0.09	0.19 (0.15)	0.04	1.17 (0.68)	0.19	1.24 (0.95)	0.16
Follow up/Initiation	0.04 (0.07)	0.01	0 (0.00)	0	1.62 (0.79)	0.27	2.21 (0.79)	0.28
Communicative functions								
Requestive	0.09 (0.08)	0.02	0.19 (0.33)	0.04	3.51 (1.41)	0.46	5.16 (1.09) *	0.54
Informative	2.53 (1.05) †	0.57	1.34 (1.29)	0.29	2.09 (0.34)	0.27	2.72 (0.47)	0.28
Acknowledgement	0 (0.00)	0	0.02 (0.05)	0	1.55 (0.99)	0.20	1.19 (0.84)	0.13
Confirmation/denial	0.68 (0.92)	0.15	1.47 (2.22)	0.33	0.38 (0.39)	0.05	0.47 (0.46)	0.05
Self-shared expression	0.65 (0.90)	0.15	0.58 (0.64)	0.12	0.15 (0.15)	0.02	0.07 (0.11)	0.01
Unintelligible	0.52 (0.54)	0.12	0.98 (0.54)	0.21	0	0	0	0

RPM = rate per minute. Two-way ANOVA and Bonferroni post hoc analysis to compare the differences of communicative turns in the EGAT and the NEGAT conditions between two groups. Parametric paired t-tests to compare the differences of moves and communicative functions between two conditions in each group. * $p < 0.05$, † $p < 0.1$.

3.2.1. Interactional Structure

Turns. The communication partners produced more communicative turns within the interaction compared to children/youths with complex needs ($F = 13.87, p = 0.001$). The difference in turns between the partners and children was not significant in the EGAT condition (estimated mean difference = 1.71, $p = 0.56$) but was significant in the NEGAT condition (estimated mean difference = 3.15, $p = 0.04$) from the Bonferroni analysis.

Moves. Slightly more initiations were found when children used EGAT in communication compared to the NEGAT condition (mean = 1.16 vs. 0.43, $t = 2.26, p = 0.07$). However, according to Table 5, R/I and F/I were not frequently found in the children, probably because of the difficulties these children had in conducting dual-purpose moves. Therefore, we collapsed I, R/I, F/I into a category representing all "initiations" because these moves all introduced a topic and/or requested responses of their own, and "initiations" were one of the most important aspects of communication for these children. Children made significantly more "initiations" when they used EGAT compared to the NEGAT condition (mean = 1.30 and 0.43, respectively, $t = 2.60, p = 0.0485$). In addition, the results of the analysis indicated that children made fewer response moves in the EGAT condition compared to the NEGAT condition (mean = 2.41 and 3.87, $t= -4.76, p = 0.005$). The partners made significantly fewer initiations (mean rate per minute = 1.97 vs. 3.87, $t= -2.74, p = 0.04$) in the EGAT condition compared to the NEGAT condition.

3.2.2. Communicative Functions

No significant differences were found in the frequency of different categories of communicative functions used by children between the two conditions. However, of marginal significance was a finding that showed children had higher frequencies of providing information in the EGAT condition compared to the NEGAT condition (mean = 2.53 vs. 1.34, t = 2.04, p = 0.097). The partners made significantly fewer requests (mean = 3.51 vs. 5.16, t= −3.37, p = 0.02) in the EGAT condition compared to the NEGAT condition. The results also showed that they mostly dominated the conversation by asking closed-ended questions (mean = 2.56 vs. 4.26 in the EGAT and NEGAT conditions, respectively).

3.2.3. Modes of Communication: EGAT and Other Modes

The analysis revealed a dominance of using EGAT as a means in communication (63%), followed by gestures (27%) for children in the EGAT condition. In the NEGAT condition, the results showed considerable variations in mode use, with gestures as the most frequent mode (48%), followed by low-tech devices in combination with gestures or vocalization (27%).

3.3. Analysis at the Intermediate Level

3.3.1. Strength of Patterns

As seen in Table 6, most cases followed the group results, including most children making more initiations, demonstrating lower rates of response moves and higher rates of provision of information in communication in the EGAT condition compared to the NEGAT condition. In addition, the partners made fewer turns, initiations and requests in the EGAT condition compared to the NEGAT condition. However, there were a few exceptional cases. Laura demonstrated slightly lower rates of provision of information in the EGAT condition compared to the NEGAT condition (rater per minute = 1.57 vs. 1.95), which was an opposite trend from the group pattern. Her communication partner showed similar and high rates of communicative turns (rater per minute = 7.22 vs. 7.50 in the EGAT and NEGAT conditions) and made similar requests in both conditions (rater per minute = 5.83, 5.55). The other exception was Peter who showed no initiations in either condition.

Table 6. Validation of group patterns by individuals at the intermediate level.

Group Patterns: Compare EGAT Condition to NEGAT Condition	Individuals					
	Jane	Laura	Peter	Molly	Sarah	Anne
Turns						
(1) Communication partners made fewer communicative turns	Yes	No	Yes	Yes	Yes	Yes
Moves						
(1) Children made more initiations	Yes	Yes	Neutral	Yes	Yes	Yes
(2) Children made fewer response moves	Yes	Yes	Yes	Yes	Yes	Yes
(3) Communication partners made fewer initiations	Yes	Yes	Yes	Yes	Yes	Yes
Communicative functions						
(1) A marginal significance that children made more provision of information	Yes	No	Yes	Yes	Yes	Yes
(2) Communication partners made fewer requests	Yes	No	Yes	Yes	Yes	Yes
Modes of communication in children and youths						
(1) In EGAT condition, a dominance of using EGAT, followed by gestures	Yes	Yes	Yes	Yes	Yes	Yes
(2) In NEGAT condition, using gestures most frequently, followed by low-tech devices in combination with gestures or vocalization	No. Low-tech with G/V, then G	No. Low-tech with G/V, then G	Yes	Yes	No. G, V, then G + V	No. G, then G + V

Yes: follow group pattern; No: deviate from group pattern; Neutral: no initiations. Abbreviations: G = Gestures, V = Vocalization.

In modes of communication, EGAT or conjointly with gestures and vocalization (range of proportions = 0.46–0.96) was used most by all children, and the second most commonly used mode was gestures (0.04–0.45). In the NEGAT condition, three of six children used gestures as the dominant channel (proportion = 0.53–0.73), two cases used low-tech devices conjointly with gestures or vocalization more frequently (proportion = 0.47–0.63), and one used nearly equivalent multi-methods involving gestures and vocalization.

In summary, the raw data in most cases validated the group results substantially, except the mode of communication in the NEGAT condition. A few exceptional cases existed, as seen particularly in the result of communicative interaction by Laura and her communication partner, who showed several incongruences from the group results.

3.3.2. Interrelationship Analysis of Moves, Communicative Functions, and Modes of Communication

As shown in Figure 3a, in the EGAT condition, most children tended to provide provision of information in their initiations (mean rate per minute = 0.98), whereas in NEGAT condition, fewer initiations and individual variations without explicit patterns were found. In the children's responses, provision of information was the highest communicative function in the EGAT condition (mean rate per minute = 1.24), while confirmation/denial represented the highest communicative function in the NEGAT condition (mean rate per minute = 1.44). The communication partners made almost twice the amount of requests in their initiations with higher rates in NEGAT compared to the EGAT condition (mean rate per minute = 2.84 vs.1.50).

In relation to modes, as shown in Figure 3b, the children provided information by means of EGAT primarily in their communicative turns (mean proportion = 0.94) and conveyed confirmation/denial or self-shared expression mostly by gesture (mean proportion = 0.70, 0.91). In the NEGAT condition Figure 3c, they predominantly used gestures for varied communicative functions (mean proportion = 0.57–1) except for the provision of information that they equally used gestures and a combination of low-tech devices and natural modes (mean proportion = 0.40, 0.41). The partners engaged in communicative functions predominantly by means of speech in both conditions (mean proportion = 0.56, 0.57).

3.4. Individual Case Studies: Analysis at the Molecular Level

One child typical of the group (Jane) and one atypical youth (Laura) who demonstrated the same diagnosis and severity of motor functions but varied in interactive patterns, were selected for further analysis. As shown in Table 6, Jane showed congruent results with most of the group patterns whereas Laura demonstrated several incongruent results.

As shown in Table 3, Jane had relatively high eye-gaze performance when using EGAT whereas Laura showed lower eye control skills (accuracy in Compass [32] = 100% vs. 36%, respectively). Jane had normal vision, and Laura had astigmatism but her performance on the Compass test was not impacted by her visual impairment, according to the report from the AT specialist. Both participants had communication abilities primarily in the level III unconventional communication [33]. However, Jane had more emerging abilities in conventional communication and concrete symbols (percent in the levels of Communication Matrix = 50%, 14.3%, respectively) compared to Laura (17.9%, 5%, respectively). Both participants used EGAT or low-tech AAC at the school or preschool.

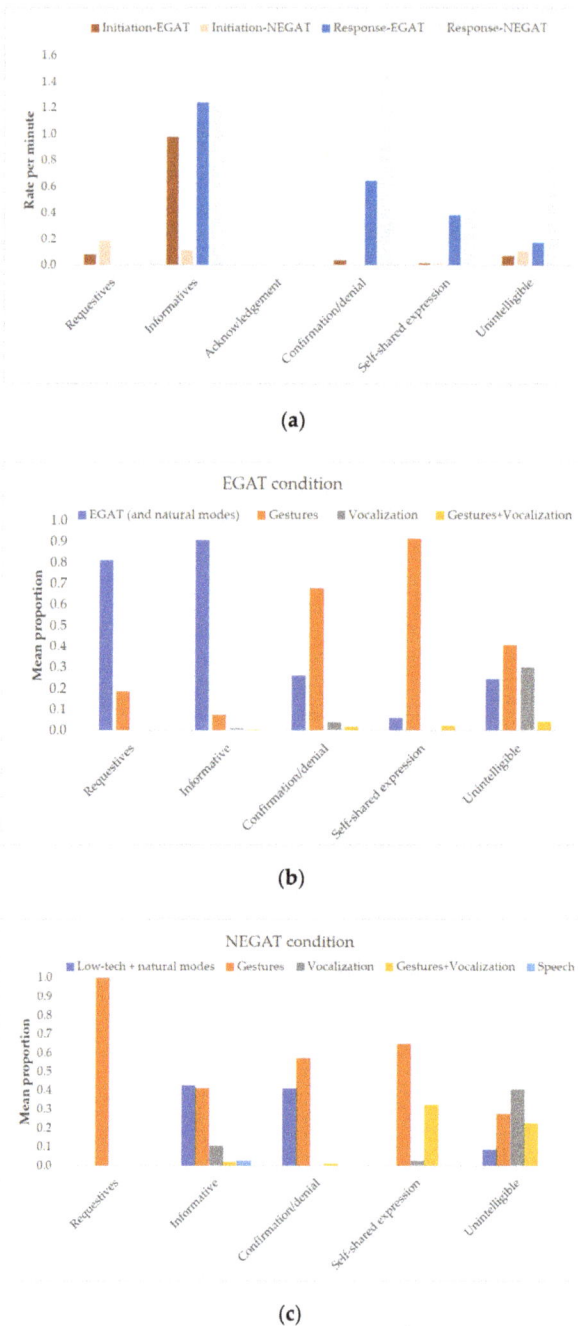

Figure 3. Interrelationships between moves, communicative functions and modes in children and youths with complex needs: (**a**) Interrelationships between moves (initiation and response) and communicative functions in the eye-gaze assistive technology (EGAT) and the non eye-gaze assistive technology (NEGAT) conditions; (**b**,**c**) Interrelationships between communicative functions and modes in the EGAT (**b**) and the NEGAT (**c**) conditions.

Their film clips demonstrated different communicative interaction activities, play activities in Jane and school cognitive tasks in Laura (Table 4). In the structured school task, Laura's teacher dominated the interaction by taking many turns in both the EGAT and NEGAT conditions (rate per minute = 7.22, 7.50), focusing on instruction and question-answer activity and requesting information, actions or clarification. Laura in turns showed quite few initiations (rate per minute = 0.37 and 0.29) but high rates of responses to answer the task (rater per minute= 1.85 and 2.82). Due to insufficient eye control skills at the early learning stage, she spent much effort operating/navigating the eye-gaze controlled computer (rate per minute = 2.04, the highest among all participants). She also showed a substantial frequency of unintelligible communicative functions particularly in the NEGAT condition (rate per min = 1.17), which might influence dyadic interaction in that the teacher would ask more questions or request clarification to receive a clear answer (see the Supplementary Materials Tables S1 and S2 for detailed data).

In summary, the individual case analysis indicated that, although Jane and Laura had similar health conditions, the form and purpose of the communication tasks in the environment (opportunities for children to take the initiative) seemed to be an essential factor for dyadic communicative interactions. Communication partners might demonstrate more directiveness in structured learning tasks than in play activities. In addition, insufficient eye control skills and communication abilities in pupils might contribute to the consequences of fewer initiations and limited information provision even when EGAT was provided.

4. Discussion

The central purpose of this study was to investigate the characteristics of the communicative interactions between children/youths with complex needs and their communication partners in the EGAT condition compared to the NEGAT condition. A systematic video coding was conducted to examine the interactional structure and communicative functions used by the dyads when EGAT is or is not used. The results demonstrated that when using EGAT, the children/youths initiated a conversation more frequently and tended to provide more information during the communicative interactions, while their communication partners made fewer communicative turns, initiated less frequently, and made fewer requests compared to the NEGAT condition. These findings, strengthened by a three-tiered method of analysis, indicated that when EGAT was provided, the children/youths could make a greater contribution to the communicative interaction compared to the NEGAT condition. This study supported that children as young as four could benefit from using this high technology to increase the power of communication during social interactions.

4.1. Initiations and Information Provision by Children in Communicative Interaction

The results of an increasing frequency of initiations in children/youths when using EGAT was encouraging. Previous video-coding research [5,14,15] showed that children with complex needs more frequently act as respondents than initiators. Their messages through body movements or gestures might be difficult to be correctly interpreted as potentially communicative by the communication partners, and their minimal movements restrict their opportunities to access many aided AAC options [5,6]. Stronger control over communicative interactions may be gained by initiating communicative interaction. Gaining more control is critical in this population in order to enjoy shared participation and build self-efficacy in communicative interaction [23]. This study demonstrated that even though these participants practiced EGAT for only three to six months, they could use it to initiate communicative interactions during play or school learning tasks. EGAT could serve as an effective method for them to gain opportunities to initiate a topic, express their opinions and increase social interactions with fewer physical demands and precisely shared referent. As a consequence, their roles as active participants could be enhanced.

The findings showed that the children/youths tended to provide information in their initiations by means of EGAT, which revealed that it could be easier for them to introduce a topic and enlarge the extent of a conversation via this AT. In contrast, in the NEGAT condition, children initiated less frequently and provided less information via gestures, vocalization or in a combination of low-tech devices. Based on the results, it is possible to inform practice that use of EGAT has the potential to provide the children/youths with better communication situations and to facilitate sharing information through age-appropriate interactions in daily life, for example, play or learning. Recent research has highlighted that the scope of communication needs to go beyond the expressions of needs and wants, and extends to development of social relationships, exchange of information and participation in social etiquette routines [42,43]. Therefore, communication partners need to facilitate access to various communication opportunities [25,44], and encourage the use of EGAT for a wider range of communicative functions in daily contexts.

4.2. Turns, Initiations, and Requests by Communication Partner in Communicative Interactions

As in previous studies, the result of this study revealed that communication partners showed dominance in the dyadic conversation by occupying more communicative turns, e.g., exhibiting a high frequency of initiations and requests to encourage the involvement of children in conversation in both the EGAT and NEGAT conditions. They dominated the conversation, probably as a means to scaffold and facilitate the children's contributions according to their available repertoires [5]. Such patterns were particularly strong in structured instruction activities, for instance, as in the atypical case, Laura. However, the findings showed that in the EGAT condition, most communication partners took fewer turns and made fewer initiations and requests compared to the NEGAT condition. Because previous articles have seldom compared the communicative interactions with and without for both communicative partners and children using aided AAC, this finding adds knowledge to how eye-gaze AT could influence dyadic interactions and ameliorate the communication asymmetry. As mentioned earlier, children showed a higher frequency of initiations and information provision when using EGAT, which might reduce the burden on communicative partners in conversations. The use of EGAT may decrease the need to refer to contextual clues and prior knowledge of the children, and facilitate the interpretation of their communicative utterances [45,46]. Conversation is a bi-directional interaction, and when communication intelligibility increases in children, the efforts by communication partners to engage children in topics or clarify the content of their expression could be alleviated.

Another possible explanation for the differences seen between the conditions is that the communication partners were aware that their children were learning to use EGAT and needed time to develop their operation skills and therefore, intentionally extended the duration of waiting and encouraged children to respond or initiate their own topic using EGAT. This argument is supported by the result that more symmetrical turns in dyadic interactions were demonstrated when these children used EGAT. Since communication partners have an influence on the interactional process, their use of sensitive responding and interaction strategies (e.g., providing an expectant delay, modeling the use of communication modes, open-ended question-asking) could have positive impacts on communicative interaction for children/youths using AAC [44,47]. Further research to address the interaction strategies that communication partners use when children use EGAT or other modes could provide more insights and guide communication partner coaching on enhanced communication technologies.

4.3. Pros and Cons of Using Eye-Gaze AT in Communicative Interaction

This study demonstrated that EGAT could provide opportunities for children with complex needs to initiate a conversation with minimal movements and engage in a wider range of communication demands, for instance, providing explicit information to others or making comments where the natural modes of communication could not be achieved. Increasing communication intelligibility could also reduce the burden of guessing for communication partners and make the co-construction of conversation easier. This innovative technology on the children's interactions with others could enhance a child's control in communication and potentially increase the long-term opportunities in social participation.

Despite the advantages, the severe motor impairments in children/youths with complex needs necessitate assistance from communication partners to set up an eye-gaze controlled computer and adapt AAC content to meet their changing needs in communication [16]. Moreover, these children might take a longer time to operate/navigate computers compared with using gestures or vocalizations, particularly when they are novice users. Insufficient eye control skills at early stages of learning and cognitive demands might cause the children to tire easily which could decrease the efficiency of EGAT use over time [48]. Recent research showed children with complex needs normally used EGAT for up to two hours per day [17], which means they might use other modes of communication in communicative interactions in daily contexts more often. It is important to develop strategies and means for increasing the frequency that children are exposed to EGAT every day, i.e., embed opportunity to use EGAT in everyday activities in natural contexts, according to a newly developed clinical guideline [49]. As of today, the time spent using EGAT is too low to allow children to use the whole communicative potential.

As AAC is certainly multimodal [13], children/youths utilize multiple communication methods, by which they think fast and efficiently to fulfill communication needs depending on the communication contexts and demands. This study supported previous research [5,14,15] by showing these children demonstrated preferences using gestures or vocalizations in communicating social routines such as greetings, responding yes–no answers, or expressing affection, probably because these natural modes might be faster and more accessible for them. Thus, the findings indicated the importance of supporting their functional use of the multimodal approach in everyday contexts [50] and echoed the statement by Light and McNaughton [23] that the central focus of AAC intervention is the communication needs of children/youths with complex needs, rather than the devices.

4.4. Strengths and Limitations

A major strength of this study is that as far as we know, it is one of the few articles using video-coding to investigate the impacts of eye-gaze AT on communicative interaction between dyads. Using a system-based approach to coding guided by the foundation of previous research enables the meaning construction of the dyadic communicative behaviors in the EGAT and NEGAT conditions. The acceptable to good inter-rater reliability increased the credibility of this study. Higher kappa values were found in the EGAT condition compared to the NEGAT condition, indicating that the behaviors in communicative interactions were easier to observe and reach the consensus when the children/youths used EGAT compared to the other condition. Moreover, this study applied a three-tiered method, combining group, intermediate and individual analysis to validate group results and reduced the bias in that extreme cases could be hidden by group patterns [8]. Individual case studies enhanced understanding of typical and atypical individual patterns and provided a preliminary reference for further clinical implications.

Several limitations of the present study should be acknowledged. First, the small samples due to the low prevalence rates, the vulnerable health conditions [2,51], and accessibility to EGAT of our target group affect generalizability. The results should be interpreted with caution. In addition, the videos were collected from parents or teachers in order to observe their communication in natural contexts. Although instruction checklists for film clips were provided, we were finally able to use only 12 videos from six dyads for coding analysis. There were several reasons for excluding videos, for instances, technical issues, lack of information or visible behaviors in communicative interactions, or dissimilar activities in the EGAT and NEGAT conditions, which made comparisons difficult and meaningless. To reduce the likelihood of biased results from small samples, a three-tiered method was used to validate group results and provide clinically useful information. Future research could consider including trained researchers to collect film clips and, if possible, recruit more participants to consolidate the findings and shed more light on this field of knowledge. However, the time expenditure required for video-coding analysis and inter-coder training might be necessary to take into consideration.

Another limitation is that we chose the best two videos in each dyad, which could represent the communicative interactions in a specific activity. The momentary observations based on videos might not be fully representative of the dyadic communicative interactions across various daily activities. Researchers could consider a combination of different methodologies to strengthen the research findings [51], for instance, integrating interviews with proxies to triangulate quantitative data and provide a comprehensive picture of the dyadic communicative interactions in daily life.

5. Conclusions

The results demonstrated that the children/youths increased initiations on communicative interactions, and the communication partners decreased dominance in communicative turns and made fewer initiations in the interactional structure when using EGAT compared to the NEGAT condition. Moreover, in communicative functions, children/youths tended to provide more information using EGAT, and the communication partners made fewer requests to direct children's responding behaviors, in contrast to the interaction in the NEGAT condition. The communication activities and the structure of the environment (e.g., play or school lessons), eye-control skills, and communication abilities could influence the dyadic interaction.

EGAT shows the potential to increase communication intelligibility, enable children/youths with complex needs gain power of communication, and facilitate the sharing of information in natural contexts. More research is needed, enrolling more participants and combining different research methods to improve generalization, and examining interactive strategies used by communication partners to support children's communication behaviors while using EGAT to guide future interventions.

Supplementary Materials: The following are available online at https://www.mdpi.com/article/10.3390/ijerph18105134/s1, Table S1: Turns, moves, communicative functions and modes of communication in communication partners, Table S2: Turns, moves, communicative functions and modes of communication in children and youths with complex needs.

Author Contributions: Conceptualization, H.H. and M.B.; Methodology, H.H., M.B., M.G. and Y.-H.H.; Formal analysis, Y.-H.H.; Investigation, M.B., D.G. and J.M.; Resources, H.H.; Writing—original draft preparation, Y.-H.H.; Writing—review and editing, H.H., M.G., A.-W.H., M.B., J.M., D.G. and Y.-H.H.; Supervision, H.H., M.G. and A.-W.H.; Funding acquisition, H.H. and M.B. All authors have read and agreed to the published version of the manuscript.

Funding: This research was funded by Vetenskapsrådet/Swedish Research Council (Dnr 2015-02427).

Institutional Review Board Statement: The study was conducted according to the guidelines of the Declaration of Helsinki, and approved by the ethical review boards in Sweden (Dnr 2018/1809-32), Dubai (DSREC-11/2017_10), and the USA (protocol ESSP-02).

Informed Consent Statement: Informed consent was obtained from all subjects involved in the study.

Data Availability Statement: The data presented in this study are available in Supplementary Materials here.

Acknowledgments: We thank all participating children and youths, parents, teachers and therapists. We thank the chiefs and the teams in Swedish assistive technology centers, and special schools in Dubai and the USA for assisting data collection and making this study possible. We are grateful to Helena Vandin at Uppsala University for contribution to the inter-rater reliability, and to the Ministry of Education in Taiwan for internal funding to support the first author's work.

Conflicts of Interest: The authors declare no conflict of interest.

Abbreviations

EGAT	Eye-gaze assistive technology
NEGAT	Non eye-gaze assistive technology
AT	Assistive technology
AAC	Augmentative and alternative communication
I	Initiation
R	Response
R/I	Response/Initiation
F/I	Follow up/Initiation
RE	Requestive
IN	Informative

Appendix A

Table A1. Coding frameworks of communicative interaction and definition for each code.

Category Code	Sub-Code	Definition
Turns		A succession of communicative signs with the boundary between turns a two-second gap supported by the presence of other communicative behaviors
Moves		Comprise single or strings of utterances/non-verbal communicative signals produced by one speaker within a conversational turn
(P) Preparation		Make ready self or other person for communicative interaction
(ON) Operation/Navigation		Operate or navigate pages on computer screen using eye-gaze technology or low-tech devices
(I) Initiation		Open the conversation, introduce a topic and could solicit a response
(R) Response		Reply to an Initiation (I) or Response/Initiation (R/I)
(R/I) Response/Initiation		Reply to an I or R/I, but also require a response of its own
(F) Follow-up		Optional, acknowledge the previous utterance and require no response
(F/I) Follow-up/initiation		Acknowledge previous move and require a response of its own
Communicative functions		Coded to represent the intentions and purpose of the speaker's communicative act
(RE) Requestive	Request joint attention	Require a listener's attention to an object, action or the speaker
	Request information	Attempt to elicit information from a listener by using closed-ended or open questions
	Request object/action	Speaker expresses the desire for an object, activity or physical action
	Request clarification	Speaker expresses that they have not understood previous utterance and require clarification
(IN) Informative	Provision of information	Speaker makes comments about objects, actions, events, internal states, or answers to requests for information, except for confirmation/denial

Table A1. Cont.

Category Code	Sub-Code	Definition
	Provision of clarification	Speaker clarifies a previous utterance or turn by repetition or revision of original message
(ACK) Acknowledgement		Response or convey understanding to previous utterance or action
(CD) Confirmation-denial		Affirmation, agreement, rejection, or disagreement to yes/no questions or to the partner's comments
(SSE) Self or shared expression		Demonstrate the speaker's personality, or express emotional states and feelings
(U) Unintelligible		Unintelligible utterances or illocutionary force, which may not be understood by a listener or coder
Modes of communication		The manner in which communicative functions are transmitted
(S) Speech		Intelligible or unintelligible speech, which may or may not be understood by a listener or coder
(V) Vocalization		Vocal sounds not intended to be speech, but which have communicative meaning interpreted by the listener
(G) Gesture		Use eye pointing, facial expression, hand-arm gesture or body language which has illocutionary force
(Lt) low-tech AAC		Use low-tech devices, e.g., communication board by means of direct or indirect selections
(EG) EGAT		Use eye gaze assistive technology (EGAT) as a means of communication

Note. Definition for each code based on previous video-coding research [5,14,15,27].

References

1. Raghavendra, P.; Virgo, R.; Olsson, C.; Connell, T.; Lane, A.E. Activity participation of children with complex communication needs, physical disabilities and typically-developing peers. *Dev. Neurorehabilit.* **2011**, *14*, 145–155. [CrossRef]
2. Dhondt, A.; Van Keer, I.; Van Der Putten, A.; Maes, B. Communicative abilities in young children with a significant cognitive and motor developmental delay. *J. Appl. Res. Intellect. Disabil.* **2019**, *33*, 529–541. [CrossRef]
3. Van Keer, I.; Colla, S.; Van Leeuwen, K.; Vlaskamp, C.; Ceulemans, E.; Hoppenbrouwers, K.; Desoete, A.; Maes, B. Exploring parental behavior and child interactive engagement: A study on children with a significant cognitive and motor developmental delay. *Res. Dev. Disabil.* **2017**, *64*, 131–142. [CrossRef]
4. Tan, S.S.; Van Gorp, M.; Voorman, J.M.; Geytenbeek, J.J.; Reinders-Messelink, A.H.; Ketelaar, M.; Dallmeijer, A.J.; Roebroeck, E.M.; Dallmeijer, A.; Gorp, M.; et al. Development curves of communication and social interaction in individuals with cerebral palsy. *Dev. Med. Child. Neurol.* **2019**, *62*, 132–139. [CrossRef] [PubMed]
5. Bunning, K.; Smith, C.; Kennedy, P.; Greenham, C. Examination of the communication interface between students with severe to profound and multiple intellectual disability and educational staff during structured teaching sessions. *J. Intellect. Disabil. Res.* **2011**, *57*, 39–52. [CrossRef] [PubMed]
6. Ogletree, B.T.; Bartholomew, P.; Wagaman, J.C.; Genz, S.; Reisinger, K. Emergent Potential Communicative Behaviors in Adults With the Most Severe Intellectual Disabilities. *Commun. Disord. Q.* **2012**, *34*, 56–58. [CrossRef]
7. Lipscombe, B.; Boyd, R.N.; Coleman, A.; Fahey, M.; Rawicki, B.; Whittingham, K. Does early communication mediate the relationship between motor ability and social function in children with cerebral palsy? *Res. Dev. Disabil.* **2016**, *53–54*, 279–286. [CrossRef]
8. Olsson, C. The Use of Communicative Functions among Pre-school Children with Multiple Disabilities in Two Different Setting Conditions: Group Versus Individual Patterns. *Augment. Altern. Commun.* **2005**, *21*, 3–18. [CrossRef]
9. Pennington, L. Speech and communication in cerebral palsy. *East. J. Med.* **2012**, *17*, 171–177.
10. United Nations. The Convention on The Rights of Persons with Disabilities. 2006. Available online: https://www.un.org/development/desa/disabilities/convention-on-the-rights-of-persons-with-disabilities.html (accessed on 30 October 2020).
11. Brady, N.C.; Bruce, S.; Goldman, A.; Erickson, K.; Mineo, B.; Ogletree, B.T.; Paul, D.; Romski, M.A.; Sevcik, R.; Siegel, E.; et al. Communication Services and Supports for Individuals with Severe Disabilities: Guidance for Assessment and Intervention. *Am. J. Intellect. Dev. Disabil.* **2016**, *121*, 121–138. [CrossRef]
12. Cook, A.M.; Polgar, J.M. *Assistive Technologies: Principles and Practice*, 4th ed.; Elsevier: St. Louis, MO, USA, 2015; pp. 1–15.

13. Beukelman, D.R.; Mirenda, P. *Augmentative & Alternative Communication: Supporting Children & Adults with Complex Communication Needs*, 4th ed.; Paul H. Brookes Pub. Co.: Baltimore, MD, USA, 2013; pp. 203–224.
14. Clarke, M.; Kirton, A. Patterns of interaction between children with physical disabilities using augmentative and alternative communication systems and their peers. *Child. Lang. Teach. Ther.* **2003**, *19*, 135–151. [CrossRef]
15. Pennington, L.; McConachie, H. Mother-child interaction revisited: Communication with non-speaking physically disabled children. *Int. J. Lang. Commun. Disord.* **1999**, *34*, 391–416. [CrossRef]
16. Borgestig, M.; Sandqvist, J.; Ahlsten, G.; Falkmer, T.; Hemmingsson, H. Gaze-based assistive technology in daily activities in children with severe physical impairments–An intervention study. *Dev. Neurorehabil.* **2016**, *20*, 129–141. [CrossRef]
17. Hemmingsson, H.; Borgestig, M. Usability of Eye-Gaze Controlled Computers in Sweden: A Total Population Survey. *Int. J. Environ. Res. Public Health* **2020**, *17*, 1639. [CrossRef] [PubMed]
18. Karlsson, P.; Allsop, A.; Dee-Price, B.-J.; Wallen, M. Eye-gaze control technology for children, adolescents and adults with cerebral palsy with significant physical disability: Findings from a systematic review. *Dev. Neurorehabil.* **2017**, *21*, 497–505. [CrossRef] [PubMed]
19. Lariviere, J.A. Eye tracking: Eye gaze technology. In *International Handbook of Occupational Therapy Interventions*; Söderback, I., Ed.; Springer: New York, NY, USA, 2014; pp. 339–362.
20. Karlsson, P.; Bech, A.; Stone, H.; Vale, C.; Griffin, S.; Monbaliu, E.; Wallen, M. Eyes on communication: Trialling eye-gaze control technology in young children with dyskinetic cerebral palsy. *Dev. Neurorehabil.* **2018**, *22*, 134–140. [CrossRef] [PubMed]
21. Vessoyan, K.; Steckle, G.; Easton, B.; Nichols, M.; Siu, V.M.; McDougall, J. Using eye-tracking technology for communication in Rett syndrome: Perceptions of impact. *Augment. Altern. Commun.* **2018**, *34*, 230–241. [CrossRef]
22. Borgestig, M.; Sandqvist, J.; Parsons, R.; Falkmer, T.; Hemmingsson, H. Eye gaze performance for children with severe physical impairments using gaze-based assistive technology—A longitudinal study. *Assist. Technol.* **2015**, *28*, 93–102. [CrossRef]
23. Light, J.; McNaughton, D. Communicative Competence for Individuals who require Augmentative and Alternative Communication: A New Definition for a New Era of Communication? *Augment. Altern. Commun.* **2014**, *30*, 1–18. [CrossRef]
24. Rytterström, P.; Borgestig, M.; Hemmingsson, H. Teachers' experiences of using eye gaze-controlled computers for pupils with severe motor impairments and without speech. *Eur. J. Spéc. Needs Educ.* **2016**, *31*, 506–519. [CrossRef]
25. Perfect, E.; Hoskin, E.; Noyek, S.; Davies, T.C. A systematic review investigating outcome measures and uptake barriers when children and youth with complex disabilities use eye gaze assistive technology. *Dev. Neurorehabil.* **2019**, *23*, 145–159. [CrossRef]
26. Borgestig, M.; Al Khatib, I.; Masayko, S.; Hemmingsson, H. The impact of eye-gaze controlled computer on communication and functional independence in children and youths with complex needs-a multicenter intervention study. *Dev. Neurorehabil.* **2021**. [CrossRef]
27. Light, J.; Collier, B.; Parnes, P. Communicative interaction between young nonspeaking physically disabled children and their primary caregivers: Part I—Discourse patterns. *Augment. Altern. Commun.* **1985**, *1*, 74–83. [CrossRef]
28. Porter, H.; Tharpe, A.M. Hearing loss and Down syndrome. *Int. Rev. Res. Dev. Disabil.* **2010**, *39*, 195–220.
29. Light, J. Do augmentative and alternative communication interventions really make a difference?: The challenges of efficacy research. *Augment. Altern. Commun.* **1999**, *15*, 13–24. [CrossRef]
30. Palisano, R.J.; Rosenbaum, P.; Bartlett, D.; Livingston, M.H. Content validity of the expanded and revised Gross Motor Function Classification System. *Dev. Med. Child. Neurol.* **2008**, *50*, 744–750. [CrossRef]
31. Eliasson, A.-C.; Krumlinde-Sundholm, L.; Rösblad, B.; Beckung, E.; Arner, M.; Öhrvall, A.-M.; Rosenbaum, P. The Manual Ability Classification System (MACS) for children with cerebral palsy: Scale development and evidence of validity and reliability. *Dev. Med. Child. Neurol.* **2006**, *48*, 549–554. [CrossRef]
32. Koester, H.H.; Simpson, R.C.; Spaeth, D.; LoPresti, E. Reliability and validity of Compass software for access assessment. In *Proceedings of RESNA 2007 Annual Conference, Phoenix, AZ*; RESNA Press: Arlington, VA, USA, 2007.
33. Rowland, C.; Fried-Oken, M. Communication Matrix: A clinical and research assessment tool targeting children with severe communication disorders. *J. Pediatr. Rehabil. Med.* **2010**, *3*, 319–329. [CrossRef]
34. Van Keer, I.; Ceulemans, E.; Bodner, N.; Vandesande, S.; Van Leeuwen, K.; Maes, B. Parent-child interaction: A micro-level sequential approach in children with a significant cognitive and motor developmental delay. *Res. Dev. Disabil.* **2019**, *85*, 172–186. [CrossRef] [PubMed]
35. Haidet, K.K.; Tate, J.; Divirgilio-Thomas, D.; Kolanowski, A.; Happ, M.B. Methods to improve reliability of video-recorded behavioral data. *Res. Nurs. Heal.* **2009**, *32*, 465–474. [CrossRef]
36. Bellieni, C.V.; Cordelli, D.M.; Caliani, C.; Palazzi, C.; Franci, N.; Perrone, S.; Bagnoli, F.; Buonocore, G. Inter-observer reliability of two pain scales for newborns. *Early Hum. Dev.* **2007**, *83*, 549–552. [CrossRef]
37. Freidlin, B.; Miao, W.; Gastwirth, J. On the Use of the Shapiro-Wilk Test in Two-Stage Adaptive Inference for Paired Data from Moderate to Very Heavy Tailed Distributions. *Biom. J.* **2003**, *45*, 887–900. [CrossRef]
38. Pritschet, L.; Powell, D.; Horne, Z. Marginally Significant Effects as Evidence for Hypotheses. *Psychol. Sci.* **2016**, *27*, 1036–1042. [CrossRef]
39. Tobii Dynavox LLC. Assistive Technology for Communication. Available online: https://www.tobiidynavox.com/en-US/?redirect=true (accessed on 20 October 2020).
40. Smartbox Assistive Technology. Available online: https://thinksmartbox.com/ (accessed on 20 October 2020).

41. Ablenet. Speech Generating Devices. Available online: https://www.ablenetinc.com/technology/speech-generating-devices (accessed on 20 October 2020).
42. De Leo, G.; Lubas, M.; Mitchell, J.R. Lack of Communication Even When Using Alternative and Augmentative Communication Devices: Are we Forgetting about the Three Components of Language. *Autism Open Access* **2012**, *2*, 109. [CrossRef]
43. Light, J.; McNaughton, D.; Beukelman, D.; Fager, S.K.; Fried-Oken, M.; Jakobs, T.; Jakobs, E. Challenges and opportunities in augmentative and alternative communication: Research and technology development to enhance communication and participation for individuals with complex communication needs. *Augment. Altern. Commun.* **2019**, *35*, 1–12. [CrossRef]
44. McNaughton, D.; Light, J.; Beukelman, D.R.; Klein, C.; Nieder, D.; Nazareth, G. Building capacity in AAC: A person-centred approach to supporting participation by people with complex communication needs. *Augment. Altern. Commun.* **2019**, *35*, 56–68. [CrossRef]
45. Goldbart, J.; Chadwick, D.; Buell, S. Speech and language therapists' approaches to communication intervention with children and adults with profound and multiple learning disability. *Int. J. Lang. Commun. Disord.* **2014**, *49*, 687–701. [CrossRef]
46. Hostyn, I.; Daelman, M.; Janssen, M.J.; Maes, B. Describing dialogue between persons with profound intellectual and multiple disabilities and direct support staff using the scale for dialogical meaning making. *J. Intellect. Disabil. Res.* **2010**, *54*, 679–690. [CrossRef] [PubMed]
47. Kent-Walsh, J.; Murza, K.A.; Malani, M.D.; Binger, C. Effects of Communication Partner Instruction on the Communication of Individuals using AAC: A Meta-Analysis. *Augment. Altern. Commun.* **2015**, *31*, 271–284. [CrossRef] [PubMed]
48. Majaranta, P.; Donegan, M.; Aoki, H.; Hansen, D.W.; Hansen, J.P.; Hyrskykari, A.; Räihä, K.-J. Introduction to Gaze Interaction. In *Gaze Interaction and Applications of Eye Tracking*; IGI Global: Hershey, PA, USA, 2012; pp. 1–9.
49. Karlsson, P.; Griffiths, T.; Clarke, M.T.; Monbaliu, E.; Himmelmann, K.; Bekteshi, S.; Allsop, A.; Pereksles, R.; Galea, C.; Wallen, M. Stakeholder consensus for decision making in eye-gaze control technology for children, adolescents and adults with cerebral palsy service provision: Findings from a Delphi study. *BMC Neurol.* **2021**, *21*, 1–24. [CrossRef] [PubMed]
50. Fried-Oken, M.; Granlund, M. AAC and ICF: A Good Fit to Emphasize Outcomes. *Augment. Altern. Commun.* **2012**, *28*, 1–2. [CrossRef] [PubMed]
51. Maes, B.; Nijs, S.; Vandesande, S.; Van Keer, I.; Arthur-Kelly, M.; Dind, J.; Goldbart, J.; Petitpierre, G.; Van Der Putten, A. Looking back, looking forward: Methodological challenges and future directions in research on persons with profound intellectual and multiple disabilities. *J. Appl. Res. Intellect. Disabil.* **2021**, *34*, 250–262. [CrossRef] [PubMed]

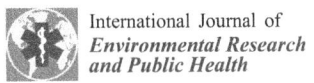

Article

Validation of the Infant and Young Child Development (IYCD) Indicators in Three Countries: Brazil, Malawi and Pakistan

Melissa Gladstone [1,*], Gillian Lancaster [2], Gareth McCray [2], Vanessa Cavallera [3], Claudia R. L. Alves [4], Limbika Maliwichi [5], Muneera A. Rasheed [6], Tarun Dua [3], Magdalena Janus [7,†] and Patricia Kariger [8,†]

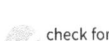

1   International Child Health and Neurodevelopmental Paediatrics, Department of Women and Children's Health, Institute of Life Course and Medical Sciences, University of Liverpool, Liverpool L12 2AP, UK
2   School of Medicine, Keele University, Keele ST5 5BG, UK; g.lancaster@keele.ac.uk (G.L.); g.mccray@keele.ac.uk (G.M.)
3   Brain Health Unit in Department of Mental Health and Substance Use, World Health Organization (WHO), 1202 Geneva, Switzerland; cavallerav@who.int (V.C.); duat@who.int (T.D.)
4   Pediatrics Department, Medicine School, Universidade Federal de Minas Gerais (UFMG), Belo Horizonte 30130-100, Brazil; lindgren@medicina.ufmg.br
5   Department of Psychology, University of Malawi, Zomba P.O. Box 280, Malawi; lmaliwichi@cc.ac.mw
6   Centre for International Health, Department of Global Public Health and Primary Care, University of Bergen, 5007 Bergen, Norway; muneera.rasheed@uib.no
7   Offord Centre for Child Studies, Department of Psychiatry and Behavioural Neurosciences, McMaster University, Hamilton, ON L8S 4KI, Canada; janusm@mcmaster.ca
8   Center for Effective Global Action (CEGA), School of Public Health, University of California, Berkeley, CA 94704, USA; patriciakariger@gmail.com
*   Correspondence: melglad@liverpool.ac.uk
†   Co-last authors.

Abstract: Background: The early childhood years provide an important window of opportunity to build strong foundations for future development. One impediment to global progress is a lack of population-based measurement tools to provide reliable estimates of developmental status. We aimed to field test and validate a newly created tool for this purpose. Methods: We assessed attainment of 121 Infant and Young Child Development (IYCD) items in 269 children aged 0–3 from Pakistan, Malawi and Brazil alongside socioeconomic status (SES), maternal educational, Family Care Indicators and anthropometry. Children born premature, malnourished or with neurodevelopmental problems were excluded. We assessed inter-rater and test-retest reliability as well as understandability of items. Each item was analyzed using logistic regression taking SES, anthropometry, gender and FCI as covariates. Consensus choice of final items depended on developmental trajectory, age of attainment, invariance, reliability and acceptability between countries. Results: The IYCD has 100 developmental items (40 gross/fine motor, 30 expressive/receptive language/cognitive, 20 socio-emotional and 10 behavior). Items were acceptable, performed well in cognitive testing, had good developmental trajectories and high reliability across countries. Development for Age (DAZ) scores showed very good known-groups validity. Conclusions: The IYCD is a simple-to-use caregiver report tool enabling population level assessment of child development for children aged 0–3 years which performs well across three countries on three continents to provide reliable estimates of young children's developmental status.

Keywords: child development; measurement; indicators; global health; validation; cross-cultural; cross-linguistic

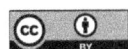

1. Introduction

Global efforts through the Millennium Development Goals have been very successful in ensuring many more children survive the perinatal period. However, this has not led to sustained thriving of those same children [1] Estimates now indicate that over 250 million children in low- and middle-income countries (LMICs) are at risk of not reaching their developmental potential by five years of age [2]. Early child development (ECD), especially the period from birth to 3 years, is a period of rapid brain development when children are most susceptible to environmental influences, making it the most critical period of development during the lifespan [3]. In many world regions, the very first indication that children are not thriving is registered at the time of school entry, which is much too late for early intervention.

Clearly, more needs to be done to ensure that very early development, in the first 1000 days [4], is better supported to ensure that optimal developmental trajectories are attainable in these children. Those first years are particularly sensitive because of the intensity of brain development. In the early years of life, the brain is extremely responsive both to positive influences, such as stimulating environment and adequate nurturing care, as well as to negative influences, such as poor nutrition, recurrent infections, lack of responsive and secure parenting, lack of early educational support and unstable economic situations. Many early intervention programs have focused on these factors, and some have demonstrated that giving children a good early start in life can critically influence brain development [3] and thus potentially optimize children's future economic and social well-being.

One of the obstacles in promoting policies and programs to effectively support children is the lack of validated and reliable measurement tools that could be used to monitor progress for the youngest age groups. While a number of individual and population-level assessments, validated for use in diverse contexts, exist for children at preschool [5], school entry [6] and primary grades [7,8], there is only a small pool of global tools available for children under 3 years. These are mainly developed in Western settings and so costly to implement in low resource settings (e.g., Ages and Stages) or need direct assessment [9], which may require substantial training (Bayley III, Griffiths), making them infeasible for monitoring at the population level. A further challenge is cultural adaptation. If a tool has been specifically developed for a particular country context [10,11], then it may not be readily applied across countries without extensive cultural adaptation, for example, to ensure accurate translation or in the use of relevant props. While some new tools have been created concurrently with the work reported here (e.g., Caregiver Reported Early Developmental Index and Survey of Wellbeing of Young Children) [12], none of them have been developed using an extensive database of child assessments gathered from low- and middle-income countries (LMIC) through a rigorous statistical process [13].

To address these challenges, we recently analyzed 14 datasets comprising 21,083 children; data were collected using seven tools in 10 LMIC countries to identify items that may reliably work across contexts and settings [13]. The resulting prototype tool that we created, the Indicators of Infant and Young Child Development (IYCD), was tested for feasibility of implementation across three sites (Brazil, Malawi and Pakistan) on three continents [14]. At the beginning of this study, the prototype tested comprised 121 items. This tool was created as a simple caregiver-reported tool that was created using tablet-based technology for gathering data (Open Data Kit (ODK)), and it included simple audio/visual media to support understanding of the developmental milestones against which children from 0–3 years were tested.

The present paper outlines the main field testing and final selection of cross-culturally neutral items to validate the WHO IYCD tool across the same three countries, to determine the feasibility of these assessments and to finalize its content. In this study we aimed to determine the performance of the final version of the tool by examining the reliability, ages of attainment and developmental trajectories of each of the IYCD items across countries, as well as in rural and urban settings, in order to ensure that all items in the tool performed consistently across multiple sites, contexts and settings. We also conducted cognitive interviews after to explore language meaning and interpretation in more depth.

2. Materials and Methods
2.1. Population, Setting and Sampling
2.1.1. Settings and Recruitment

The study was conducted in three countries: Brazil, Malawi and Pakistan. We chose these three countries due to their spread across three continents, the cultural diversity, the feasibility of conducting assessments in both low- and middle-income and rural and urban settings and the availability and interest of the country teams to work with us within a limited time scale. In each country, caregivers of babies and infant children were approached for participation in varying ways depending on the setting.

- Brazil. Children and caregivers were recruited by the research team from primary care health centers when parents and children were coming for routine visits or to access any other service such as immunization, pharmacy, dentistry, etc., both in rural and urban areas of Minas Gerais state. The urban sample also included children recruited in a daycare center for children of Sofia Feldman Hospital's staff. While this daycare can be attended by children of all hospital employees, the cleaners, cooks, administrative staff and technicians constitute the majority of parents.
- Malawi. Children and caregivers were recruited by Health Surveillance Assistants (community health workers) from urban Blantyre and semi-rural Bangwe regions from primary health care centers when children and their caregivers were attending routine visits (the under-5 clinic).
- Pakistan. Children and caregivers were recruited through the random sampling of lists of children registered with respective Lady Health Workers.

2.1.2. Informed Consent

Research procedures were approved by local Ethics Committees. Full information on the study was provided in the local language before requesting consent, with frequent back-checking to ensure understanding. Participants were informed of the security procedures used to ensure confidentiality and the organizational provisions for data storage and archiving. Informed consent forms were written to be easily understood by lay persons, enabling them to understand the aims, procedures and potential risks of participation. All information was read aloud, in the presence of an adult witness, to participants who were illiterate. Respondents who decided to participate completed a written consent form, and for participants who were illiterate, a witnessed oral consent and a thumbprint in lieu of a signature was requested. All participants were informed that taking part was voluntary and that they were free to withdraw at any time. It was also made clear that taking part or not taking part would in no way affect care for their child. This consent procedure followed WHO recommendations. Once they agreed to participate, caregivers in each country were given a participant information document and were consented by different cadres of workers who had received in-depth training on the informed consent process through Good Clinical Practice (GCP). This included pediatricians, occupational therapists and physiotherapists (Brazil), nurses (Malawi) and Lady Health Workers (Pakistan). Families were recruited between 1 August 2016 and 1 December 2016.

2.1.3. Sampling

As this was a validation study, it was important that we sampled enough children from across the entire age range in order to adequately test all the items in each age group. In order to achieve adequate representation of children at the higher ages, we sampled children up to 42 months for analysis purposes. A stratified sampling frame was drawn up to quota sample children within eight age group strata (3-month intervals from 0 to 12 months and 6-month intervals from 13 to 42 months) by gender and from urban and rural settings. The sampling grid contained $8 \times 2 \times 2 = 32$ cells with children to be sampled in each cell ($n = 96$ per country) (see File S1). To create subsamples for reliability and cognitive interviews, one caregiver of a child from each cell ($n = 32$ per country) was randomly selected and invited to take part in the reliability testing, and three caregivers from different cells in each age stratum per country (*n* = 24 per country) were randomly selected for cognitive interviews.

2.2. Exclusion Criteria

The exclusion criteria were informed by existing evidence on health factors that may have affected developmental progress of children in the study. Children who had a mid-upper arm circumference (MUAC) of <12.5 [15] and infants less than six months old with a MUAC of <13 [16] at recruitment were excluded (Figure 1). Children who were unwell on the day of assessment or who had other chronic health needs (including neurodevelopmental disorders, HIV or those with recurrent infections) were excluded from the study prior to recruitment.

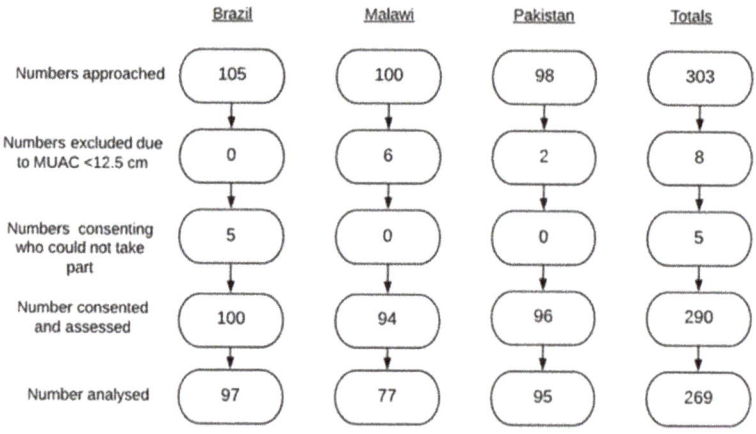

Figure 1. Flow chart demonstrating recruitment to IYCD validation study.

2.3. Measures

2.3.1. Child Development (IYCD)

The IYCD tool version 1.1 implemented in this study included 121 items: 46 motor (22 fine, 24 gross), 40 language (24 expressive, 16 receptive), and 35 socio-emotional items, which resulted from the feasibility study [14]. The tool was created for use on a tablet-based system using ODK (open data kit) with parent report items. The tool contains items such as: "Does your child reach for and hold objects at least for a few seconds?" (motor) or "Does your child use two words together in a meaningful phrase/speak in short two-word sentence? For example, 'mama go', 'give mama', 'daddy gone'." (language) or "Does your child ever try to imitate your actions around the house?" (socio-emotional). In each country, all items were translated by two local translators who knew the subject and then were back translated by two different language experts with consensus gained at each stage. Back translations in all countries were then checked by the subject matter expert team (M.G., P.K., M.J.) and were streamlined as much as possible between countries.

In the preliminary study, all children were assessed for all items despite their age, enabling us to determine the age at which 50% of children could achieve each item. For this main study, each item of the tool was then placed in order by the age at which approximately 50% of children could achieve it from these preliminary data. A starting point for asking each item was determined using the age of children first achieving the skills based on our previous meta-data synthesis and feasibility work [13,14]. In order to facilitate understanding of the items by caregivers, photos, videos or sounds were provided as appropriate (e.g., a sound example for "Does your child make single sounds like "buh" or "duh" or "muh"?). These were first selected and reviewed to consensus by the authors, then finalized based on feedback from the field teams, who also provided some of the photos and videos. They were presented to the caregivers on tablets for each item that was highlighted in the tool as needing a prompt (Figure 2).

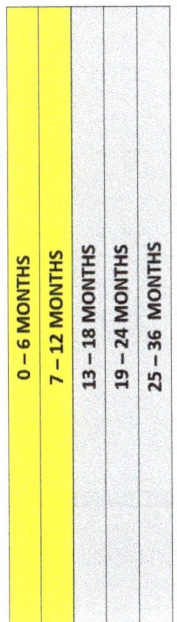
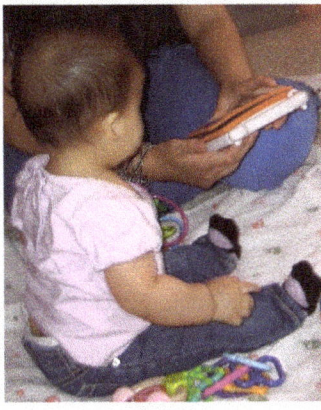

Figure 2. Example of items with prompts.

2.3.2. Anthropometry

Anthropometric measurements of every child (weight, height, MUAC and head circumference) were collected as per standard WHO protocols [17]. Children were weighed with an electronic infant scale or an electronic adult weighing scale with reading increments of 10 g. Height or length was taken using an infantometer, recorded to the nearest 1 mm, and head circumference was also measured (using non-stretchable plastic tapes, recorded to the nearest 1 mm). Mid-upper arm circumference was obtained using a standard tape measure to the nearest 1 mm. These measures were used to create a height-for-age z-score (HAZ), weight-for-age z-score (WAZ) and a weight-for-height z-score (WHZ) for each child.

2.3.3. Socioeconomic Status and Family Information

Socioeconomic status (SES) variables included wealth index and maternal education, which were assessed using Demographic & Health Survey (DHS) items standardized for each country [18]. The wealth index comprised 21 items as recommended for multiple assets analysis (water source, fuel use, assets, transportation, animals owned, toilet facilities etc.). Information on the stimulation and learning opportunities offered by the child's home environment was collected with the family care indicators (FCI) [19] items included in the UNICEF Multiple Indicators Cluster Survey.

2.4. Training and Procedures for Data Collection

Training was provided by the local team members/co-authors (Brazil C.R.L.A., Malawi L.M.S., Pakistan M.A.R.), with a consistency check visit by one of the other co-authors (Brazil P.K., Malawi M.G., Pakistan V.C.). Training took place over a period of 2–3 days at each site and was conducted in person at each site. The cost of the training depended on the cost of the trainer visit, hiring a room and transport costs to the training location for children and families attending. The training procedures were monitored so a formal "training the trainer" package could be developed. Training materials are available through the IYCD website (https://ezcollab.who.int/iycd, accessed on 2 June 2021).

Once trained, the country teams conducted assessments with caregivers. Generally, the IYCD assessment was conducted first, followed by the physical measurement of the child. In seven cases in Brazil, three in Malawi and none in Pakistan, the IYCD assessment had to be ceased and reprised on another occasion. The majority of the interviews were recorded using tablets run on Open Data Kit software [20].

2.4.1. Reliability Testing

At the initial assessment, a random subsample (n = 96; 32 from each of the three sites) was invited to come back for a second assessment to test consistency of measurement. Inter-rater reliability (two different assessors within the same day at a different time and test-retest reliability (same assessor 3–7 days apart) were conducted in the same setting where the child was seen originally (in Brazil and Malawi, this was done in the health centers, and in Pakistan this was done in homes).

2.4.2. Cognitive Interviews

Nine cognitive interviews in each setting were conducted to establish whether caregivers understood each item. They were also asked how they would explain the question back to the interviewer [21]. Responses were recorded and transcribed verbatim into a spreadsheet for review. All comments were translated into English. Translated responses from cognitive interviews were collated into one document and reviewed by the core team (G.L., G.Mc.C., M.G., M.J., P.K., T.D., V.C.). Input was requested from local investigators (C.R.L.A., L.M.S., M.A.R.) during a teleconference. The results were used to inform decisions to revise wording or retain/delete items as described in the results to ensure optimal clarity of the formulation of all items chosen in the final tool. No formal qualitative analyses were conducted.

2.5. Procedures for Finalization of the IYCD

In order to finalize the tool, firstly, each core team member reviewed the evidence of the items' performance based on 4 criteria: (i) universality (whether the age at which 50% of children passed each item was similar across countries in terms of location) and discrimination (whether the plotted curve trajectories (slopes) adequately demonstrated increasing attainment by age), as described in Lancaster et al. [13], (ii) inter-rater and test-retest reliability, and (iii) responses from the cognitive interviews (verbatim). Secondly, a joint full team meeting was conducted with the core and country teams. This meeting, which included M.G. (neurodevelopmental pediatrician), T.K. (developmental psychologist), M.J (developmental biologist), G.L. (biostatistician), V.C. (pediatric neurologist), T.D. (pediatric neurologist), M.R. (psychologist), C.R.L.A. (pediatrician) and L.S. (psychologist), was convened to reach consensus as to which items were to be included in the final version of the IYCD.

2.6. Sample Size

In order to enable item response theory (IRT) methods to be used in the analysis, which was important for building the scoring algorithm [22], we established that a sample of approximately 300 children was required. Considering the time needed to carry out the assessments and collect all the data, as well as available funding and feasibility of assessments in the countries, the sample size was set at 96 children per country, 288 in total. This also allowed us to devise a quota sampling scheme with equal allocation of children to each cell (see File S1). For the IRT model used (2PL), 250 children are considered a sufficient sample size [23] and 288 children gives us an 80% power at a two-sided 0.05 alpha to detect as significant a Pearson's correlation of 0.16 or higher of the tool score against other contextual variables. Thus, we felt the sample size sufficient for the purpose of tool validation.

2.7. Statistical Analyses

2.7.1. IYCD Item-by-Item Analyses

An exploratory item-by-item analysis was conducted using logistic regression with the log odds of the probability of passing regressed on the natural logarithm of age to determine how well each item performed across countries. The age at which 50% of children passed an item and the slope of the curve were extracted for each country, and both empirical- and model-based probabilities of passing an item were plotted against age to provide a graphical representation of item trajectories for each country.

2.7.2. Demographic and Contextual Covariates

The demographic profile of the countries was summarized using mean and standard deviation (SD) for continuous data and count (percentage) for categorical data. The age of the child was computed by subtracting the date of birth of the child from the date of administration of the first application of the measure. Decimal age was used throughout, whereby 1 year is equal to 1, 6 months is equal to 0.5 and 3 months is equal to 0.25, and so on. Weight-for-age z-scores (WAZ), height-for-age z-scores (HAZ) and weight-for-height z-scores (WHZ) were constructed according to the WHO 2006 standards [24,25]. They were computed in R using code provided from WHO Anthrostat [26]. In order to make the FCI score comparable across different ages, a generalized partial credit model (GPCM) was used in the R package MIRT [27]. Maternal education was divided into four main categories: no school, primary only, secondary only, and above secondary. In order to make the responses between the DHS wealth index data comparable across countries, we also constructed a two-parameter logistic IRT model using MIRT [27] to create a socioeconomic status (SES) score. The generation of the FCI and SES scores are detailed elsewhere [28].

2.7.3. Missing Data

Missing IYCD item responses (1.6%) were not imputed as the IRT model uses full maximum likelihood estimation. Missing covariate data were imputed using the R package MICE [29]. The numbers of missing data points for covariates were: HAZ $n = 29$; WAZ $n = 23$; maternal education $n = 5$; sex $n = 1$; FCI $n = 6$; SES $n = 6$; urban/rural $n = 0$.

2.7.4. Reliability Analyses

Inter- and intra-rater reliability were calculated for each item using a raw agreement proportion (the proportion of pairs of ratings that agree exactly), Cohen's kappa statistic as well as Gwet's AC1 [30], which provides more stable estimates [31] of agreement in situations where there is high trait (pass/fail) prevalence.

2.7.5. Creation of a Development-for-Age z-Score (DAZ)

Once the final items had been selected, a scoring system for the final tool was set up. A generalized partial credit model (GPCM) [32] using an empirical histogram prior [33,34] to account for the non-normality in the ability (development) distribution was fitted to the data using the R [35] package MIRT [27]. As the data contained a mixture of binary and three ordinal category responses, a polytomous IRT model was required. Taking the latent scores for each child from the IRT model, the LMS (lambda, mu, sigma) [36,37] method of centile estimation was used to remove the effect of age to create age contingent z-scores, which we termed "development-for-age z-scores", or DAZ for short.

2.7.6. Validation

The DAZ scores were plotted against the demographic and contextual variables to explore known-groups construct validity of the tool by comparing countries, maternal education categories and gender. Differences in mean scores were tested using a t-test or analysis of variance (ANOVA). Concurrent validity with respect to FCI scores, SES scores, WAZ, HAZ and WHZ was examined using Pearson or Spearman correlation coefficients. A more detailed analysis is described elsewhere [28].

2.7.7. Patient and Public Involvement

We did not directly include patient and public involvement in this study, but all community activities were discussed with health clinic staff and leaders in study areas prior to starting the study. The study team leads received feedback from the local assessors on a regular basis about any problems or difficulties in recruitment within the communities. No issues were reported, and there were no major issues with recruitment.

3. Results

Complete data were available for 269 children (Table 1): 97 in Brazil, 77 in Malawi (due to issues with the tablets not functioning appropriately and not saving data) and 95 in Pakistan (Figure 1). Recruitment was generally high in all locations, was always during working hours and was not problematic. Most caregivers consented to their children being included in the study; however, 5 of the 105 caregivers consented but were unable to be assessed in Brazil due to lack of time. In Pakistan, there were no refusals during recruitment. The Pakistan team in particular found recruitment easy as data collectors were from the same community, they spoke the same language and they already had a strong relationship with the community. Similarly, the staff from Malawi College of Medicine worked closely with the health surveillance teams in the local health centers, where recruitment for studies is common and with most parents willing to take part. Only eight (2.7 %) of all children approached did not meet stringent criteria of having a MUAC greater than 12.5 cm (two from Pakistan and six from Malawi). Seventeen children in Malawi and three from Brazil had missing data on developmental milestones, mainly due to issues with the tablets not functioning, missing birth date data and problems uploading data properly. There were low proportions of missing data (0–2%) for maternal education (5), sex (1), urban/rural (6), FCI score (6) and SES (6) and slightly higher numbers for HAZ (29), WAZ (23) and WHZ (29) (9–11%). Missing data were imputed for all covariates.

Table 1. Table of children recruited and included in the validation of the Indicators of Young Child Development (IYCD).

Country		Brazil			Malawi			Pakistan			Total
Setting of Those Who Had Data Analyzed		Rural		Urban	Rural		Urban		Rural		Urban	
Sex of Participants		M	F	M	F	M	F	M	F	M	F	M	F	
Age band of participants (months)	0–2	3	2	2	5	2	2	2	2	3	3	3	3	32
	3–6	3	3	3	4	3	2	4	2	3	4	3	3	38
	6–9	3	3	3	1	2	2	3	3	3	3	2	3	31
	9–12	3	3	4	3	2	4	2	2	3	3	3	2	34
	12–18	4	4	2	4	3	0	3	3	3	3	3	3	35
	18–24	3	3	3	3	2	5	2	2	3	2	3	3	34
	24–36	3	3	3	2	2	2	3	2	3	3	3	3	32
	36–42	2	4	3	3	4	3	1	1	3	4	3	3	33
	Total		97				77				95			269

3.1. Sample

Sample characteristics are shown in Table 2. In our sample, almost all (98%) Brazilian mothers had completed secondary education or above and generally had a higher SES index (0.59) and FCI score (0.25) than in other settings. The Brazilian children had HAZ (-0.28) and WAZ (0.05) closest to the WHO standards. In the Malawi sample, very few caregivers went beyond secondary education, with most evenly split between those who completed primary or secondary education; the mean children's HAZ and WAZ were somewhat below the WHO normal standards (-0.85 and -0.06 respectively). Our Pakistan sample was the least educated, with only a third (36.8%) of mothers completing secondary school education or above. It also had the highest number of children with a low mean HAZ and WAZ (mean −1.1 and −0.92 respectively).

Table 2. Demographic features of children in IYCD sample across countries.

Country	Brazil n = 97	Malawi n = 77	Pakistan n = 95	Total n = 269
Demographics				
Age	1.33 (1.01)	1.30 (0.97)	1.34 (1.03)	1.33 (1.00)
M/F	47/50	40/37	47/48	134/135
Anthropometry				
Mean HAZ *** (SD)	−0.28 (1.11)	−0.85 (1.17)	−1.08 (1.0)	−0.72 (1.14)
Mean WAZ **** (SD)	0.05 (1.14)	−0.06 (1.17)	−0.92 (1.04)	−0.31 (1.22)
Maternal education (% total per country)				
No School	0	3 (3.9)	21 (22.1)	24 (8.9)
Primary (%)	2 (2.1)	34 (44.1)	39 (41.1)	75 (27.9)
Secondary (%)	70 (72.2)	36 (46.8)	18 (18.9)	124 (46.1)
Above (%)	25 (25.8)	4 (5.2)	17 (17.9)	46 (17.1)
SES *				
Mean (SD)	0.59 (0.59)	−0.12 (0.59)	−0.47 (0.51)	−0.30 (0.92)
MCS FCI **				
Mean (SD)	0.25 (0.62)	−0.14 (0.72)	−0.15 (0.37)	0.0 (0.61)

* Socioeconomic status index score created from DHS using a two-parameter logistic IRT model. ** Family care indicator index score created from Family Care Indicators using a two-parameter logistic IRT model and GAMLSS for age correction. *** HAZ—height for age z score. **** WAZ—weight for age z score

3.2. Item Performance

Figure 3 illustrates examples of different item response trajectories.

Plots for all items tested are available in the second supplementary file (File S2). Approximately 90% of items fell into the patterns demonstrated in Figure 3a,b, with well-marked developmental progression in item attainment among children within and between each country. Two examples of poor items are illustrated by lines that are very flat (Figure 3e) or that show too much variation in progression between countries (Figure 3f).

A number of items (11/121) did not show a clear developmental trajectory. Nine of eleven poorly performing items belonged to the socio-emotional domain (representing 9/35 or 26% of the items in that domain), and one each belonged to the gross motor and expressive language domains (representing 1/24 or 4% of items in each domain). Items that showed considerable differences in terms of attainment across countries and the poorly performing items were subjected to expert review by the core and country teams. During the review (reported below), it was ascertained whether the item was likely to be exhibiting bias (due for example to misunderstanding or poor translation), or true differences between countries, and therefore whether it should be retained or deleted from the finalized tool.

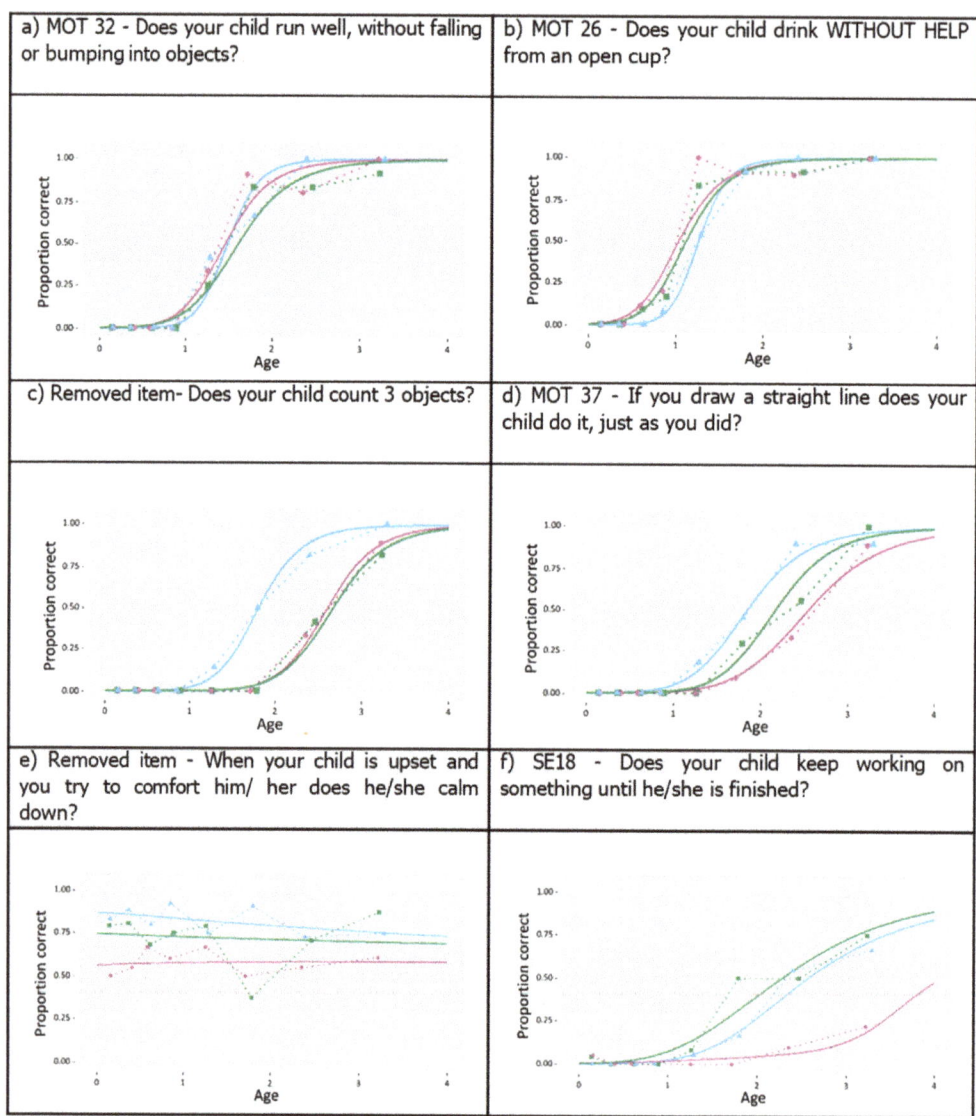

Figure 3. Examples of logistic regression of items. The first two plots, (**a**,**b**), show clear developmental trajectories by age for each country, with agreement between countries. The next two plots, shown in (**c**,**d**), display items that have good developmental trajectories but also some differences between countries. Examples of two poorly performing items are shown in (**e**,**f**). Green—Pakistan, Blue—Malawi, Pink—Brazil.

3.3. Reliability

Inter-rater and test-retest reliability statistics were calculated for all 121 items tested. The results are shown for the 90 well-performing items that were eventually retained in the finalized tool (Table 3) and the 33 removed items. We report statistics as a whole across all countries, as numbers for individual countries were too small due to sample sizes. The raw proportion of agreement (RAP) is reported as well as frequencies of items with statistics less than 0.6 (poor/fair/moderate reliability), between 0.61 and 0.80 (good) and above 0.81 (very good) for Cohen's kappa and Gwet's AC1 [31]. As it can be seen from the table, the majority of items showed very good reliability, with poorest outcomes in the socio-emotional domain and highest reliability values in the motor domain. Inter-rater reliabilities by domain for the retained items ranged from 0.78 to 0.95. Intra-rater (or test-retest) demonstrated excellent reliabilities, with a range of mean reliability by domain from 0.84 to 0.96.

Table 3. Reliability frequencies by domain for WHO IYCD items for the 90 retained items and the 33 removed items.

Domain of Development	Type of Reliability Assessed	Mean RAP ***	Kappa <0.6	Kappa >0.6 & <0.8	Kappa >0.8	AC1 <0.6	AC1 >0.6 & <0.8	AC1 >0.8	Total Number of Items	
			Number of items retained meeting the criteria							
Motor	Inter	0.95	3	8	29	0	1	39	40	
	Intra	0.96	0	6	34	0	0	40		
Language and Cognitive	Inter	0.89	5	7	18	2	8	20	30	
	Intra	0.94	0	7	23	0	0	30		
Socio-emotional	Inter	0.78	11	8	1	6	9	5	20	
	Intra	0.84	5	12	3	0	10	10		
Total items									90	
			Removed Items **							
Motor	Inter	0.96	1	2	3	0	0	6	6	
	Intra	0.96	2	0	4	0	0	6		
Language and Cognitive	Inter	0.88	2	5	2	1	2	6	9	
	Intra	0.94	2	2	5	0	1	8		
Socio-emotional	Inter	0.71	17	1	0	10	7	1	18	
	Intra	0.79	6	12	0	4	9	5		
Total removed									33	

** NOTE: Of the items removed, 9 had inter-rater reliability kappa statistics < 0.40, and 6 had intra-rater reliability kappa statistics < 0.40. These include the 10 behavior items showing no developmental trajectories that were later added to the final tool as important non-scoring items. RAP ***—Raw Agreement Proportion, Kappa—Kappa statistic of agreement, AC1—Gwet's AC1 agreement statistic.

3.4. Cognitive Interviews

Twenty-seven caregivers (nine in each country) were interviewed and in all cases, generally demonstrated a good understanding of the questions that were asked of them. The feedback they provided was used to revise wording of a few items. The four items that showed the highest degree of misunderstanding were: "Does your child walk backwards, two or more steps without any support?" (GRO20), "When you say 'no', does your child stop what they are doing?" (REC7), "Can your child complete a five piece puzzle?" (EXP23) and "Can your child understand on first try what is being said to him/her?" (SE12). All these items were removed as shown in Table 4 with item numbers as in Prototype 1 [14].

3.5. Finalisation of the Tool

The tool was reviewed and finalized according to the four criteria described in the methods. After the review of items' performance, including the feedback from cognitive interviews, 100 hundred items were retained, 23 items were marked for deletion (Table 4) and 10 were retained as important non-scoring items (see below). Four of the twenty-three items were revealed to have extensive overlap in the range of age of attainment, and two were therefore deleted. The main reasons for item deletion were, therefore: poor developmental trajectories, poor reliability, wide differences in age attainment between countries and issues with clarity of meaning from cognitive testing. These are listed together with item wording in Table 4. Two additional items were added for the higher ages to fill gaps: LAN19 "Does your child say at least six words?" and LAN22 "Does your child identify at least seven objects?" Agreement was reached by the team to finalize the IYCD. The final list of items is in the Supplementary Materials and has 100 items with 90 of them in 3 domains of development (40 motor items, 30 language and cognitive items and 20 socio-emotional items). Ten behavioral items that showed no or very poor developmental progression on the socio-emotional scale were also retained as important but were not to be scored as part of the IYCD final score.

Table 4. Table of items in IYCD prototype removed and reasons why.

Domain	Item Number from Prototype 1 *	Item Wording	Reason for Removal
Motor	FIN1	Does your child look at your face with interest and attention?	Same age attainment as adjoining items and slightly confusing when translating and back translating.
	FIN24A	Does your child write the first letter of his/her name?	(This item was added in phase I/II.) Item age attainment too advanced for 0- to 36-month children.
	GRO2	When you hold your child in a sitting position, does he/she hold his head steady?	Same age attainment as adjoining items, therefore no need for this item
	GRO3	When pulling your child from lying down on his or her back to sitting, does your child hold his/her head steady?	Same age attainment as adjoining items, therefore no need for this item.
	GRO20N	Does your child walk backwards, two or more steps WITHOUT any support?	Same age attainment to adjoining item; "stands on one foot with support", which was more understandable on cognitive testing. Reliability not high.
	GRO23	While standing, does your child CATCH a ball and hold on to it, for at least a few seconds?	Same age attainment to GRO21 (Does your child stand on one foot without any support for at least a few seconds?), which requires fewer props.
Language	REC1	Does your child respond or startle when a loud sound is made?	Not related to age (poor developmental trajectory).
	REC2	Does your child respond to your voice or someone else's voice even if you are not talking to the child directly?	Same age attainment to REC3 (Does your child turn his/her head toward your voice or some noise?) but less consistent across different countries
	REC7	When you say "no", does your child stop what they are doing?	Same age attainment as adjoining items. Confusing item; not easy to ask on cognitive testing.
	REC18N	If you ask your child "Where is the boy/girl/baby/cow/chicken/etc.?" can your child POINT TO or look at the right picture?)	Same age attainment as REC10 (When you ask "where is the ball/ spoon/ cup/ cloth/ door/ plate/ bucket etc." does your child look at or point to (or even name) the object? How many objects can your child identify?) but more variability between countries. Very variable direct vs. parent report
	EXP17	When looking at pictures or watching others, can your child tell you what ACTION is taking place (for example running, playing, sleeping etc.)	Same age attainment as adjoining items, and some countries not happy that this item was culturally acceptable.
	EXP18	How many objects can your child name?	Same age attainment as adjoining items, therefore no need for this item.
	EXP22	Can your child explain correctly what the following are used for? Cup (eating/drinking), spoon (eating), knife (cutting), matches (lighting fire, burning things), torch (light), broom	Same age attainment as adjoining items and some cultural differences across countries, making the item less consistent
	EXP25A	Does your child count three objects?	Same age attainment as adjoining items, therefore no need for this item.
	EXP28	Does your child know a song or rhyme from memory?	Attained at a later age, and confusing item for assessors
Socio-emotional	SE3	When your child is upset and you try to comfort him/ her does he/she calm down?	Not related to age (poor developmental trajectory).
	SE7	When you leave your child with a family member, does your child go with that person easily?	Not related to age (poor developmental trajectory).
	SE14	Does child pretend to drink from a cup, or eat with a spoon?	Not related to age (poor developmental trajectory).

Table 4. Cont.

Domain	Item Number from Prototype 1 *	Item Wording	Reason for Removal
	SE16	Does your child care for a doll or stuffed animal as if it were a person (for example by feeding and bathing it)?	Not related to age (poor developmental trajectory).
	SE24	Is your child easily distracted, that is has trouble sticking to any activity?	Not related to age (poor developmental trajectory).
	SE29	When child is very upset, can he/she calm self quickly?	Not related to age (poor developmental trajectory).
	SE30	Would you say that your child bullies or is mean to others at times?	Not related to age (poor developmental trajectory).
	SE32	When you send your child to get something, does he/she forget what he/she was supposed to get?	Not related to age (poor developmental trajectory).

* Please note the item numbers shown here are the item codes from the previous version of the tool.

3.6. Validation of IYCD Score Using the DAZ Scoring System

Graphs depicting the 10th, 25th, 50th, 75th and 90th centiles of attainment of each item within a domain were constructed (Figure 4).

Figure 5 shows a density plot of the DAZ scores across countries.

The plots show clear differences between countries in DAZ scores, with Brazil achieving slightly higher developmental scores overall than Pakistan and Malawi. Malawi in turn is slightly ahead of Pakistan in terms of the children in our samples. Mean (SD) DAZ scores by country were Brazil = 0.52 (0.86), Malawi = −0.13 (0.91), Pakistan = −0.43 (0.98), and these were found to be statistically significantly different ($F(2,266) = 26.87$, $p < 0.001$). Table 5 shows that DAZ scores were highly correlated with HAZ, WAZ, maternal education, SES and family environment (FCI). Some example density plots are shown in Figure 5b–d. Figure 5b shows the relationship between DAZ scores by WAZ tercile, which was significant ($F(2,243) = 5.657$, $p = 0.004$), mean (SD) DAZ score for lower tercile = −0.16 (1.10), middle tercile = −0.08 (0.86), and upper tercile = 0.31 (0.91). Figure 5c shows the significant relationship between SES tercile by DAZ scores ($F(2, 260) = 27.00$, $p < 0.001$), lower tercile = −0.38 (0.88), middle tercile = −0.21 (1.03), upper tercile = 0.56 (0.77). However, as expected the relationship between sex and DAZ was not significant ($t(266) = −0.66$, $p = 0.51$), mean (SD) DAZ score for males = −0.05 (0.98) and females = 0.03 (1.01) (Figure 5d).

Table 5. Correlation matrix of main variables.

	DAZ	AGE	SEX	HAZ	WAZ	MAT_ED	SES	FCI
DAZ								
AGE	0.01							
SEX	0.04	0.00						
HAZ	0.25 ***	−0.04	0.13					
WAZ	0.25 ***	−0.06	0.24 ***	0.56 ***				
MAT_ED	0.37 ***	0.10	−0.01	0.29 ***	0.27 ***			
SES	0.36 ***	0.04	0.04	0.25 ***	0.10	0.56 ***		
FCI	0.22 ***	0.74 ***	0.04	0.00	0.00	0.25 ***	0.24 ***	
URB/RUR	0.15 *	−0.05	−0.02	−0.03	0.00	0.20 **	0.22 ***	0.05

Correlation involving an ordinal variable uses Spearman's correlation coefficient; all others use Pearson's. SEX: Male = 1, SEX: Female = 2; URB/RUR: rural = 1, URB/RUR: urban = 2. * $p < 0.05$, ** $p < 0.01$, *** $p < 0.001$. DAZ—development-for-age z score, HAZ—height for age z score, WAZ—weight for age z score, MAT_ED—maternal education, SES—socioeconomic status, FCI—family care indicators.

The final version of the tool (IYCD version 1.2) is shown in File S2. The tool and all related training materials are available on the WHO IYCD website (https://ezcollab.who.int/iycd, accessed on 2 June 2021).

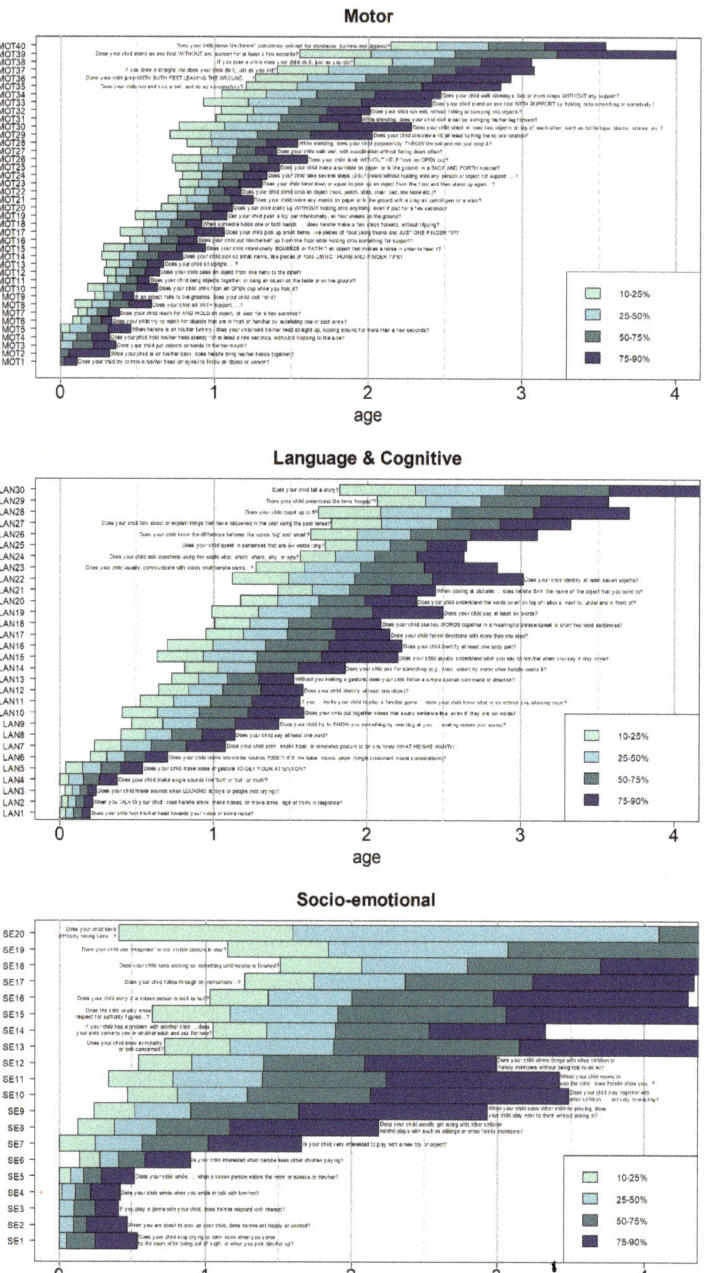

Figure 4. Domains of development with age succession of items with bars showing 10th, 25th, 50th, 75th and 90th centile for attainment across countries.

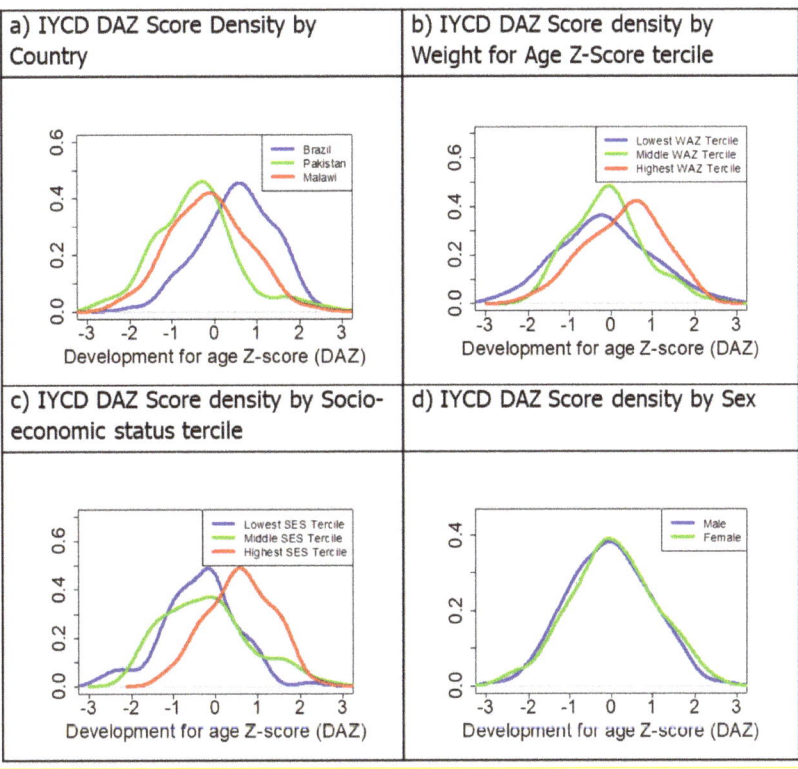

Figure 5. Density plots of development-for-age z-scores (DAZ) by country, WAZ, SES and Sex. (**a**) Development for age z score by country, (**b**) development for age z score varying by weight for age z scores broken into terciles, (**c**) development for age z score by socioeconomic status broken up into terciles and (**d**) development for age z score by sex.

4. Discussion

The WHO 0–3 indicators of Infant and Young Child Development (IYCD) tool is a parent report tool with 100 items (40 fine motor and gross motor, 30 language, 20 socio-emotional and 10 non-scored behavior items) that shows very good reliability, clear developmental trajectories and minimal variability across countries. Through this process, we have established a set of items for children under 3 years of age that can reliably monitor children's achievement of developmental milestones at approximately the same age across countries. We have further demonstrated that these items can be reported reliably by parents and that the items reflect well the development of children in three countries on three different continents.

Our analyses showed clear developmental trajectories comparable across the three different sites for all items within the motor (gross and fine) and language domains of development. There were fewer items that followed clear developmental trajectories in the socio-emotional development domain. Moreover, some items, though deemed important for healthy development, did not follow the age-based developmental trajectory in the same way as items in the motor and language domain. In response to this, the socio-emotional domain in the IYCD was limited to 20 items that met the developmental criteria. Ten remaining items, due to their relevance and associations with other critical variables, were retained in a separate scale whose scoring is not included in the development-for-age (DAZ) final score.

Recent developments in the field have demonstrated similar results to our own. For example, the results of the study on the Guide for Monitoring Child Development—a more detailed practitioner interview with a parent of a child under 3 years—demonstrated clear and comparable developmental trajectories on milestones across four countries [38] Moreover, research evidence from another new tool created for the same purpose as IYCD, the Caregiver Reported Early Development Instrument (CREDI), has also demonstrated developmental progression of young children's skills across countries [12] and strong association with family socioeconomic status [39]. This work was conducted concurrently to IYCD, and the teams are now harmonizing for future stages of work [40]. Even though the development of Ages and Stages Questionnaire has been largely based on US-based samples, and it combines observation with parent report, thus not directly comparable with our methodology nor as feasible for large-scale monitoring, results of cross-cultural use support our findings [41]. While all the tools mentioned above have specific advantages, to our best knowledge, none of them used a theoretical framework combined with such an extensive empirical database in the way that the IYCD has.

Despite the diversity of our sample, which came from three countries from three continents with diverse language, culture and customs, our analyses revealed item performance remarkably similar across the sites. We believe that the detailed operating procedures developed prior to the study and closely adhered to throughout supported this outcome. For example, the process of exact translation and back translation from the English to each local language to retain the meaning of items as closely as possible across sites, supported by the local investigators and at least two other team members for each country, ensured high quality control. In following the standard guidelines, we also used exactly the same very specific operating procedures across all sites in assessment of developmental milestones, anthropometry, socioeconomic status and family care. All difficulties and country-specific adjustments were discussed to consensus to ensure that any amendments were within the accepted margins. Our study demonstrated that it is possible to maintain such processes in the measurement of very early child development and that it leads to results comparable across countries. It is our intent to make the procedures available so that they can be utilized on a wider scale in the future.

Despite these strengths, our study had some important limitations. The sample for this study was limited to 269 participants. The next stage in this work would be to conduct a full large-scale validation study across numerous countries and settings to enable us to ensure validity and normal reference values across settings. With the recent nurturing care framework and strategic development goals promoting the need for measurement of early child development as an outcome for programmatic and population level studies [42,43], it is important that efforts to establish valid and comparable developmental monitoring tools move to the next stage. In view of the recently increased interest and volume of evidence on development of children in the first 3 years, the next stages in this work will be to compare and harmonize tools to create one version of a tool that can be upscaled, validated and standardized across multiple countries in order to provide clarity for the international community. This next step is presently underway through the harmonization of work conducted by the CREDI, IYCD and D-Score teams [40]. Our detailed study processes described here in this paper and elsewhere will support these next stages of work ([13,44] Lancaster et al., 2020).

Even though 93% of the original recruited sample was included in the final analysis, there were also data missing due to some inaccuracy in birthdate data collection. As this is so crucial to the creation of developmental trajectories, future studies should attempt to avoid this difficulty, for example, by checking the age and birthdate on several occasions during data collection as an added check to ensure accuracy. Another method to ensure accuracy of age, corrected gestational age and birthdate would be to utilize large birth cohorts for the next stage of work in conducting a wider validation of a tool for global use. We aim to use these types of cohorts for our next stages of work [40]. For this study, we used a paper version to collect data, only using the electronic sources for item demonstrations (e.g., audio sounds or photos or videos illustrating items). In the process of creation of the IYCD, we developed a tablet version that is available for use and can be obtained through the IYCD research team.

5. Conclusions

The IYCD has shown excellent reliability and validity to be used in population level measurement of early child development in low-income settings. Further testing is required to ascertain its ability to detect the effects of intervention. Through the detailed process of its development, we created a blueprint for a global adaptation of parent-reported measure of development of children under 3 years of age.

Supplementary Materials: The following are available online at https://www.mdpi.com/article/10.3390/ijerph18116117/s1, File S1: Table demonstrating sampling framework for each country/. File S2: Final IYCD tool with 100 items.

Author Contributions: M.G. wrote the first draft of the paper and revised the paper. M.G., G.L., T.D., P.K., V.C., and M.J. conceived the study. All authors contributed to protocol development and refinement. All authors were involved with data collection, but M.A.R., C.R.L.A. and L.M. led data collection in each country. G.L. and G.M. led and conducted the analysis. All authors contributed to final analysis and conclusions from data. M.G. led the writing of the manuscript, but all authors discussed the results and contributed to the final manuscript. All authors have reviewed and consented for publication of the manuscript and have certified the authorship list and contributions. All authors have read and agreed to the published version of the manuscript.

Funding: This study has been supported by Grand Challenges Canada and The Bernard van Leer Foundation—grants provided to the World Health Organisation (WHO). G.L. and G.M. had full access to the data, and all authors had final responsibility for the decision to submit for publication. The funders had no role in study design, data collection and analysis, decision to publish, or preparation of the manuscript.

Institutional Review Board Statement: The study protocol complied with the principles of the Helsinki Declaration. The study received ethical approval from the WHO ethical review committee (ERC 0002747) as well as in-country ethics approval from Aga Khan University, Pakistan (4139-Ped-ERC-16), Federal University of Minas Gerais, Brazil (CAAE: 53888416.6.3001.5132), the College of Medicine Research Ethics Committee University of Malawi (P.03/16/1916) and the McMaster University, Hamilton (Canadian) Ethics Review Board (HiREB 1613). Approval was also acquired from all local health organizations where recruitment took place. All families who were recruited were provided with verbal and written information regarding the study, and all caregivers signed the approved consent form.

Informed Consent Statement: Informed consent was obtained from all subjects involved in the study.

Data Availability Statement: The dataset supporting the conclusions of this article is available upon request from the WHO team and can be requested through Vanessa Cavallera; cavallerav@who.int.

Acknowledgments: We would like to thank all those children and families who gave their time to take part in this study. We would also like to thank the research assistants and teams from each of the three countries (Brazil, Malawi, Pakistan) who worked tirelessly to ensure that this study happened with as much detail as it did.

Conflicts of Interest: M.G., P.K., M.J., G.L., C.R.L.A., M.A.R., L.M. and V.C. were all provided with funding to support running of the study from the WHO as a central body for the grants provided by G.C.C. and Bernard van Leer. The authors alone are responsible for the views expressed in this article, and they do not necessarily represent the views, decisions or policies of the institutions with which they are affiliated.

List of Abbreviations

IYCD	Infant and Young Child Development
DAZ	development-for-age z-score
LMIC	Low- and middle-income country
MUAC	Mid-upper arm circumference
HIV	Human immunodeficiency virus
HAZ	height-for-age z-score
WAZ	weight-for-age z-score
WHZ	weight-for-height z-score
SES	Socioeconomic status
DHS	Demographic & Health Survey
FCI	Family care indicators
UNICEF	United Nations International Childrens Fund
LMS	Lambda, mu, sigma
MIRT	Multidimensional item response theory
GPCM	Generalised partial credit model
ANOVA	Analysis of variance
RAP	Raw proportion of agreement

References

1. Victora, C.; Requejo, J.; Boerma, T.; Amouzou, A.; Bhutta, Z.A.; Black, R.E.; Countdown, T. Countdown to 2030 for reproductive, maternal, newborn, child, and adolescent health and nutrition. *Lancet Glob. Health* **2016**, *4*, e775–e776. [CrossRef]
2. Black, M.M.; Walker, S.P.; Fernald, L.C.H.; Andersen, C.T.; DiGirolamo, A.M.; Lu, C.; McCoy, D.C.; Fink, G.; Shawar, Y.R.; Shiffman, J.; et al. Early childhood development coming of age: Science through the life course. *Lancet* **2017**, *389*, 77–90. [CrossRef]
3. Shonkoff, J.P. From neurons to neighborhoods: Old and new challenges for developmental and behavioral pediatrics. *J. Dev. Behav. Pediatr.* **2003**, *24*, 70–76. [CrossRef]
4. Daelmans, B.; Darmstadt, G.L.; Lombardi, J.; Black, M.M.; Britto, P.R.; Lye, S. Lancet Early Childhood Development Series Steering. Early childhood development: The foundation of sustainable development. *Lancet* **2017**, *389*, 9–11. [CrossRef]
5. Loizillon, A.; Petrowski, N.; Britto, P.; Cappa, C. *Development of the Early Childhood Development Index in MICS Surveys*; UNICEF: New York, NY, USA, 2017.
6. Janus, M.; Offord, D. Development and psychometric properties of the Early Development Instrument (EDI): A measure of children's school readiness. *Can. J. Behav. Sci.* **2007**, *39*, 1–22. [CrossRef]
7. Dubeck, M.M.; Gove, A. The early grade reading assessment (EGRA): Its theoretical foundation, purpose, and limitations. *Int. J. Educ. Dev.* **2015**, *40*, 315–322. [CrossRef]
8. RTI International. Early Grade Mathematics Assessment (EGMA) Toolkit. 2014. Available online: https://ierc-publicfiles.s3.amazonaws.com/public/resources/EGMA%20Toolkit_March2014.pdf (accessed on 9 April 2021).
9. Boggs, D.; Milner, K.M.; Chandna, J.; Black, M.; Cavallera, V.; Dua, T.; Lawn, J.E. Rating early child development outcome measurement tools for routine health programme use. *Arch. Dis. Child.* **2019**, *104* (Suppl. 1), S22–S33. [CrossRef]
10. Abubakar, A.; Holding, P.; van Baar, A.; Newton, C.R.; van de Vijver, F.J. Monitoring psychomotor development in a resource-limited setting: An evaluation of the Kilifi Developmental Inventory. *Ann. Trop. Paediatr.* **2008**, *28*, 217–226. [CrossRef] [PubMed]
11. Gladstone, M.; Lancaster, G.A.; Umar, E.; Nyirenda, M.; Kayira, E.; van den Broek, N.R.; Smyth, R.L. The Malawi Developmental Assessment Tool (MDAT): The creation, validation, and reliability of a tool to assess child development in rural African settings. *PLoS Med.* **2010**, *7*, e1000273. [CrossRef]
12. McCoy, D.C.; Sudfeld, C.R.; Bellinger, D.C.; Muhihi, A.; Ashery, G.; Weary, T.E.; Fink, G. Development and validation of an early childhood development scale for use in low-resourced settings. *Popul. Health Metr.* **2017**, *15*, 3. [CrossRef] [PubMed]
13. Lancaster, G.A.; McCray, G.; Kariger, P.; Dua, T.; Titman, A.; Chandna, J.; Janus, M. Creation of the WHO Indicators of Infant and Young Child Development (IYCD): Metadata synthesis across 10 countries. *BMJ Glob. Health* **2018**, *3*, e000747. [CrossRef]
14. Kariger, P.; Janus, M.; Dua, T.; Gladstone, M.; Lancaster, G. Measurement of Child Development Birth through Age Three. In Proceedings of the Annual Conference of the Comparative and International Education Society, Vancouver, BC, Canada, 6–10 March 2016.
15. De Onis, M.; Onyango, A.W.; Van den Broeck, J.; Chumlea, W.C.; Martorell, R.; Wijnhoven, T.M.; Wang, T.; Bjoerneboe, G.-E.A.; Bhandari, N.; Lartey, A.; et al. Measurement and Standardization Protocols for Anthropometry Used in the Construction of a New International Growth Reference. *Food Nutr. Bull.* **2004**, *25*, S27–S36. [CrossRef]
16. Kerac, M.; Mwangome, M.; McGrath, M.; Haider, R.; Berkley, J.A. Management of acute malnutrition in infants aged under 6 months (MAMI): Current issues and future directions in policy and research. *Food Nutr. Bull.* **2015**, *36* (Suppl. 1), S30–S34. [CrossRef]

17. Borghi, E.; de Onis, M.; Garza, C.; Van den Broeck, J.; Frongillo, E.A.; Grummer-Strawn, L. Construction of the World Health Organization child growth standards: Selection of methods for attained growth curves. *Stat. Med.* **2006**, *25*, 247–265. [CrossRef]
18. Rutstein, S. The DHS Wealth Index: Approaches for Rural and Urban Areas. 2008. Available online: http://pdf.usaid.gov/pdf_docs/PNADN521.pdf (accessed on 9 April 2021).
19. Kariger, P.; Frongillo, E.A.; Engle, P.; Britto, P.M.; Sywulka, S.M.; Menon, P. Indicators of family care for development for use in multicountry surveys. *J. Health Popul. Nutr.* **2012**, *30*, 472–486. [CrossRef]
20. Hartung, C.; Lerer, A.; Anokwa, Y.; Tseng, C.; Brunette, W.; Borriello, G. *Open Data Kit: Tools to Build Information Services for Developing Regions*; Association for Computing Machinery: London, UK, 2010.
21. Collins, D. *Cognitive Interviewing Practice*; SAGE: Los Angeles, CA, USA, 2015.
22. Cappelleri, J.C.; Lundy, J.J.; Hays, R.D. Overview of Classical Test Theory and Item Response Theory for Quantitative Assessment of Items in Developing Patient-Reported Outcome Measures. *Clin. Ther.* **2014**, *36*, 648–662. [CrossRef]
23. Wyse, A.E. R.J. DE AYALA (2009) The Theory and Practice of Item Response Theory. *Psychometrika* **2010**, *75*, 778–779. [CrossRef]
24. W.H.O. Multi-Growth Reference Standards Group. W.H.O Growth Standards. *Acta Paediatrica* **2006**, *95*, 5–101.
25. Mei, Z.; Grummer-Strawn, L.M. Standard deviation of anthropometric Z-scores as a data quality assessment tool using the 2006 WHO growth standards: A cross country analysis. *Bull. World Health Organ.* **2007**, *85*, 441–448. [CrossRef] [PubMed]
26. W.H.O. Multi-Growth Reference Standards Group. Anthrostat Software. 2008. Available online: http://www.who.int/childgrowth/software/en/ (accessed on 2 June 2021).
27. Chalmers, R.P. mirt: A multidimensional item response theory package for the R environment. *J. Stat. Softw.* **2012**, *48*, 1–29. [CrossRef]
28. McCray, G.; Lancaster, G.A. *WHO 0–3 Child Development Indicators Project: Statistical Report for Phase 2 Pilot Study*; Institute of Primary Care and Health Sciences: Keele, UK, 2017.
29. Buuren, S.V.; Groothuis-Oudshoorn, K. mice: Multivariate imputation by chained equations in R. *J. Stat. Softw.* **2010**, *45*, 1–68. [CrossRef]
30. Gwet, K.L. *Handbook of Inter-Rater Reliability: The Definitive Guide to Measuring the Extent of Agreement among Raters*; Advanced Analytics, LLC.: Gaithersburg, MD, USA, 2014.
31. Wongpakaran, N.; Wongpakaran, T.; Gwet, K.L. A comparison of Cohen's Kappa and Gwet's AC1 when calculating inter-rater reliability coefficients: A study conducted with personality disorder samples. *BMC Med. Res. Methodol.* **2013**, *13*, 61. [CrossRef]
32. Muraki, E. A Generalized Partial Credit Model: Application of the EM Algorithm. *Appl. Psychol. Meas.* **1992**, *1992*, 30.
33. Bock, R.D.; Aitkin, M. Marginal maximum likelihood estimation of item parameters: Application of an EM algorithm. *Psychometrika* **1981**, *46*, 443–459. [CrossRef]
34. Mislevy, R. Estimating latent distributions. *Psychometrika* **1984**, *49*, 359–381. [CrossRef]
35. Development Core Team, R. *R: A Language and Environment for Statistical Computing*. 2.13.1; R Foundation: Vienna, Austria, 2010.
36. Cole, T.J. Fitting smoothed centile curves to reference data (with discussion). *J. R. Stat. Soc. Ser. A* **1988**, *151*, 385–418. [CrossRef]
37. Cole, T.J.; Green, P.J. Smoothing reference centile curves: The LMS method and penalized likelihood. *Stat. Med.* **1992**, *11*, 1305–1319. [CrossRef] [PubMed]
38. Ertem, I.O.; Krishnamurthy, V.; Mulaudzi, M.; Sguassero, Y.; Balta, H.; Gulumser, O.; Bilik, B.; Srinivasan, R.; Johnson, B.; Gan, G.; et al. Similarities and differences in child development from birth to age 3 years by sex and across four countries: A cross-sectional, observational study. *Lancet Glob. Health* **2018**, *6*, e279–e291. [CrossRef]
39. Fink, G.; McCoy, D.C.; Yousafzai, A. Contextual and socioeconomic variation in early motor and language development. *Arch. Dis. Child.* **2020**, *105*, 421–427. [CrossRef] [PubMed]
40. GSED Team. The Global Scale for Early Development (GSED). 2019. Available online: https://earlychildhoodmatters.online/2019/the-global-scale-for-early-development-gsed/ (accessed on 1 March 2021).
41. Squires, J.; Bricker, D. *Ages & Stages Questionnaires®Third Edition (ASQ®-3) A Parent-Completed Child Monitoring System*; Paul H. Brookes Publishing Co., Inc.: Baltimore, MD, USA, 2009.
42. Dua, T.; Tomlinson, M.; Tablante, E.; Britto, P.; Yousfzai, A.; Daelmans, B.; Darmstadt, G.L. Global research priorities to accelerate early child development in the sustainable development era. *Lancet Glob. Health* **2016**, *4*, e887–e889. [CrossRef]
43. Richter, L.; Black, M.; Britto, P.; Daelmans, B.; Desmond, C.; Devercelli, A.; Vargas-Baron, E. Early childhood development: An imperative for action and measurement at scale. *BMJ Glob. Health* **2019**, *4* (Suppl. 4), e001302. [CrossRef]
44. Lancaster, G.; Kariger, P.; McCray, G.; Janus, M.; Gladstone, M.; Cavallera, V.; Dua, T.; Alves, C.R.; Rasheed, M.; Senganimalunje, L. *Conducting a Feasibility Study in a Global Health Setting for Constructing a Caregiver-Reported Measurement Tool: An Example in Infant and Young Child Development*; Lancaster, G.A., Ed.; Sage: London, UK, 2020. [CrossRef]

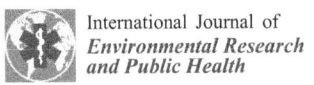

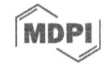

Perspective

Crisis Brings Innovative Strategies: Collaborative Empathic Teleintervention for Children with Disabilities during the COVID-19 Lockdown

Verónica Schiariti [1,*] and Robin A. McWilliam [2]

1 Division of Medical Sciences, University of Victoria, Victoria, BC V8W 2Y2, Canada
2 Department of Special Education and Multiple Abilities, The University of Alabama, Tuscaloosa, AL 35405, USA; theramgroup0@gmail.com
* Correspondence: vschiariti@uvic.ca; Tel.: +1-250-472-5500

Citation: Schiariti, V.; McWilliam, R.A. Crisis Brings Innovative Strategies: Collaborative Empathic Teleintervention for Children with Disabilities during the COVID-19 Lockdown. *Int. J. Environ. Res. Public Health* **2021**, *18*, 1749. https://doi.org/10.3390/ijerph18041749

Academic Editor: William Douglas Evans

Received: 10 January 2021
Accepted: 7 February 2021
Published: 11 February 2021

Publisher's Note: MDPI stays neutral with regard to jurisdictional claims in published maps and institutional affiliations.

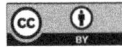

Copyright: © 2021 by the authors. Licensee MDPI, Basel, Switzerland. This article is an open access article distributed under the terms and conditions of the Creative Commons Attribution (CC BY) license (https://creativecommons.org/licenses/by/4.0/).

Abstract: *Background:* While coronavirus disease 2019 (COVID-19) continues to spread across the globe, public health strategies—including the social distancing measures that many countries have implemented— have caused disruptions to daily routines. For children with disabilities and their families, such measures mean a lack of access to the resources they usually have through schools and habilitation or rehabilitation services. Health emergencies, like the current COVID-19 pandemic, require innovative strategies to ensure continuity of care. The objective of this perspective paper is to propose the adoption of two innovative strategies for teleintervention. *Methods:* The novel strategies include: (1) to apply the principles of the Routines-Based Model beyond the early years of development, and (2) to adopt My Abilities First—which is a novel educational tool promoting an abilities-oriented approach in healthcare encounters. *Results:* In the context of COVID-19, and using accessible language, the content of the paper highlights what is important for families and individuals with disabilities, and how the proposed novel strategies could be useful delivering remote support. *Conclusions:* The principles of the Routines-Based Model and My Abilities First are universal and facilitate collaborative, empathic, family-centered teleintervention for children and youth with disabilities during and post the COVID-19 lockdown.

Keywords: COVID-19; functioning; participation; Routines-Based Model; family-centered; child; pandemic; teleintervention; abilities; rights

1. Crisis Brings Innovative Strategies

The coronavirus disease 2019 (COVID-19) is causing a global crisis, not only because of the rapid spread of the virus but also the impact of public health strategies currently in place, aiming to stop human-to-human transmission. The social distancing measures that many countries have implemented have caused huge disruptions to daily routines. Children with or without disabilities are no longer playing outside, as playgrounds are currently closed in most countries and lockdown restricts outings. Families are no longer getting together, celebrating, or sharing key milestones with extended family members, and children are not seeing their grandparents, cousins, or uncles and aunts. Almost 90% of children are not attending schools around the world; that is, 1.5 billon children are not receiving regular education [1]. For children with disabilities and their families, social distancing measures mean a lack of access to the resources they usually have through schools and habilitation or rehabilitation services [2,3]. This shows the need for a change in service provision to ensure continuity of care for children with disabilities.

During a crisis, like the COVID-19 pandemic, it is essential to prioritize inclusion, collaboration, diversity, and equity. Most important, in our opinion, for the habilitation and rehabilitation of children with disabilities, the COVID-19 crisis may facilitate the global adoption of innovative strategies in remote service provision. Some examples of changes that can be accelerated during and after the COVID-19 pandemic—at a global level—are as follows: setting collaborative and meaningful goals; focusing on abilities; empowering families; emphasizing children's rights to express their feelings and opinions; fostering emotional and nurturing connections among professionals and families; changing attitudes towards disability; and improving distance service provision by applying early intervention principles beyond the age of five years.

While the COVID-19 pandemic continues to spread across the globe, children with or without disabilities continue to grow and develop. Children's development is a dynamic process by which the child moves progressively from dependency on everyday functioning towards maturity and independence. In this dynamic process, the child's functioning depends on continuous interactions with the family or other caregivers. These interactions frame the acquisition of various skills, showing the importance of seeing the child in the context of the family [4]. For children with disabilities who need habilitation and rehabilitation, service delivery models that base their interventions on the children's natural contexts to support them in their daily routines and functioning are essential.

2. Proposed Innovative Strategies Using Remote Support

Based on our experience working in the field of early child development and childhood disability in different countries and embracing the global academic solidarity that the COVID-19 crisis has generated, in this paper we share selected innovative strategies to support continuity of care for children with disabilities from birth to transition to adulthood. As such, the objective of this perspective paper is to propose the adoption of two innovative strategies for teleintervention for children and youth with disabilities and their families. Specifically, using remote or virtual support, we propose: (1) to apply the Routines-Based Model (RBM) beyond the early years of development, and (2) to adopt My Abilities First in healthcare encounters. These strategies promote collaborative, empathic, family-centered teleintervention for children with disabilities during and post the COVID-19 lockdown.

The RBM is a collection of practices that, together, provide a unified approach to working with young children aged 0 to 5 years with disabilities and their families [5]. It emphasizes (a) children's functioning in their everyday routines and (b) supporting families. The RBM practices are well defined, have implementation checklists, and are supported by research. The model has three main components: needs assessment and intervention planning; a consultative approach; and a method for running classrooms. RBM is based on a simple premise: all the intervention occurs between visits. This premise means that the visit should be based on building the caregiver's capacity. RBM is implemented in many different cultures, continents, and contexts [5].

My Abilities First is an open access educational tool promoting an abilities-oriented approach to disability evaluation and intervention [6]. This e-tool educates professionals and the general public about the importance of having a positive attitude towards disability, acknowledging that people with disability have the right to attain the highest standard of health care, without discrimination. My Abilities First encourages the systematic identification of strengths and limitations performing everyday routines, as well as barriers and facilitators influencing functioning.

As shown in Figure 1, RBM and My Abilities First share guiding principles for delivering comprehensive services for children with disabilities and their families, including the dynamic role of child–environment interactions, the importance of delivering child/family-centered care, the adoption of a biopsychosocial and a rights-based approach for needs assessments, planning and interventions, and the ultimately goal of empowering families and children to make decisions about their care, among others.

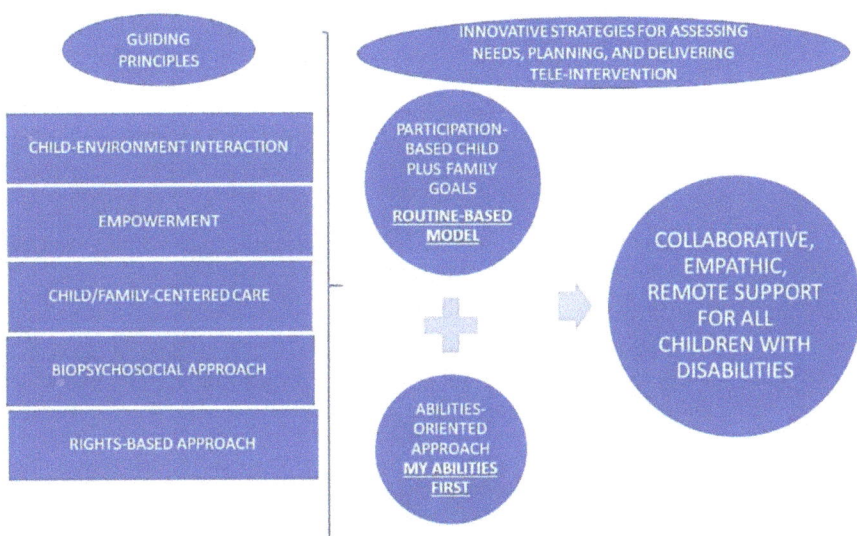

Figure 1. Innovative strategies for delivering remote support for all children with disabilities.

3. The Need for New Service Delivery Strategies during COVID-19

3.1. What Is Important?

Firstly, using the principles of RBM, this article addresses what is different during the lockdown, how to assess needs with a conversation, the importance of emphasizing meaningful functioning and participation in a support plan, using family consultation in virtual visits, and the need for professionals to look after themselves. Secondly, this paper introduces the novel My Abilities First and highlights the importance of adopting a rights-based approach during the COVID-19 pandemic. Importantly, this paper invites the readers to reflect on their current practices and consider new strategies for delivering teleconsultation and/or teleintervention, celebrating strengths and abilities in natural environments where children live and grow.

3.2. What Is Different during COVID-19?

During the lockdown, professionals who typically work in schools, clinics, or other service delivery environments now find themselves making videoconferencing calls to children and their families. This strange situation allows us to learn lessons from early intervention (birth to five), where professionals have been visiting homes for decades [5,7]. They therefore have methods for working with families in the context of everyday routines. These methods, if done correctly, are largely transferable to videoconference calls. By done correctly, we mean using the visits to build the family's capacity to "intervene" with their child throughout the week [7]. Incorrect home visits would be professionals working directly with the child for, say, an hour and expecting that tiny dose to be generalized and applied to the rest of the week. The older a child is, the more that kind of tutorial-type visit could work. With young children, it does not. The RBM has numerous strategies that have already been disseminated as applicable in early intervention through virtual visits in several countries [8]. In this paper, the authors propose to expand RBM for families of children with disabilities of all ages.

Virtual visits during the lockdown are different from home visits at other times for a few reasons. First, the adults often get no break: they are forced to be at home with their children with no additional help. Weekends are great but the longest weekend ever is not! Especially vulnerable to this stress are adults who are caring for and entertaining children alone, such as single parents or the partners of essential workers. Similarly, for some siblings, having no time away from their brothers or sisters can be exhausting. This situation is obviously exacerbated if one of the children has challenging behaviors. Second, in many households, privacy is unobtainable. Third, life can be boring at home, with day after day of no change, especially children who have difficulties with attention or independent play or who are simply the products of the modern age can become easily bored—and every parent knows how trying it is to have children who say they are bored.

The lockdown has created a quite-different environment, but professionals working with children of all ages with disabilities are trying to support children and families through videoconferencing. One place to begin is to reassess needs.

3.3. Assess Needs with a Virtual Conversation

During the lockdown, technology is fundamental to carry on everyday life. Everyday life is what this article is about, and technology is our way of connecting with families' everyday lives.

With children's and families' lives disrupted by the lockdown, the functioning needs of the child and the families' needs are different. We can consider a routines-based conversation, family-level questions, and support the family to choose their goals.

Professionals can ask families about their day-to-day life, beginning with waking up and all the way to adults' going to bed. At each time of the day (i.e., routine, as we define it), we ask the family to describe the child's engagement, independence, and social relationships in that routine. Structuring the conversation by routines is natural, in that families can walk you through their day, and contextual: we hear about children's functioning, and when and where the skills are needed. We ask families what children are interested in as well as what they can do. When those abilities and interests do not match the demands of the routine, we have diminished functioning. We note these concerns as we are talking to families, but they are not goals. If we have a good, in depth conversation we will uncover many such concerns—more than needed for our goal plan—and the Routines-Based Model is notorious for already having long lists of goals. The routines-based conversation is based on the well-known, evidence-based Routines-Based Interview (RBI) [9–11]. During this Routines-Based Conversation, if the child in question is old enough to participate meaningfully, this contribution can add to the richness of the discussion. The family should make the determination whether the child's participation would be helpful or disruptive. One of the tenets of the RBM is the question "Whose child is it?".

In addition to the conversation about child functioning in routines, the conversation can include the time, worry, and change questions, a hallmark of the RBI: do you have enough time for yourself or yourself and another person? When you lie awake at night, worrying, what do you worry about? If you could change anything in your life, what would it be?

These powerful questions have two benefits. First, they show the family that you care enough to ask these questions about the adults' well-being. You can also ask them of the child, if appropriate. Second, they go beyond daily routines to deeper, more emotional needs, which is precisely why some professionals try to avoid them—professionals who are not used to dealing with emotions or who mistakenly think that they need to fix any need mentioned. As we said earlier, families at this point are not choosing goals.

After asking the time, worry, and change questions, we might recap the conversation so far, in just a few minutes, to remind the family of the concerns. This is a reminder: it is not a time to rehash the whole discussion or to try to make the family feel good about their routines. The purpose of a recap is to remind them of concerns.

3.4. Set Goals Addressing Meaningful Participation

The family then chooses goals for their child and themselves. The child can participate in this process, as appropriate, and the family has editing power, meaning the family has the last say in what goals are decided upon. The professional can help the family by looking at the notes and reminding the family of concerns that arose during the routines-based conversation. Typically, the RBI produces 10–12 goals, both child and family goals. The routines-based conversation might produce fewer but should still be six or more goals.

The professional reads or shows, perhaps through a shared screen, the goals the family has chosen and asks them to put these into order of importance. If appropriate, the child can participate in this process. Once the professional has this importance prioritization, he or she can create a Goal x Routine matrix, such as shown in the RBM resource page (Access to RBM resource page available here http://eieio.ua.edu/uploads/1/1/0/1/110192129/intervention_matrix_completed_english.pdf (accessed on 2 April 2020)).

Once we know the child's and family's needs, we should develop a plan. Research has shown that having goals is better than not having goals [12]. Next, we discuss the importance of child goals addressing meaningful participation (Access to RBM resources provided in Supplementary Material S1).

3.5. Emphasize Meaningful Participation in a Plan

Participation has come to be acknowledged as a critical dimension in the definition of disability [4]. The impairment in a person is only as handicapping to that person as it affects the person's ability to function meaningfully (i.e., participate) in his or her environment [4,13]. We therefore take needs the family identifies and develop them into participation-based goals and family goals.

Participation-based goals put the emphasis or purpose of a skill the child needs to achieve on engagement in a routine. For example, if a parent says she/he wants the child to use two-word combinations, in the RBM, this would have come from a discussion about a need in one or more routines. A goal like this could be for a young child or an older child with significant communication delays. An important point is that the need came from a need for meaningful participation in a routine. Needs in routines should be authentic.

A participation-based goal might therefore read as "Javier will participate in breakfast time, going outside time, and hanging out time by using two-word combinations." This goal tells us the skill, using two-word combinations, and the purpose: to participate in those three routines. It is a perfect participation-based goal but it is not measurable. When professionals want goals to be measurable, they can keep the goal and add acquisition, generalization, and maintenance criteria, as in "We will know he can do this when he uses three two-word combinations at breakfast time, going outside time, and one hanging-out time in one day for four consecutive days." The acquisition criterion is the frequency of two-word combinations: three. The generalization criterion is the routines: three of them. The maintenance criterion is amount of time: four consecutive days.

In addition to child goals, the list of goals must include at least one family goal. Family goals are necessary because of what, in the RBM, we call the two-bucket principle: a mother can fill her child's bucket only to the extent her bucket is full. Some family goals are related to the child, such as getting information about the child's disability. Other family goals are not directly related to the child, such as time for parents alone or fulfilling individual dreams.

Planning is important, and then professionals help families with that plan. The next section addresses how to help families tackle that plan.

3.6. Use Family Consultation in Virtual Visits

How do you help families confined with their children with special needs? If you have been using the RBM, this process is not a big challenge, because the RBM is all about building families' capacities to meet child and family needs: it is not about direct, hands-on work. This section describes how the virtual visit is focused on a plan, develops strategies with caregivers, and involves three types of action.

The videoconference visit is focused on the previous visit and on goals. By the end of the previous visit, the professional had documented what the parents had decided to try, as strategies, with their child. For older children, it might be what the child was going to try doing, with or without assistance. Families, including the child, if appropriate, had also determined what they wanted the focus of this visit to be.

Therefore, the professional would know what the topic was. Families should also be given the opportunity, however, to determine the agenda for the visit, so professionals should ask two questions: how have things been going (a general question)? Has anything new happened since our last talk?

These questions allow the family to bring up topics that might not have been previously planned. If the family has something they want to talk about, that sets at least the beginning of the agenda. If they do not, the professional reminds the family about (a) strategies they were going to work on since the last meeting and (b) what the family said they wanted the focus of this visit to be on.

When discussing what the family had been doing, they reflect on how the intervention has been going. This discussion might lead to the family and the professional tweaking the strategy. The amount of context the professional had had previously would predict how many questions he or she would ask during this strategy tweaking: if the professional had much context, he or she might not need to ask many questions. If the professional did not have much context, he or she should ask many questions to ensure his or her suggestions were relevant. Some children with disabilities are trying strategies themselves, but they are still functioning in home contexts, during this quarantine time. So, families are still integrally involved in the execution of these strategies.

Professionals' suggestions are the result of finding solutions or problem solving. Traditionally, professionals made recommendations to families quickly, based on good will and experience: Most of us professionals are quick to come up with helpful suggestions for families (Example of professional recommendations provided here https://naturalenvironments.blogspot.com/2014/07/self-regulation-in-working-with-families.html (accessed on 4 April 2020)). We should ask questions before making suggestions, and this process can involve the child, if appropriate (Access to RBM resources provided in Supplementary Material S1).

While determining solutions (i.e., developing strategies) we can incorporate, in virtual visits, three types of action. First, we can see what the child does. The family can show us what the child typically does or is now doing. In addition, the child might say, "Look what I can do", or the professional might ask the child to show what he or she is doing in that routine. Second, the family can show what they are doing or are considering doing. For example, the family might say, "Look what I've been trying to do when I take Ted to the grocery store", and they show a video clip of a trip to the grocery store. Third, the professional describes a strategy, after asking at least four questions. The professional can be as explicit as possible about the idea and can even demonstrate with a doll. Importantly in the RBM, we always check in with the family with two questions, especially important online: Do you think this strategy will work? As busy as you are at these times of the day, do you think you'll be able to carry out these strategies you've chosen?

Before hanging up, the professional and family, including the child, if appropriate, review what was discussed on this virtual visit, review what the family is going to do between this visit and the next, and the family says what they want the focus of the next virtual visit to be. At this point, the professional can use a Goals x Routines matrix to remind the family of the goals on the plan. In the RBM this information is recorded on the Next-Steps Form (NSF).

We have just discussed two pieces of paper, the NSF and the matrix. When visits are through videoconferencing, the professional and the family will need to work out the best method of seeing this paperwork and other materials. If they are using Zoom or Skype, they can share screens. They might take screen shots, scans, or photographs and send them via email or other social media.

Family consultation, therefore, can work well in a virtual visit, focusing on the family's agenda and on goals they have selected. Nevertheless, supporting families virtually can be stressful and exhausting. Hence, the following section, address the importance of looking after yourself.

3.7. Look after Yourself

Professionals themselves are on lockdown, so they might have their own children at home, who they are caring for and helping with school work. They are in virtual visits with families, hearing about their difficulties and worries. Many families' struggles are not about things professionals can necessarily help with. Family-centered professionals can problem solve (solution find, in RBM language) with families, but families might, especially now, just need someone to listen—and listening to difficult situations can be draining.

It is important, therefore, for professionals to keep their expectations appropriate. They should approach each virtual visit with a goal of providing encouragement, a listening ear, and some information, not of solving a problem.

The NSF can help professionals feel a sense of control over what sometimes seems a chaotic way of supporting families. If you know you are going to have to write down what we did today, you will record and reflect on the major topics of your virtual visit. Furthermore, the commitment the family makes, even if it is only one strategy—maybe even one they are continuing—again helps you feel the visit was productive. Finally, with a few or many visits a day, a professional should tell someone about a success, preferably the professional's success, not simply the child's or family's. You could tell a family member, a friend, a colleague, or a supervisor. With a supervisor, you could say, "I'm not seeking advice or help. I simply want you to hear about a success I had because you understand my work." Looking after yourself by keeping expectations appropriate, using the NSF, and telling someone about a success will help you keep up your strength to help families.

Professionals might also need to engage in self-care: What do you do for yourself, to refill your bucket and to stave away the anxiety of the lockdown, the coronavirus, the changed home environment, and the problems of families? If you cannot think of something healthy to do for yourself, find something. One of us has taken to walking for an hour up and down hills in the woods every morning. What you do for yourself does not have to be about work. Can you say to yourself, "You are a great home/virtual visitor, this is hard, and you are a caring person"? We are all different and what fills our bucket differs, but this is a time where we need to be aware of our own needs and whether we are meeting those needs.

3.8. Focus on "My Abilities First"

The COVID-19 pandemic might accelerate a global change towards inclusive and empathic healthcare encounters, using telemedicine or in person. A change about views of disability and how healthcare services are provided is needed globally [14,15]. Individuals experiencing disabilities have often voiced their unsatisfying and emotionally detached interactions with healthcare professionals [14].

A recently created electronic tool—called My Abilities First—breaks with the traditional view of disability and educates about the experience of living with a disability [6]. The rationale for the need of developing this novel abilities-oriented approach tool was based on lessons learned from a qualitative study that sought children's opinions about their strengths and limitations in performing day-to-day activities [16]. Overall, children and youth with disabilities focused primarily on their abilities and strengths, cheering age-appropriate interests [16]. As a result, My Abilities First was created allowing children and youth with disabilities to use their own words to describe themselves and their functional needs. Moreover, My Abilities First operationalizes a rights-based approach in medical education and practice, emphasizing that users' opinions about themselves and their needs should be routinely sought [17].

My Abilities First can be accessed from mobile devices and it can be used in telehealth during or post the COVID-19 lockdown. Information gathered using this electronic tool can start a conversation with children and adults with disabilities about their needs for interventions or teleintervention.

My Abilities First could be used along the RBM strategies with families of all children with disabilities, regardless the age or underlying health condition. The web-based animations included in My Abilities First educate healthcare students, professionals, and the general public, changing common societal, incorrect assumptions about disability [16,18], thus enhancing the global impact of using a positive language in healthcare. As such, the global adoption of My Abilities First—during and post COVID-19 lockdown—could bring shared purpose, proximity, empowerment, trust, and joy in healthcare.

Specifically, My Abilities First consists of three web-based animations [6] (Access to animations provided in Supplementary Material S1). The first video introduces how to apply an abilities-oriented approach in healthcare encounters. It proposes the creation of a "my abilities identification card" which can be included in every health record. The target audience of this video includes health and health- allied professionals (My Abilities identification card animation available here https://youtu.be/WyW6ey3kHvM (accessed on 24 April 2020)).

The second web-animation included in My Abilities First describes the personal experience of a person living with a chronic health condition during healthcare encounters. This animation highlights the importance of applying a holistic approach in routine healthcare encounters, asking questions to identify the strengths of the person and capabilities performing daily routines. The audience of this video includes clinicians, researchers, educators, administrators, and students (My Abilities First—Getting to know me animation available here https://youtu.be/Dnn_-0IEe_Q (accessed on 1 May2020)).

Finally, the third video promotes a change in attitudes towards disability from a child's perspective. In this animation, a typical developing child advocates for social inclusion of children with disabilities, illustrating the importance of focusing on abilities and changing societal attitudes towards disability. The target audience of this video is the general public, school-aged children, and peers (My Abilities First for peers animation available here https://youtu.be/myHFKggNeGc (accessed on 1 May 2020)).

4. Global Impact of Routines-Based Model and My Abilities First

RBM has been implemented in 10 countries over the past 30 years. The model provides actual practices for implementing a family-centered approach in person or virtually [5,8,19]. The model has been modified to include cultural adaptations in different countries and RBM tools are available in languages other than English.

Professionals applying RBM reported improved goals, in terms of functionality and measurability, improved team functioning, and more collaborative consultation [9,20]. Moreover, the short and long-term effectiveness of the RBM collaborative interventions has been shown in randomized controlled trials [21–23].

On the other hand, My Abilities First was recently created; it was published in April 2020 [6]. Since its publication, the e-tool has received global attention; it has been downloaded more than 800 times from all continents. It is currently being translated into Spanish, Portuguese, Chinese, and Polish. A pilot study checking satisfaction and change in healthcare attitudes using My Abilities First is underway in Taiwan (led by Professor Hua-Fang Liao, from the National Taiwan University) and in Brazil (led by Professor Egmar Longo, from the Federal University of Rio Grande do Norte). Furthermore, My Abilities First has been included in the pool of innovative resources listed in the International Alliance of Academies of Childhood Disability (IAACD) COVID-19 Task Force page (IAACD COVID-19 Task Force page https://iaacd.net/iaacd-covid-19-task-force/ (accessed on 5 July 2020)). This international initiative is collecting and sharing information related to the impact of COVID-19 on people with disabilities around the world. Finally, My Abilities First has been selected as the theme of a global campaign launched by the European Academy of Childhood Disability (EACD), inviting children and young adults with disabilities—from around the globe—to share their abilities and major facilitators influencing optimal functioning. This campaign is part of the Global Partnership Day (Global Partnership Day, EACD, My Abilities First https://eacd2021.com/my-abilities-first/ (accessed on 30 January 2021)) organized by the EACD in 2021.

Implementation Challenges

The implementation of new strategies can be exciting, but it involves change. Due to the current restrictions related to COVID-19, children with disabilities, their families, and professionals had to accommodate to different ways of receiving and delivering services. Accommodating to new ways of doing things is inherently difficult. Implementation challenges related to RBM have been well-described [20], for example changing professionals' service delivery approach from a medical model to a truly family-centered approach, where families make meaningful decisions about goals, what to work on in between visits and what to focus on. Implementation challenges related to My Abilities First include barriers to change in practice at the organizational or individual level, as adopting an abilities-oriented approach—in person or virtually—means a different way to collect information, plan and deliver interventions in healthcare encounters. Education highlighting the importance of adopting new approaches based on rights, child and family-centered care is essential to ameliorate these implementation challenges.

5. Conclusions

The COVID-19 lockdown has changed our personal and professional routines. This historical event has united the globe. We believe this is a good time to expand good practices (i.e., RBM beyond early intervention, for older children with disabilities), to adopt innovative tools (i.e., routine remote teleintervention for vulnerable populations globally), to change attitudes towards disability and adopt a universal rights-based approach in healthcare encounters with children and adults with disabilities (i.e., adopting My Abilities First, combined RBM teleintervention with My Abilities First).

In summary, it is possible to leverage the COVID-19 crisis by adopting innovative strategies in the field of childhood disability, like RBM teleintervention for all children with disabilities beyond the early years of life, and by facilitating access to the universal inclusive educational tools discussed in this paper.

Supplementary Materials: The following are available online at https://www.mdpi.com/1660-4601/18/4/1749/s1, Routine Based Model (RBM) Intervention Matrix; RBM professional recommendations; links to My Abilities First web animations; IAACD COVID-19 Task Force page; 33rd EACD annual meeting—Global Partnership Day page—My Abilities First campaign.

Author Contributions: Conceptualization and methodology, V.S. and R.A.M.; writing—original draft preparation, R.A.M. and V.S.; resources and writing—review and editing, R.A.M. and V.S.; visualization, V.S. and R.A.M.; project administration, R.A.M.; Animations design and creation My Abilities First, V.S. All authors have read and agreed to the published version of the manuscript.

Funding: This paper received no external funding.

Institutional Review Board Statement: This perspective paper did not require ethics review.

Informed Consent Statement: This perspective paper did not require informed consent.

Data Availability Statement: Data sharing is not applicable to this article as this is an opinion paper.

Acknowledgments: R.A. McWilliam is the creator of the Routines-Based Models for Early Intervention (Birth to Five years). Verónica Schiariti is the developer of the open access e-tool My Abilities First.

Conflicts of Interest: The authors declare no conflict of interest.

References

1. World Health Organization (WHO). COVID-19 Situation Report #77. 2020. Available online: https://www.who.int/docs/default-source/coronaviruse/situation-reports/20200406-sitrep-77-covid-19.pdf?sfvrsn=21d1e632_2 (accessed on 17 April 2020).
2. Lee, J. Mental health effects of school closures during COVID-19. *Lancet Child. Adolesc. Health* **2020**, *4*, 421. [CrossRef]
3. Wim Van, L.; Zachary, P. COVID-19, School Closures, and Child Poverty: A Social Crisis in the Making. *Lancet Public Health* **2020**, *5*, e243–e244.
4. World Health Organization (WHO). *International Classification of Functioning Disability and Health Children*, 4th ed.; World Health Organization: Geneva, Switzerland, 2007.
5. McWilliam, R.A. *Family-Centered Intervention Planning: A Routines-Based Approach*; Communication Skill Builders: Tucson, AZ, USA, 1992.
6. Schiariti, V. MY ABILITIES FIRST: Positive language in health care. *Clin. Teach.* **2020**, *17*, 272–274. [CrossRef] [PubMed]
7. Dunst, C.J.; Bruder, M.B.; Espe-Sherwindt, M. Family capacity-building in early childhood intervention: Do context and setting matter? *Sch. Community J.* **2014**, *24*, 37–48.
8. McWilliam, R.A. Tele-Intervention and the Routines-Based Model. 2020. Available online: http://naturalenvironments.blogspot.com/2020/03/tele-intervention-and-routines-based.html (accessed on 7 April 2020).
9. Boavida, T.; Aguiar, C.; McWilliam, R.A.; Correia, N. Effects of an in-service training program using the routines-based interview. *Top. Early Child. Spec. Educ.* **2016**, *36*, 67–77. [CrossRef]
10. Hughes-Scholes, C.H.; Gavidia-Payne, S.; Davis, K.; Mahar, N. Eliciting family concerns and priorities through the Routines-Based Interview. *J. Intellect. Dev. Disabil.* **2017**. [CrossRef]
11. McWilliam, R.A.; Casey, A.M.; Ashley, D.; Fielder, J.; Rowley, P.; DeJong, K.; Votava, K. Assessment of family-identified needs through the routines-based interview. In *Young Exceptional Children Monograph Series No. 13: Gathering Information to Make Informed Decisions*; McLean, M.E., Snyder, P., Eds.; The Division for Early Childhood of the Council for Exceptional Children: Missoula, MT, USA, 2011; pp. 64–78.
12. Locke, E.; Latham, G. Goal-setting theory. In *Organizational Behavior 1: Essential Theories of Motivation and Leadership*; Miner, J.B., Ed.; Routledge: New York, NY, USA, 1994; pp. 159–183.
13. Granlund, M.; Bjorck-Akesson, E. Inservice training of pre-school consultants in family-oriented intervention—Training process and outcome. *Br. J. Dev. Disabil.* **1996**, *42 Pt 1*, 1–23. [CrossRef]
14. Shakespeare, T.; Iezzoni, L.I.; Groce, N.E. Disability and the training of health professionals. *Lancet* **2009**, *374*, 1815–1816. [CrossRef]
15. World Health Organization (WHO). Disability and Health 2018. Available online: https://www.who.int/news-room/fact-sheets/detail/disability-and-health (accessed on 1 April 2019).
16. Schiariti, V.; Sauve, K.; Klassen, A.F.; O'Donnell, M.; Cieza, A.; Masse, L.C. 'He does Not See Himself as being Different': The Perspectives of Children and Caregivers on Relevant Areas of Functioning in Cerebral Palsy. *Dev. Med. Child. Neurol.* **2014**, *56*, 853–861. [CrossRef] [PubMed]
17. Schiariti, V. The human rights of children with disabilities during health emergencies: The challenge of COVID-19. *Dev. Med. Child. Neurol.* **2020**, *62*, 661. [CrossRef] [PubMed]
18. Schiariti, V. Focus on functioning: Let's apply the ICF model. *Clin. Teach.* **2016**, *13*, 378–380. [CrossRef] [PubMed]
19. McWilliam, R.A. Metanoia in early intervention: Transformation to a family-centered approach. *Rev. Latinoam. Educ. Inclusiva* **2016**, *10*, 155–173.
20. McWilliam, R.A.; Boavida, T.; Bull, K.; Cañadas, M.; Hwang, A.W.; Józefacka, N.; Lim, H.H.; Pedernera, M.; Sergnese, T.; Woodward, J. The Routines-Based Model Internationally Implemented. *Int. J. Environ. Res. Public Health* **2020**, *17*, 8308. [CrossRef] [PubMed]
21. Hwang, A.-W. *The Long-Term Effectiveness of Implementing a Participation-Based Early Intervention Program. for Children with Developmental Delay: A Cluster-Randomized Controlled Trial*; Final Report (Project NO.: MOST-105-2314-B-182-012); Ministry of Science and Technology: Taipei, Taiwan, 2017.
22. Hwang, A.-W.; Chao, M.; Liu, S. A randomized controlled trial of routines-based early intervention for children with or at risk for developmental delay. *Res. Dev. Disabil.* **2013**, *34*, 3112–3123. [CrossRef] [PubMed]
23. Hsieh, Y.H.; Liao, H.F.; Jeng, S.F.; Tseng, M.H.; Schiariti, V.; Tsai, M.Y.; Sun, S.C. Collaborative Home-Visit Program for Young Children with Motor Delays in Rural Taiwan: A Pilot Randomized Controlled Trial. *Phys. Ther.* **2020**, *100*, 979–994. [CrossRef] [PubMed]

MDPI
St. Alban-Anlage 66
4052 Basel
Switzerland
Tel. +41 61 683 77 34
Fax +41 61 302 89 18
www.mdpi.com

International Journal of Environmental Research and Public Health Editorial Office
E-mail: ijerph@mdpi.com
www.mdpi.com/journal/ijerph